Colposcopy of the
Cervix, Vagina, and Vulva

Colposcopy of the Cervix, Vagina, and Vulva

A COMPREHENSIVE TEXTBOOK

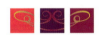

Michael S. Baggish, M.D.

Chairman
Department of Obstetrics and Gynecology
Good Samaritan Hospital

Director
Obstetrics and Gynecology Resident Education
Good Samaritan Hospital
Bethesda North Hospital

Professor
University of Cincinnati College of Medicine
Cincinnati, Ohio

Illustrations by **Joe Chovan**

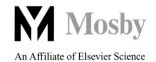

Mosby

An Affiliate of Elsevier Science

Mosby
An Imprint of Elsevier Science

The Curtis Center
Independence Square West
Philadelphia, Pennsylvania 19106

NOTICE

Medicine is an ever-changing field. Standard safety precautions must be followed, but as new research and clinical experience broaden our knowledge, changes in treatment and drug therapy may become necessary or appropriate. Readers are advised to check the most current product information provided by the manufacturer of each drug to be administered to verify the recommended dose, the method and duration of administration, and contraindications. It is the responsibility of the licensed prescriber, relying on experience and knowledge of the patient, to determine dosages and the best treatment for each individual patient. Neither the publisher nor the author assumes any liability for any injury and/or damage to persons or property arising from this publication.

Acquisitions Editor: Stephanie Donley
Publishing Services Manager: Joan Sinclair

Printed in China

Last digit is the print number: 9 8 7 6 5 4 3 2 1

This book is dedicated to the four women in my life:

Leslie Ann Baggish, my wife
Julia Susan Baggish, my daughter
Cindy Beth Baggish, my daughter
Mindy Ann Baggish, my daughter

Preface

Colposcopy is a visual technique for observing disorders affecting the lower genital tract. Initially, the technique was restricted to examination of the cervix but as the title of this textbook indicates, colposcopy has proliferated to advantageous use in the vagina and vulva as well as the cervix.

The raison d'être for this work was and still is the persistent need to teach the basics to beginners, advanced principles to those with experience, and to update seasoned colposcopists. I also consider this book suitable for nurse practitioners and family practitioners who wish to practice colposcopy. The anticipated secondary goal will be fulfilled if this book continues to serve the purchaser as a ready reference over several years.

Although the subject matter appears rather narrow at first consideration, this is not the case. In fact, the rather simplistic experience of viewing the cervix via magnification has developed during the last 30 years into a study of diseases and treatments involving a significant region of female anatomy and function.

This book has been constructed from the outset to provide many color colpophotographs, visually explicit drawings, and necessary as well as practical histopathology, cytology microphotographs. The essence of the aforesaid plan was based on my personal experience first learning colposcopic techniques between 1965–1967 and subsequently teaching colposcopy from both the GME and CME perspectives. The often used expression that a picture is worth a thousand descriptive words is a true statement as it pertains to the case of colposcopy.

This book has been divided into five (5) sections to create a smooth pattern of organization and flow.

Section I deals largely with terminology, instrumentation, and the generic aspects of colposcopy.

Section II is the largest section of the book. This section focuses upon colposcopy at specific sites, i.e. cervix, vagina, vulva. The major sections are further subdivided into consistent subheadings which are designed to provide the reader with comprehensive details about that particular anatomical portion of the lower genital tract and skewed towards the viewpoint of the colposcopic examination. The final subsection under each specific site is devoted to actual case histories collected over a period of 30 years together with color colpophotographs illustrating the case's colposcopic findings.

Section III details various treatment choices for the management of intraepithelial neoplasia at various locations in the lower genital tract. The treatments are illustrated to show the technical aspects of each operation in order to assist the reader in his/her performance of these surgical procedures.

Section IV is focused on a number of special collateral conditions and/or confusing areas relative to the colposcopic role in the management of neoplastic disorders. Within this section are discussions relating to the 2001 Bethesda System for reporting cervical cytology. I have utilized two diagrams to help the reader deal with a number of clinical scenarios. The format purposely avoided reproducing the typical flow diagram monstrosity. Tree-like branching diagrams are mainly confusing. I personally find them difficult to read and most of all laborious. If the latter is the experience of other people, then it is little wonder that readers do not remember the content for future usage. Together with my artist, I have substituted a color format combined with icons to create an interesting schema to provide a guide for follow-up and necessary procedures based on outcome data.

The final section of the book contains an extensive bibliography. I have read and have in my library a number of books written on the subject of colposcopy. They have originated from several nations including: England, France, Germany, Norway, Australia, and the United States. I have attempted to emulate those books that project interesting contents and to avoid the wordiness and overkill that permeates other publications. Several books that are included in my bibliography are out of print, including Fluhman's book on the cervix and Jorden and Singer's Treatise on the same subject. Similarly, these older books contain excellent reference material, photographs, and drawings.

The extensive bibliography presented me with an excellent opportunity to sift through old and new data. The trend of many contemporary authors to subordinate material published in the past to recently published data is regrettable. I have found much in the older literature to be interesting, well researched, and accurate. It is not uncommon for "new reports" to restate known facts and "rediscover" data.

Table of Contents

CHAPTER 1B
Glossary

Acanthosis: Hyperplasia of the prickle cell layer of the squamous epithelium; alternatively, thickening and downward extension of the rete peg into the underlying dermis.

Adenosis: Mucous glandular tissue within the walls of the vagina.

Anaplasia: Loss of structural differentiation and organization that is synonymous with cancer. Cells revert to their most immature form.

Atrophy: Shrinkage, or recession, of cellular or constituent tissue elements.

Atypia: A nonspecific term often used by pathologists to describe an unusual or abnormal cellular configuration or condition or, occasionally, squamous cell hyperplasia, such as basal cell hyperplasia.

Carcinoma in situ: Abnormal cells characterized by cytologic changes within the nucleus and cytoplasm. These changes include hyperchromatism, pleomorphism, derangement of the nuclear-to-cytoplasmic ratio, increased mitotic activity, and lack of maturation and cellular organization involving the full thickness of the epithelium. A layer of hyperkeratosis or parakeratosis is not considered normal maturation and does not preclude a diagnosis of carcinoma in situ. This term is synonymous with intraepithelial neoplasia grade 3.

Condyloma: Condylomata are diagnosed microscopically when the tissue sample demonstrates papillomatosis, acanthosis, parakeratosis, or hyperkeratosis. Often, the epithelium contains koilocytes.

Condylomatous change: The presence of several, but not all, of the criteria required to make a pathologic diagnosis of condylomata within the squamous epithelium. Typically, the gross lesions are flat and white rather than papillary and fleshy. The epithelium contains koilocytes.

Dysplasia: Disturbed cellular growth or maturation characterized by abnormal cellular forms and disruption of cellular organization and orientation. These changes are limited to the epithelium. Based on the amount of epithelium involved, dysplasia is classified as mild, moderate, or severe.

Ectopy: The presence of glandular epithelium on the portio of the cervix. The term implies that the glandular cells are misplaced, or ectopic, from their normal location.

Endocervical gland: A misnomer that refers to the endocervical clefts, or tunnels, that constitute a portion of the plicated topography of the endocervical canal and the microanatomy of the endocervical mucosa.

Endocervical metaplasia: Extension of endocervical cells from their native endocervical canal to a location beyond the external cervical os and out onto the portio vaginalis. This condition usually is caused by pregnancy or the use of oral contraceptive hormones, but also may be caused by prenatal exposure to diethylstilbestrol.

Erosion: A misnomer that refers to the presence of endocervical tissue, or mucus-secreting epithelium, on the portio vaginalis of the uterine cervix. True erosion implies the loss of epithelium.

Eversion: A term that implies movement of endocervical mucosa from the canal onto the portio of the cervix.

Hyperkeratosis: Thickening of the cornified layer of stratified squamous epithelium that is characterized grossly by raised areas of white tissue. The greater the degree of hyperkeratosis, the whiter the tissue (Fig. 1-1).

Hyperplasia: An increased number of cellular or constituent tissue elements.

Hypertrophy: Enlargement of existing cellular or constituent tissue elements.

Intraepithelial neoplasia: A premalignant condition that affects the epithelium of the cervix, vagina, and vulva. Although the term is best applied and most accurately defined for these locations, the same terminology is used for other sites in the female genital tract. Dysplasia and intraepithelial neoplasia are analogous. Intraepithelial neoplasia is classified as grades 1 (mild), 2 (moderate), and 3 (severe).

Invasive carcinoma: Invasion of abnormal cells beyond the epithelium and into the underlying and surrounding stroma. Early stages of invasion often are marked by hypermaturity in reverse fashion, or downward maturation of cells into the stroma. Invasion of lymphatic and/or blood vascular structures may occur as well.

Malignancy: A virulent, life-threatening condition that is synonymous with cancer and causes local or distal invasion and destruction of normal tissue.

Microinvasion: Early stromal invasion that cannot be diagnosed by unassisted or colposcopically aided vision. The diagnosis is made only by viewing a microscopic tissue section. Typically, the invasion extends only a few millimeters (1 to 2 mm) below the basement membrane of the epithelium, and microscopic examination of multiple serial sections does not show invasion of lymphatic or vascular tissue.

Neoplasia: New growth. The term may indicate a disturbance of growth characterized by uncontrolled mitotic activity. Essentially, the nucleus is programmed or transformed to survive autonomously into perpetuity.

Original, or native, epithelium: Epithelium that occupies a specific anatomic location before shifts occur in the squamocolumnar transformation zone. The two types of native epithelium, ectocervical squamous epithelium and endocervical mucous epithelium, abut each other at the anatomic external os.

Parakeratosis: Abnormal type of keratinization in which nuclei are found in the keratinized layer (Fig. 1-1).

Squamous metaplasia: Metaplasia refers to the replacement of one cell type by another. In the cervix, a glandular cell usually is replaced by a squamous cell. The process begins below the basement membrane, where a totipotential, or reserve, cell is programmed to change its subsequent differentiation. Beneath the mucus-secreting glandular epithelium, immature squamous cells form and multiply rapidly, eventually pushing the glandular cells into the cervical canal or vagina. Squamous metaplasia occurs physiologically at three times during the female's life cycle: in the neonatal period, at puberty, and during pregnancy.

Stenosis: A severe decrease in the size of an opening, canal, or tubular structure, typically as a result of scar formation, or fibrosis.

Transformation zone: An area of the cervix where columnar epithelium coexists with squamous metaplasia in various stages of maturity. This zone typically includes the original squamocolumnar junction.

Keratosis

Parakeratosis

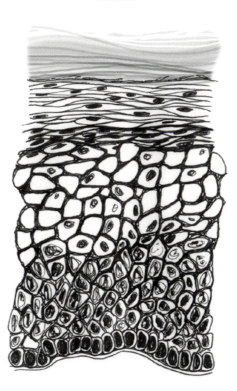
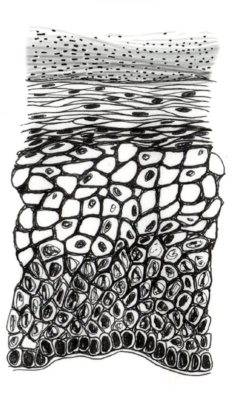

FIGURE 1-1 Normal squamous epithelium (*left*) and parakeratosis (*right*). Parakeratosis is an abnormal type of keratinization that shows nucleated cells in the keratin layer.

CHAPTER 2
The Colposcope

The colposcope is a binocular dissecting microscope. Binocular instrumentation offers the advantage of true three-dimensional vision. Coupled to the microscope is an intense halogen or xenon light source. In current models, the microscope is connected to a remote light generator via a fiberoptic cable. In older models, the light source is included within the housing of the optical system. A rheostat is used to adjust the intensity of the light. Modern colposcopes are easily adjusted up or down by means of cantilevered arms that are balanced with springs or hydraulic systems (Figs. 2-1*A* and *B*, 2-2, and 2-3).

The objective lens of the colposcope determines its focal distance. Changing the objective lens alters that distance. Most objective lenses range from 250 mm (near) to 400 mm (far). The average focal length is 300 mm (Fig. 2-4*A*). Eyepieces add additional magnification to the image (e.g., 10×). For most patients, the eyepieces are adjusted at a zero setting. The microscope may be parfocalized by setting the eyepieces on zero, sharply focusing the microscope at the highest magnification, and then switching to low magnification and focusing each eyepiece to obtain a sharp view (Fig. 2-4*B*).

Magnification ranges from scanning (0.4×) to high power (2.5×), plus the magnification provided by the eyepiece (Fig. 2-4*C*). The magnification may be increased or decreased by turning a dial on the microscope head. Some models use a zoom lens rather than preset magnification stops. Several high-quality microscopes allow the operator to separate the eyepiece from the microscope

and interpose a beam splitter (Fig. 2-4*D*). The beam splitter diverts a portion of the returning light to an attached accessory device (e.g., 35-mm, Polaroid, or television camera [Fig. 2-4*E*]). Additionally, a direct-view binocular or monocular teaching tube may be coupled to the microscope. As noted, a modern colposcope provides intense, cold light that originates from a remote generator (Figs. 2-4*F* and *G*).

To obtain the greatest advantage from colposcopy, the operator should be thoroughly familiar with the instrument. In particular, the operator should be familiar with the location of the green filter because it can help to define abnormal vascular patterns. Similarly, the operator should be familiar enough with the operating mechanics to troubleshoot problems and perform minor repairs.

In the office setting, colposcopes range from simple to elaborate. However, regardless of the type of instrument used, the key elements are multiple levels of magnification, a quality optical system, and intense light (Figs. 2-5, 2-6, and 2-7).

Colposcopy is best performed with the use of a motorized examination table that can be raised and lowered electrically. Sophisticated tables can elevate the head and foot positions separately. Attempting to perform colposcopy with a fixed examination table can cause the operator to hunch over the table in an attempt to obtain the most favorable axis for examination. In addition, positioning problems can complicate the process of performing directed biopsy.

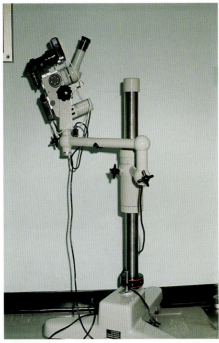
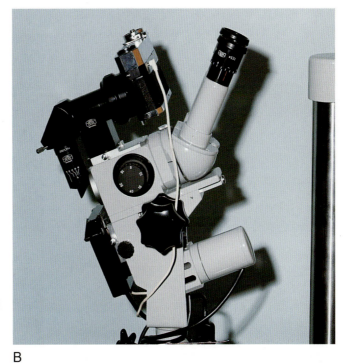

A   B

FIGURE 2-1 A, A 1960s vintage colposcope whose optical system is comparable in quality to contemporary systems. **B,** Magnification ranges from 6× to 40×, and is readily changed on the dial that is mounted on the left side of the instrument. The binocular eyepieces can be focused individually. The camera is mounted permanently on the top of the instrument. A flash unit is affixed with a dovetail fitting just below the objective lens of the microscope. Light is supplied by an incandescent bulb.

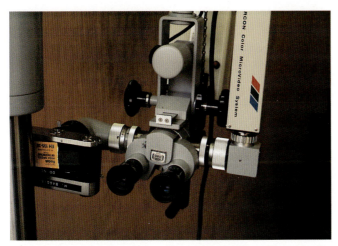

FIGURE 2-2 A 1970s colposcope with a beam splitter. A Circon television camera is mounted on the right side, and a 35-mm camera with an objective lens is attached to the left side. The sliding column of the stand is seen on the far left.

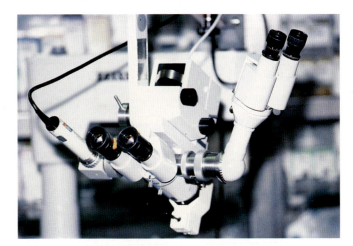

FIGURE 2-3 A 1980s colposcope equipped with a halogen light source and a binocular teaching tube attachment. The scope is mounted on a cantilevered arm that is perfectly balanced with a system of springs. Although the teaching tube has two eyepieces, the image is monocular.

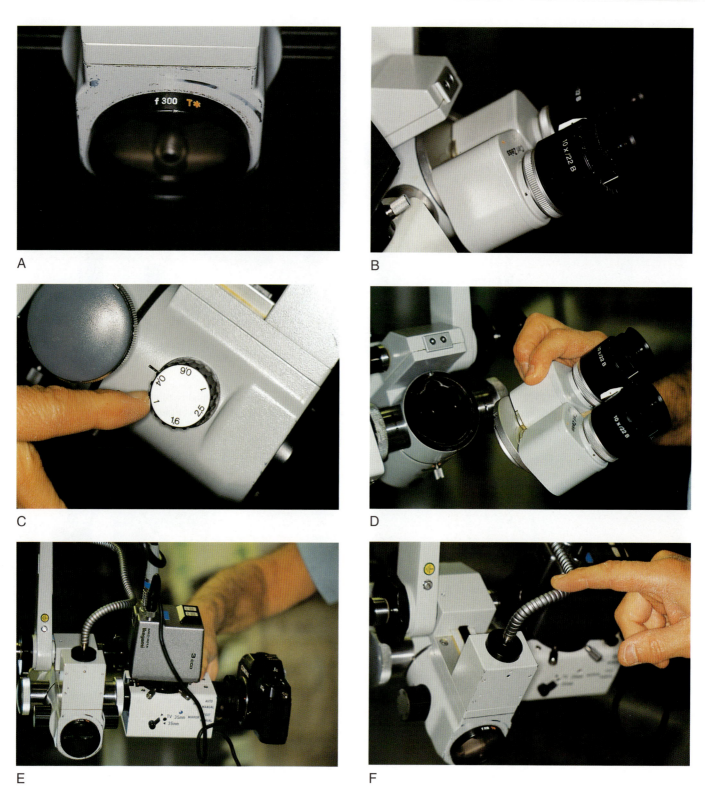

FIGURE 2-4 **A,** The focal length of the objective lens is inscribed on its periphery. In this case, the focal distance is 300 mm, which is ideal for viewing and operating on the cervix and vagina. **B,** The eyepieces magnify 10× and are individually adjustable. **C,** The adjustable magnification ranges from scanning (0.4×) to high power (2.5×). Most work is performed at a magnification of between 4× and 16×. **D,** The binocular lens is detached from the beam splitter by loosening a thumb screw. Similarly, the beam splitter may be detached from the body of the colposcope. **E,** This 1990s contemporary colposcope is mounted on an S-2 balanced stand (see Fig. 3-1*B*) and equipped with an adjustable arm and a fiberoptic light system. A 35-mm still camera and a three-chip video camera are mounted on the left side of the attached beam splitter. **F,** A fiberoptic cable is connected to the top surface of the housing, just behind the objective lens. The corrugated light cable remains cool because the generator is located remotely. *(continued)*

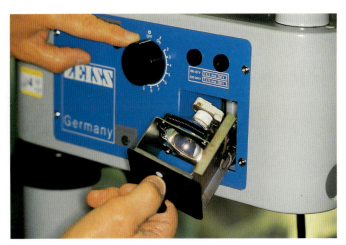

G

FIGURE 2-4 G, The light generator and halogen bulb are located within the stand and are remote from the body of the colposcope.

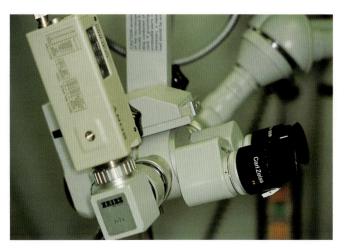

FIGURE 2-5 This office colposcope is equipped with a beam splitter. A reasonably priced single-chip camera can be attached. This system is ideal for instructional use as well as for recording patient data on slides or videotape.

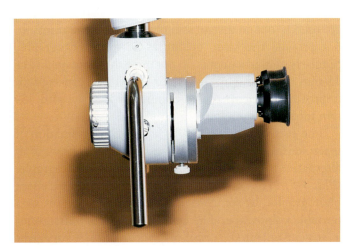

FIGURE 2-6 This simple clinic colposcope is arm-mounted for easy control. It has an excellent optical system and a fiberoptic light source.

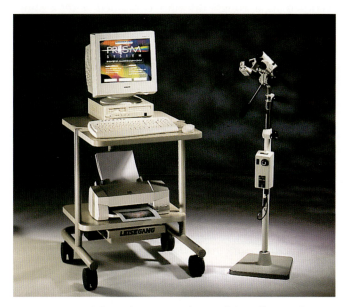

FIGURE 2-7 This colposcope is designed for office or clinic use and can be supplemented to include a computer information system and a digital photographic printer.

CHAPTER 3
Documentation of Findings

Accurate recording of data is an integral component of colposcopic examination. Most basically, data are recorded as a rough drawing combined with a short narrative or a codified legend. These types of sketches may be helpful for the originator, but are less helpful to others who need to review the patient's records. Another technique uses a template drawing together with an established set of terms to record each colposcopic procedure. If the recorder is a reasonably good artist, these records will be helpful to others who review the record (Fig. 3-1*A*).

Clearly, the best documentation includes a replica of the image seen by the examiner (Fig. 3-1*B*). A teaching tube can be coupled to the beam splitter port of the optical system to allow a second person to see the same view as the examiner. Although this tube does not provide the true three-dimensional view seen by the examiner (Fig. 3-2), this type of documentation by a second or third party is superior to a stylized drawing.

Application of late 20th century technology to the concept of the teaching tube led to the coupling of a still or television camera to the beam splitter. Since the 1970s, the resolution of video images has improved dramatically as a result of enhanced light sensitivity, size reduction, and increased lines of resolution. A television camera attachment offers several advantages. Any number of secondary viewers can see the same image as the operator (Fig. 3-3). In addition, the patient can see the field and can be shown both abnormalities and normal anatomy. Finally, the colposcopic examination can be recorded and later edited, and still pictures can be obtained digitally from the recording.

Several types of still cameras can be attached to the colposcope in a variety of configurations. The most common type of attachment is through the beam split-ter, either with or away from the television mount (Figs. 3-4*A* and *B*). Most cameras use a 35-mm format because it provides excellent detail. Although Polaroid cameras are used to obtain instant still photographs, the prints do not provide the same quality as 35-mm photographs. Similarly, digital cameras do not offer the same quality as 35-mm photography, but their quality is expected to improve and eventually to compete favorably with 35-mm microphotography.

The cervicoscope, which consists of a combination of macrolenses coupled to ring and flash illumination, is an alternative to microscope-mounted 35-mm photography (Fig. 3-5). This method provides consistently excellent photographs. In some respects, the camera serves as a portable colposcope. The camera body is mounted onto a trigger-operated, pistol-grip device. The operator focuses the camera by moving it closer to or farther away from the object to be photographed (Fig. 3-6). When the object appears in sharp focus, the operator depresses the trigger. ASA 100 or 200 color slide film is recommended for use with microscope-mounted or cervicoscope 35-mm cameras.

Linking a digital camera and a computer to the colposcope is a recent innovation. The digital camera feeds a real image of the field to the computer screen. The operator uses a mouse to superimpose captions and symbols on the image. Similarly, typed information can be incorporated into the file. The image and the report are stored in the memory of the computer and can be recalled later. When linked with a color printer, the digital photograph can be printed and attached to the patient's medical record. By marrying the drawing to the photograph, this system provides precise, detailed documentation that renders an excellent teaching and research tool (Figs. 3-7*A* and *B*).

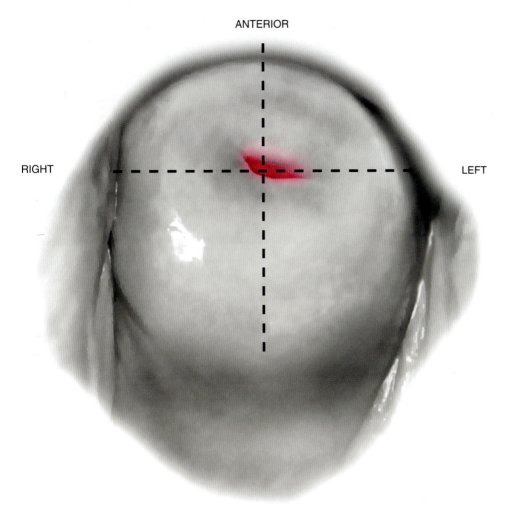

ANTERIOR

RIGHT

LEFT

POSTERIOR

Metaplasia	= MTPL
White epithelium	= WE
Abnormal transformation zone	= ATZ
Endocervix	= ENDCx
Punctation	= PUNC
Mosaic	= MOS
ATYP vessels	= ATP VES

A

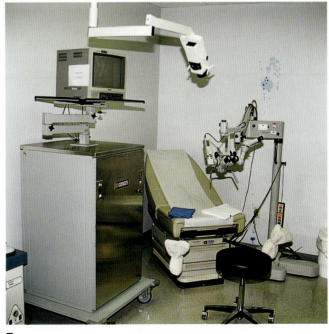

B

FIGURE 3-1 A, A schematic template provides a convenient model that the operator can use to sketch visualized lesions and document their location. A list of common abbreviations is included. **B,** This office colposcopy system provides excellent documentation with a video camera that is attached to the lens system with a beam splitter.

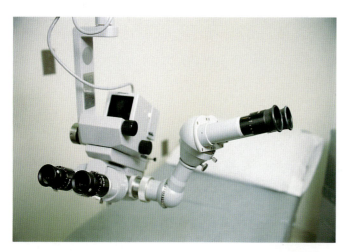

FIGURE 3-2 A binocular teaching tube is attached to the colposcope with a beam splitter. The teaching tube does not provide a three-dimensional view.

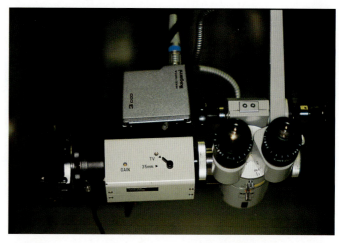

FIGURE 3-3 A three-chip television camera is attached to the colposcope with a beam splitter.

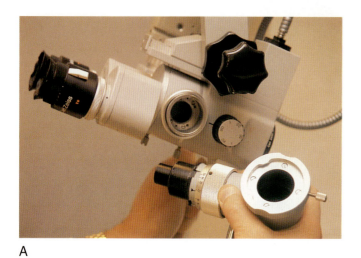

A

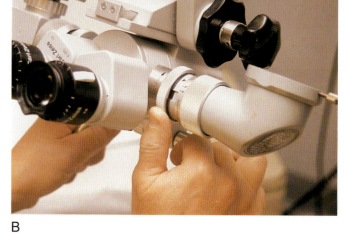

B

FIGURE 3-4 **A,** A photographic coupling device allows a 35-mm camera to be attached with a separate port. **B,** The device shown in Figure 4A is secured in place on beam splitter 2. The video camera is attached on the opposite side.

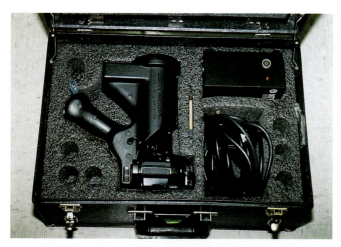

FIGURE 3-5 A complete cervicoscope system includes a 35-mm camera and a complex lens system mounted on a handheld firing device. A power transmitter and accompanying cords are included as well.

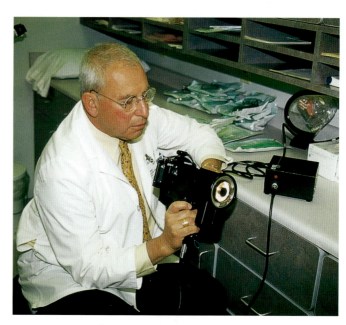

FIGURE 3-6 The camera is aimed at the cervix and focused by moving the lens closer to or farther away from the object. The ring flash provides illumination.

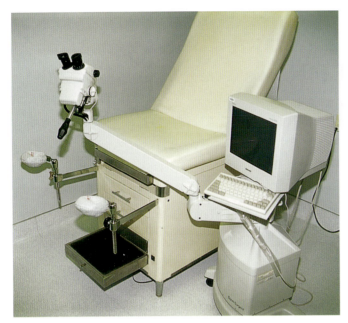

A

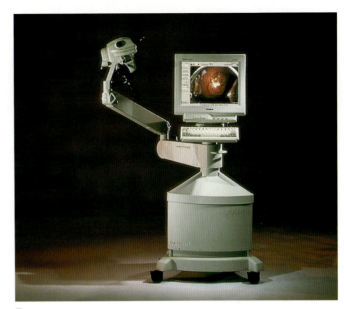

B

FIGURE 3-7 A, This computerized colposcope includes a digital file and labels that can be entered and retrieved. **B,** A digital picture is transmitted directly from a real-time video image.

CHAPTER 4
Cytology

In the past, significant confusion surrounded the clinical interpretation of cervicovaginal cytologic reports. In part, this problem was related to classification and reporting methods, which differed from laboratory to laboratory. Historically, one of the oldest classifications used a grading system of 1 to 5. Although this system lacks specificity and precision, it is still used in some places.

Class 1   Normal

Class 2   Inflammatory

Class 3   Dysplastic

Class 4   Carcinoma in situ

Class 5   Suspicion for invasive cancer

In an effort to establish a uniform system to classify and report cytologic findings, between 1988 and 1991, gynecologic pathologists established the Bethesda System. This system classifies cytologic findings into the following categories:

NORMAL CYTOLOGY
BENIGN CELLULAR CHANGES
Infection
Reactive changes
EPITHELIAL CELL ABNORMALITIES
Squamous cell abnormalities
A.   Atypical squamous cells of undetermined significance
B.   Low-grade squamous intraepithelial lesion
     Human papillomavirus lesions
     Cervical intraepithelial neoplasia grade 1, or mild dysplasia
C.   High-grade squamous intraepithelial lesion

Cervical intraepithelial neoplasia grades 2 (moderate dysplasia) and 3 (severe dysplasia, or carcinoma in situ)
D.   Squamous cell carcinoma
Glandular cell abnormalities
A.   Benign endometrial cells
B.   Glandular cells of undetermined significance
C.   Endocervical adenocarcinoma
D.   Endometrial adenocarcinoma
E.   Extrauterine adenocarcinoma

OTHER MALIGNANT NEOPLASM

In 2001, the earlier Bethesda classification was revised as System 2001. Table 4-1 shows the new Bethesda classification, which appeared in *Contemporary Obstetrics and Gynecology* in 2001. Table 4-2 shows a later, abridged format that appeared in *JAMA* in 2002.

The adequacy of cervicovaginal cytology and the accuracy of the findings are dependent on the ability of the practitioner (physician, nurse, or medical assistant) to obtain a satisfactory specimen from the cervix or vagina. A satisfactory specimen includes both squamous cells and endocervical or squamous metaplastic cells.

The cells must be well preserved to permit an accurate interpretation of the findings. Different instruments are used to obtain an accurate representation of cells from the cervix: a sample from the ectocervix is obtained with a spatula, a sample from the squamocolumnar junction is obtained with the forked end of a spatula stick, and a sample from the endocervical canal is obtained with a cytobrush.

To make an accurate diagnosis, the clinician must be familiar with both cytologic terminology and the cellular appearance associated with key disorders. The normal cervix contains three general types of squamous cells that originate in the ectocervix: superficial, or estrogen-sensitive cells (Fig. 4-1); intermediate, or progesterone-

TABLE 4-1
Proposed Bethesda System 2001

Specimen Type: *Indicate conventional (Papanicolaou) smear vs. liquid-based smear vs. other.*

Specimen Adequacy

Satisfactory for evaluation *(Describe presence or absence of endocervical or transformation zone component and any other quality indicators, e.g., partially obscuring blood, inflammation.)*

Unsatisfactory for evaluation . . . *(Specify reason.)*
  Specimen rejected or not processed *(Specify reason.)*
  Specimen processed and examined, but unsatisfactory for evaluation of epithelial abnormality because of . . . *(Specify reason.)*

General Categorization (optional)

Negative for intraepithelial lesion or malignancy
Epithelial cell abnormality: See interpretation of result *(Specify squamous or glandular.)*
Other (e.g., endometrial cells in a woman ≥ 40 years of age): See interpretation of result

Automated Review

If automated device used, specify device and result.

Ancillary Testing

Briefly describe test methods and report result clearly.

Interpretation of Result

Negative for intraepithelial lesion or malignancy *(When there is no cellular evidence of neoplasia, state this in the general categorization above or in this section, regardless of whether there are organisms or other non-neoplastic findings.)*
ORGANISMS
  Trichomonas vaginalis
  Fungal organisms morphologically consistent with *Candida* species
  Shift in flora suggestive of bacterial vaginosis
  Bacteria morphologically consistent with *Actinomyces* species
  Cellular changes associated with herpes simplex virus
OTHER NON-NEOPLASTIC FINDINGS *(optional; list not inclusive)*
  Reactive cellular changes associated with:
    Inflammation (includes typical repair)

Radiation
Intrauterine contraceptive device
Glandular cells status after hysterectomy
Atrophy

Epithelial cell abnormalities
SQUAMOUS CELL
Atypical squamous cells:
  Of undetermined significance (ASC-US)
  Cannot exclude HSIL (ASC-H)
Low-grade squamous intraepithelial lesion (encompassing human papillomavirus, mild dysplasia, and cervical intraepithelial neoplasia grade 1) (LSIL)
High-grade squamous intraepithelial lesion (encompassing moderate and severe dysplasia, carcinoma in situ, and cervical intraepithelial neoplasia grades 2 and 3) (HSIL)
  With features suggestive of invasion *(if invasion is suspected)*
Squamous cell carcinoma
GLANDULAR CELL
Atypical
  Endocervical cells *(not otherwise specified or specify in comments)*
  Endometrial cells *(not otherwise specified or specify in comments)*
  Glandular cells *(not otherwise specified or specify in comments)*
Atypical
  Endocervical cells, favor neoplastic
  Glandular cells, favor neoplastic
Endocervical adenocarcinoma in situ
Adenocarcinoma
  Endocervical
  Endometrial
  Extrauterine
  Not otherwise specified

Other

Endometrial cells in a woman ≥ 40 years of age *(Specify if negative for squamous intraepithelial lesion.)*

Other malignant neoplasms: *(Specify.)*

Educational Notes and Suggestions (optional)

Suggestions should be concise and consistent with clinical follow-up guidelines published by professional organizations. References to relevant publications may be included.

(Adapted with permission from Contemp Obstet Gynecol 46:25, 2001.)

sensitive cells (Fig. 4-2); and parabasal cells (Fig. 4-3). The endocervical component consists of columnar mucus-secreting cells that emanate from the endocervical canal (Fig. 4-4). Young, or immature (metaplastic), squamous cells inhabit the squamocolumnar junction. These cells are commonly seen in Papanicolaou smear specimens.

Newer collection techniques, particularly the thin prep technique, minimize debris and provide a more uniform monolayer of cells on the glass slide. Regardless of

the collection technique used, the specimen must be fixed immediately to avoid loss of cells. Clearly, minimizing debris and artifact leads to more accurate screening and diagnosis (Figs. 4-5A to D).

Because the vagina normally contains no glandular cells, vaginal specimens typically contain only squamous cells. However, in some women, including those who were exposed to diethylstilbestrol, adenosis is present in the vagina.

TABLE 4-2
The 2001 Bethesda System (Abridged)

Specimen Adequacy

Satisfactory for evaluation (*Note presence or absence of endocervical or transformation zone component.*)
Unsatisfactory for evaluation . . . (*Specify reason.*)
Specimen rejected or not processed (*Specify reason.*)
Specimen processed and examined, but unsatisfactory for evaluation of epithelial abnormality because of . . . (*Specify reason.*)

General Categorization (*optional*)

Negative for intraepithelial lesion or malignancy
Epithelial cell abnormality
Other

Interpretation of Result

Negative for intraepithelial lesion or malignancy

ORGANISMS
  Trichomonas vaginalis
  Fungal organisms morphologically consistent with *Candida* species
  Shift in flora suggestive of bacterial vaginosis
  Bacteria morphologically consistent with *Actinomyces* species
  Cellular changes associated with herpes simplex virus
OTHER NON-NEOPLASTIC FINDINGS (*optional; list not comprehensive*)
  Reactive cellular changes associated with:
    Inflammation (includes typical repair)
    Radiation
    Intrauterine contraceptive device

Glandular cells status after hysterectomy
Atrophy

Epithelial cell abnormalities

SQUAMOUS CELL
Atypical squamous cells (ASC)
  Of undetermined significance (ASC-US)
  Cannot exclude high-grade squamous intraepithelial lesion (ASC-H)
Low-grade squamous intraepithelial lesion (encompassing human papillomavirus, mild dysplasia, and cervical intraepithelial neoplasia grade 1) (LSIL)
High-grade squamous intraepithelial lesion (encompassing moderate and severe dysplasia, carcinoma in situ, and cervical intraepithelial neoplasia grades 2 and 3) (HSIL)
Squamous cell carcinoma
GLANDULAR CELL
Atypical glandular cells (*Specify endocervical, endometrial, or not otherwise specified.*) (AGC)
Atypical glandular cells, favor neoplastic (*Specify endocervical or not otherwise specified.*) (AGC-N)
Endocervical adenocarcinoma in situ (AIS)
Adenocarcinoma

Other (*list not comprehensive*)

Endometrial cells in a woman ≥ 40 years of age

Automated Review and Ancillary Testing (*Include as appropriate.*)

Educational Notes and Suggestions (*optional*)

(Adapted with permission from JAMA 287:2114, 2002.)

Cellular abnormalities are classified as nuclear or cytoplasmic. Atypical squamous cells of undetermined significance are more notable than those seen with immature metaplasia, but less prominent than the cellular atypia that is seen in low-grade squamous intraepithelial lesions (Figs. 4-6*A* and *B*).

Nuclear abnormalities include nuclear enlargement, abnormal nuclear shape, hyperchromatic (black) nuclei, chromatin clumping (the opposite of finely dispersed chromation), and multinucleation.

Cytoplasmic abnormalities include a reduction in the relative amount of cytoplasmic material compared with the nucleus; reversal of the nuclear-to-cytoplasmic ratio; dyskeratosis, or abnormal keratin formation; and vacuole, or halo, formation.

Criteria for Cytologic Diagnosis

Koilocytosis
This abnormal cell type is associated with human papillomavirus infection and is characterized by cytoplasmic vacuolization and nuclear abnormalities that include

abnormally shaped nuclei, multiple nucleation, and disorders of chromatin formation, or polyploidy (Figs. 4-7*A* and *B*).

Low-grade squamous intraepithelial lesion
According to the Bethesda criteria, these cells may appear singly or in sheets. Nuclear abnormalities are confined to mature cells and include increased nuclear-to-cytoplasmic ratio, binucleation, and multinucleation. Hyperchromasia is present, but chromatin usually is evenly distributed. Cell borders are distinct.

High-grade squamous intraepithelial lesion
According to the Bethesda criteria, these cells may occur singly, in sheets, or as a syncytium. Nuclear abnormalities occur in immature cells, although the cytoplasm may be densely keratinized. The nuclear-to-cytoplasmic ratio is further reduced compared with low-grade squamous intraepithelial lesions. Hyperchromatism and coarse chromatin graining are evident. Overall, cells are small compared with low-grade squamous intraepithelial lesions (Figs. 4-8*A* and *B*).

Squamous cell carcinoma

The cellular changes are an extension of the abnormalities seen in high-grade squamous intraepithelial lesions. Bizarrely shaped cells with tails that show keratosis, multinucleation, and dark, abnormally shaped nuclei suggest invasive cancer. Similarly, sheets of small, densely stained pleomorphic cells that consist almost entirely of nuclear material typically are associated with necrotic and inflammatory cells and also are characteristic of invasion.

Cells that contain abnormal mitotic figures also may be seen (Fig. 4-9*A*).

An abnormal cytology report is never diagnostic (Fig. 4-9*B*) and should prompt further investigation, including colposcopy and biopsy. When a Papanicolaou smear shows a more severe abnormality than is detected on directed biopsy, more extensive sampling, such as conization or loop excision, is indicated.

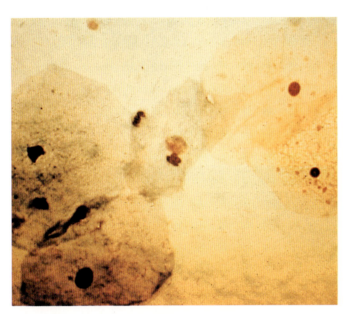

FIGURE 4-1 Normal superficial cells contain abundant orange-pink cytoplasm (eosinophilia). The single nucleus is dark and pyknotic. (Courtesy of Leo Koss, MD.)

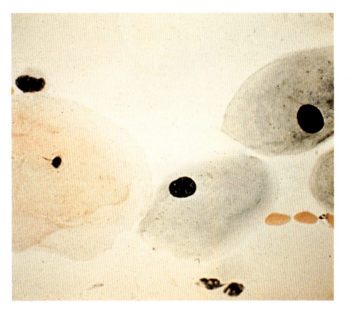

FIGURE 4-2 Intermediate cells lie deeper in the epithelial layer and are more plentiful during the progestational phase of the cycle, whereas superficial cells mirror the estrogenic phase. This basophilic (bluish) cell sometimes is referred to as a boat-shaped, or navicular, cell. The nuclei are uniform, but larger than those seen in superficial cells. (Courtesy of Leo Koss, MD.)

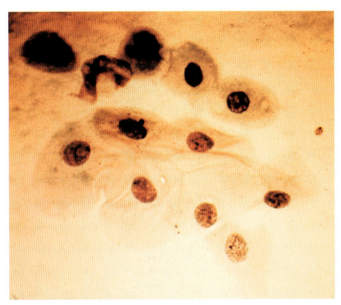

FIGURE 4-3 Parabasal cells are the deepest cells. More of these cells are shed from an atrophic (e.g., postmenopausal, or estrogen-deprived) cervix. These cells are smaller than those shown in Figures 4-1 and 4-2, with less cytoplasm and relatively larger nuclei. The nuclei are regular, and the chromation is well dispersed. (Courtesy of Leo Koss, MD.)

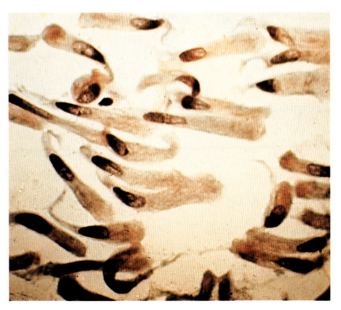

FIGURE 4-4 A normal Papanicolaou smear also contains endocervical cells. These columnar, mucus-containing cells have regular, basilar, ovoid nuclei. After staining, the cytoplasm is gray. (Courtesy of Leo Koss, MD.)

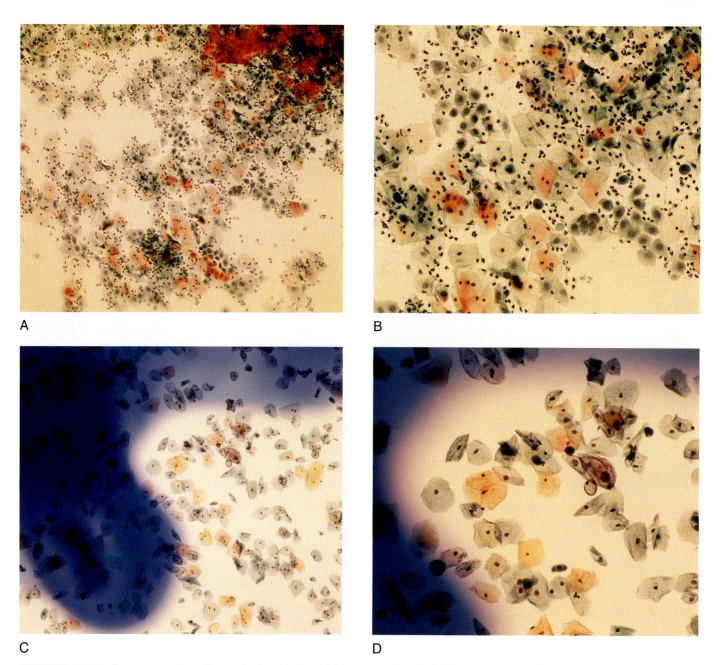

FIGURE 4-5 **A,** Low-power view of a standard cervical cytologic preparation. **B,** Higher-power view of Figure 5A. Inflammatory debris partly obscures several cells. **C,** A thin prep monolayer preparation contains less debris than the cell preparation shown in Figure 5A. **D,** The cellular clarity provided in this high-power view shows why the quality of the interpretation is superior to the standard preparation (*B*).

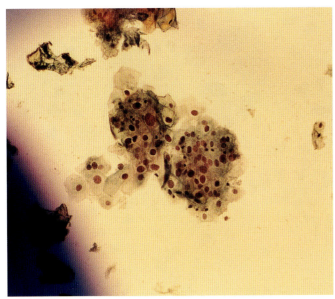
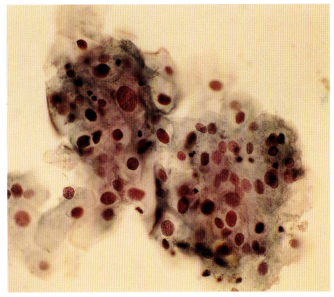

A

B

FIGURE 4-6 **A,** This low-power view shows a clump of cells with minimal cytologic and nuclear atypism. This specimen was graded as atypical squamous cells of undetermined significance. **B,** A higher-power view of Figure 6*A* shows nuclei of abnormal size and shape. Additionally, several cells are binuclear and at least three cells show changes that suggest early koilocytosis. This specimen was graded as atypical squamous cells of undetermined significance. These changes suggest a low-grade squamous intraepithelial lesion, or condylomatous atypia.

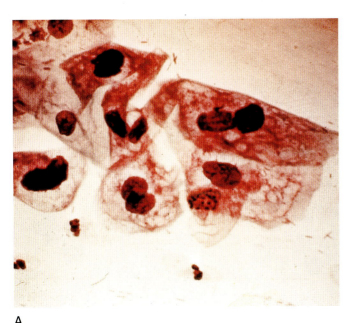
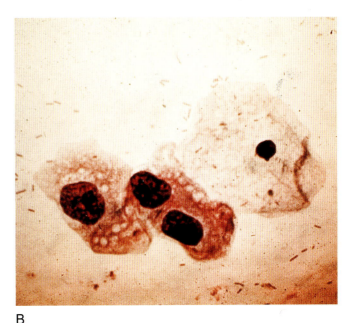

A

B

FIGURE 4-7 **A,** These dysplastic cells show hyperchromasia, binucleation, and cytoplasmic vacuolization. These changes are characteristic of human papillomavirus infection. (Courtesy of Leo Koss, MD.) **B,** These koilocytes are identified by nuclear atypia, or polyploidy; cytoplasmic vacuolization; and clearing. (Courtesy of Leo Koss, MD.)

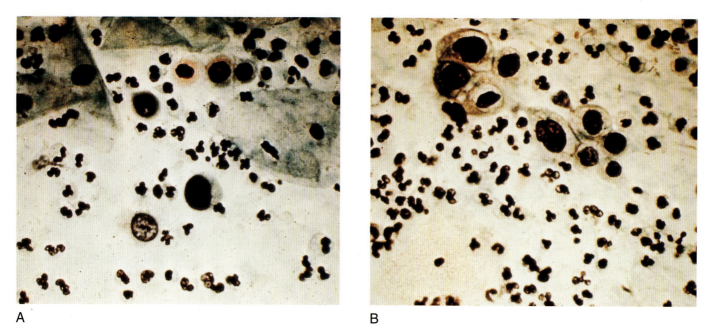

A   B

FIGURE 4-8 A, These small cells have large, hyperchromic nuclei and are characteristic of carcinoma in situ. An individually keratinized, nucleated cell is seen (*top center*). **B,** These malignant cells were shed from a carcinoma in situ lesion. They show features of human papillomavirus infection. Cytoplasmic clearing is seen around the hyperchromatic nuclei.

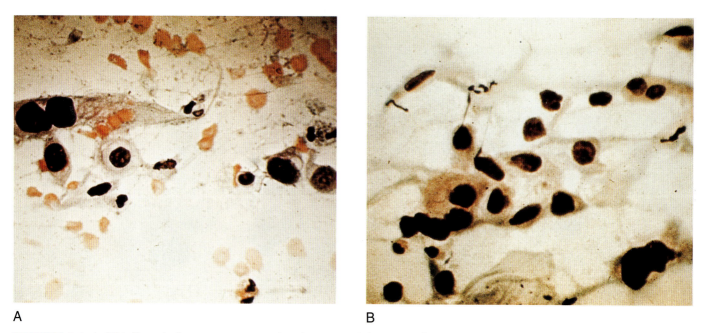

A   B

FIGURE 4-9 A, This Papanicolaou smear suggests invasive cancer. A bizarre, pollywog-like cell is seen, and its head contains two black nuclei. (Courtesy of Leo Koss, MD.) **B,** This cluster of malignant columnar cells has dark, or hyperchromatic, nuclei and cytoplasm that are suggestive of mucus formation.

CHAPTER 5
Indications

Because the colposcope, or operating microscope, provides variable magnification and intense light, it is a useful tool in the diagnosis and treatment of disorders of the lower genital tract. Clearly, colposcopy has broad applications for the diagnosis and treatment of benign, premalignant, and malignant disorders.

Cervix

The most common application of colposcopy is to diagnose suspected cervical premalignancy. In most cases, colposcopy is performed after a patient has an abnormal finding on Papanicolaou smear. Cytologic screening is a recognized technique for mass sampling of the population that is at risk for cervical malignancy. This screening permits objective identification of patients whose cervical cellular findings show premalignant changes. Cytology is a screening tool rather than a complete diagnostic tool.

Colposcopic examination is indicated in any patient whose cytologic findings show repetitive atypical squamous cells of undetermined significance, squamous intraepithelial lesions, glandular cell abnormalities, or suspected malignancy. Some investigators recommend performing "reflex" human papilloma virus DNA testing, or typing, in any patient who has cytologic evidence of atypical squamous cells of undetermined significance. Women who test positive for low risk human papillomavirus types or who have no human papillomavirus DNA can be followed annually with repeat cytologic examination. Thus, the goal of colposcopy is to identify the source of atypical cells that would not be detected by unassisted visual examination. Optical verification of specific cervical abnormalities allows the next step, directed biopsy, to be performed. To take full advantage of colposcopic localization, a biopsy specimen must be obtained while the field is observed continuously through the lenses of the colposcope. Swinging the colposcope away and performing a biopsy at the site where the operator previously viewed the abnormal cervical epithelium is less accurate and does not take full advantage of a true colposcopically directed biopsy. The purpose of the biopsy is to establish a diagnosis through histopathologic analysis of a tissue sample.

Vagina

As with the cervix, premalignant lesions of the vagina are suspected after cytologic screening yields abnormal results. Atypical vaginal findings also may be associated with atropy in estrogen-deprived postmenopausal women. Nevertheless, the prudent clinician should follow up a report of atypical vaginal findings by performing colposcopic examination of the vagina. Vaginal colposcopy requires the use of a long, fine skin hook to expose hidden recesses within the vaginal folds. As with the cervix, directed biopsy is required to make a diagnosis.

Vulva

Unlike cervical and vaginal colposcopy, vulvar colposcopy rarely is performed in response to abnormal findings on cytologic screening. Vulvar colposcopy typically is performed after a suspicious lesion is noted on the vulva. Colposcopic examination is performed to magnify the lesion to better determine its significance as well as to identify smaller lesions that are not visible to the unaided eye. Similarly, vulvar colposcopically directed biopsy is more accurate than undirected sampling. Several non-neoplastic dermatologic disorders affect the vulva, and the magnification offered by the colposcope is a distinct advantage in obtaining an accurate diagnosis.

SECTION II
Colposcopy of Specific Sites

A
Colposcopy of the Cervix

CHAPTER 6
Anatomy and Microanatomy of the Cervix

Gross Anatomy

The uterine cervix is the lowest portion of the uterus (Figs. 6-1*A* to 6-1*C*). Laypeople often refer to this structure as the neck of the womb. The cervix has two sections, the portio vaginalis cervix, or ectocervix, and the supravaginal portion of the cervix. The portio vaginalis cervix protrudes into the vagina and is surrounded by four vaginal cul de sacs, or fornices. The supravaginal portion of the cervix is not seen on vaginal examination and is located above the vaginal mucosal reflection. The cervix is cylindrical and measures approximately 3 to 4 cm in height and ranging between 1 to 3 cm in diameter. The diameter of the cervix depends on the status of the patient, whether nulliparous (1 cm) or multiparous (3 cm). The portio vaginalis cervix is clearly marked with an opening, the external os. The os roughly marks the junction between the ectocervix and the endocervix. The external os varies in size and shape depending on whether the patient has been pregnant or has undergone instrumentation (Figs. 6-2*A* and *B*). The average diameter of the nulliparous os is 3–4 mm. The ectocervix is smooth and has a rich, pink color. The endocervix is red to orange-red and has a series of papillary clusters with interspersed clefts (Fig. 6-3). The external os contains mucus that may be clear or cloudy, depending on the phase of the menstrual cycle.

At the uterine (corpal) end of the cervix is a 3-mm, sphincter-like portal known as the internal os. The internal os is the entry point into the uterine cavity (Fig. 6-4). Force is required to dilate the internal os and enter the uterine cavity. The endocervical canal joins the internal and the external os. This canal is 3.5 to 4.0 cm long and has a pattern of longitudinal folds. These folds increase the surface area of the epithelium of the mucus-secreting columnar lining cells (plica palmata) [Fig. 6-5]. Further branching folds spread out peripherally from the plica palmata, creating a palm tree–like pattern that is known as the arbor vitae. Between the folds lie holes, or

clefts, that range in depth from 1 to 2 mm to as much as 1.2 cm (Figs. 6-6*A* and *B*; 6-7).

Microscopic Anatomy

The portio vaginalis cervix is covered with stratified squamous epithelium and essentially is a mucous membrane. Unless the cervix is prolapsed and exposed to the environment, it has no keratin layer.

The portio vaginalis cervix has five layers of cell-types (Fig. 6-8*A*). The first layer is a single layer of basal cells that lie directly on the basement membrane that separates the epithelium from the underlying stroma. These cells are immature and have active mitoses and large nuclei in relation to the cytoplasm. The second layer, or prickle cell layer, consists of several layers of cells that are larger than the basal cells and have relatively more cytoplasm. The prevalence of intracellular bridges gave this layer of cells its name. As in the basal cell layer, mitosis is normal (Figs. 6-8*B* and *C*).

The third layer consists of glycogenated cells that are larger than those of the prickle cell layer. These cells appear clear because of the vacuolation of the cytoplasm. These changes must not be confused with koilocytosis. The fourth layer consists of nonvacuolated, flattened cells that have basophilic staining properties. The fifth layer, sometimes referred to as the stratum corneum (see Figs. 6-8*B* and *C*), consists of progressively flatter, elongated cells that lack vacuoles and have small pyknotic nuclei and eosinophilic cytoplasm.

The endocervix is composed of a single layer of tall, columnar, mucus-secreting epithelium with basilar nuclei (Fig. 6-9*A*). This layer lines the endocervix from approximately the level of the external os to the level of the internal os. Mucus is easily detected on tissue sections by periodic acid-Schiff stain or mucicarmine stain. The layer of mucous cells follows the course of the endocervical clefts as they descend into the underlying cervical stroma

(Fig. *6-9B*). These clefts follow a winding, complex course, and may extend to depths of greater than 1 cm (Fig. *6-10A*). When microscopic sections are prepared, the dermatome knife cuts across the clefts, orienting some in cross-section and others in frontal or longitudinal configurations (Fig. *6-10B*). The misnomer "endocervical glands" resulted from the varied microscopic orientation that created the appearance of mucus-secreting glands. These structures are not racemose mucous glands.

A variable zone of young squamous cells lies at the area of transformation between the mature, multilayered, squamous epithelium of the ectocervix and the single-layered, mucus-secreting columnar epithelium of the endocervical canal (Figs. *6-11A* to *F* and 6-12). This cellular formation has a variety of names, including squamous metaplasia, squamocolumnar prosoplasia, and reserve cell hyperplasia. Various stages of squamous metaplasia are seen in nearly every normal cervix. The mechanism of squamous metaplasia is an essential element relative to the genetics of intraepithelial neoplasia.

Fluhmann described five stages of squamous metaplasia. Stage 1 consists of squamous differentiation of subepithelial reserve cells. A single layer of cuboidal cells appears beneath the columnar cells. In Stage 2, the immature cells divide and create a layer of five to six rows of red-staining polyhedral cells that lift the columnar cells away from the basement membrane. In Stage 3, the young squamous cells form 8 to 12 layers and begin to differentiate. The glandular epithelium is cast off onto the endocervical canal. In Stages 4 and 5, differentiation continues and culminates in the formation of 20- to 30-layered mature squamous epithelium that contains the previously described five cell types (Figs. *6-13A* to *F*).

The cervical stroma consists of collagen interspersed with arterioles, venules, and lymphatic vascular channels. Deep within the stroma are glandular structures that are lined by low, cuboidal cells (see Fig. *6-10A*). Typically, one structure is larger than the surrounding structures. The larger structure is the mesonephric duct, and the smaller spaces may be remnants of the mesonephric tubules or outpouches of the duct. The mesonephric duct may persist at any point between the epoophoron and the hymen (Fig. 6-14).

A basement membrane is seen between the basal cells as well as the columnar cells and the underlying stromal connective tissue. This membrane is seen as a magenta-staining line on periodic acid-Schiff stain. Totipotential reserve cells lie under the basement membrane. This layer consists of cuboidal cells that have a clear halo surrounding a dense, round, centrally placed nucleus. This reserve cell is seen within any tissue that is derived from the müllerian ducts. The reserve cell is a descendant of the original peritoneal cell that invaginated into the mesenchyme of the coelomic cavity to form the embryonic müllerian duct. Depending on its programming, the reserve cell can form any type of cell within the müllerian-derived reproductive tract. The presence of tubal epithelium in the cervix or corpus uteri is explained by this capability. Likewise, metaplasia in the oviduct or endometrium is caused by squamous differentiation of reserve cells in those locations.

As the cranial portion of the cervix blends with the lower portion of the corpus, or isthmus, the cervical stroma contains increasing quantities of smooth muscle (see Fig. 6-14). Similarly, mucus-secreting columnar cells are interspersed with the glycogen-containing columnar cells that are typically found in the endometrium.

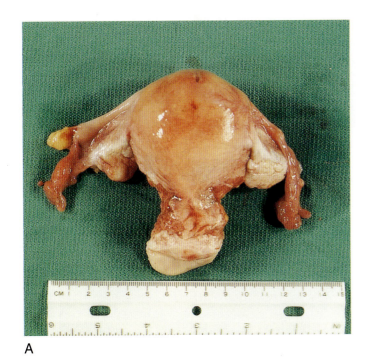

A

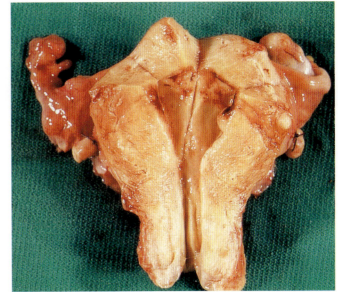

B

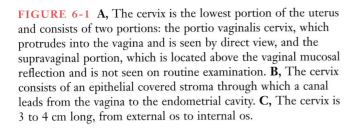

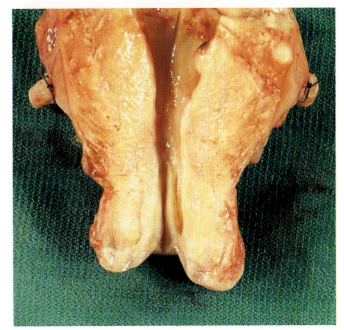

C

FIGURE 6-1 A, The cervix is the lowest portion of the uterus and consists of two portions: the portio vaginalis cervix, which protrudes into the vagina and is seen by direct view, and the supravaginal portion, which is located above the vaginal mucosal reflection and is not seen on routine examination. **B,** The cervix consists of an epithelial covered stroma through which a canal leads from the vagina to the endometrial cavity. **C,** The cervix is 3 to 4 cm long, from external os to internal os.

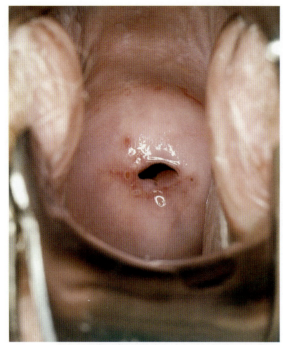

A

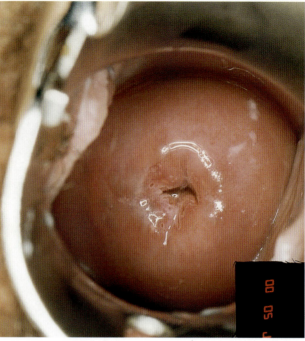

B

FIGURE 6-2 A, This normal cervix has an obvious patent, normal external os that is filled with clear (estrogenic) mucus. The squamocolumnar junction lies just inside the os. **B,** Squamous metaplasia is seen at the level of the external os. The gland openings and cloudy white epithelium are characteristic of young squamous cells (metaplasia).

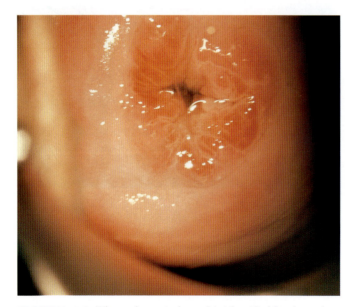

FIGURE 6-3 The endocervical canal is identified by the red-orange color of the single layer of mucous epithelium. The squamocolumnar transformation zone is seen on the portio vaginalis cervix.

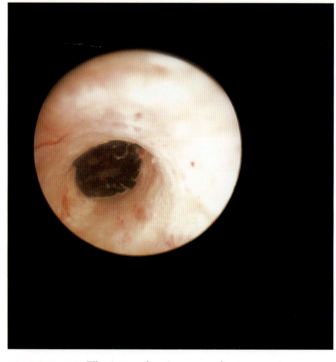

FIGURE 6-4 The internal os is seen on hysteroscopic examination. The hysteroscope is positioned in the middle portion of the cervical canal. Physiologic narrowing is seen. The supravaginal portion of the cervix can be seen only from the interior, by endoscopic examination.

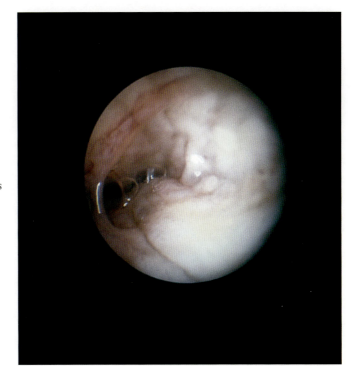

FIGURE 6-5 The pattern of papillae and clefts characteristic of the endocervical canal is seen. The lumen is seen on the reader's left and is identified by bubbles of CO_2.

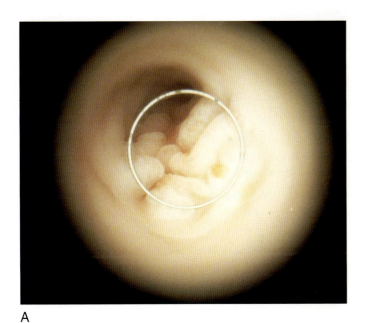

A

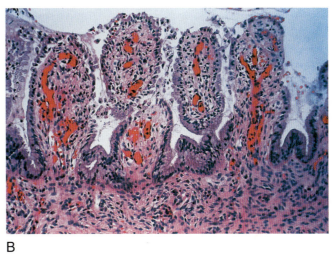

B

FIGURE 6-6 A, Folds and clefts within the endocervical canal create the arbor vitae pattern that is seen through a contact hysteroscope with a 6-mm–diameter viewing circle. **B,** A microscopic longitudinal cut of endocervical mucosa shows the papillary and vascular patterns of the mucosa. The vessels that extend to the terminus of the papillary fold are responsible for the red appearance of the endocervical mucosa.

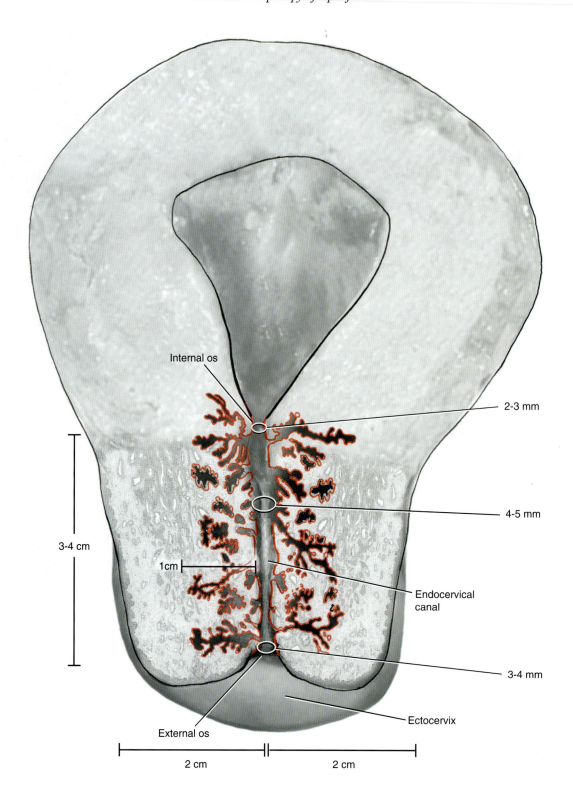

Internal os

2-3 mm

3-4 cm

4-5 mm

1cm

Endocervical
canal

3-4 mm

Ectocervix

External os

2 cm

2 cm

FIGURE 6-7 Cutaway sagittal view of a normal uterus. The detail shows the quantified schematic structure of the endocervical canal. The diameter of a multiparous cervix is approximately twice as large as that of a nulligravid cervix. The structure of the endocervical clefts is seen as they wind deeply into the underlying stroma.

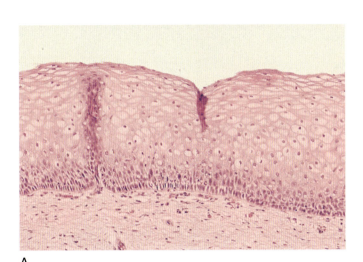

A

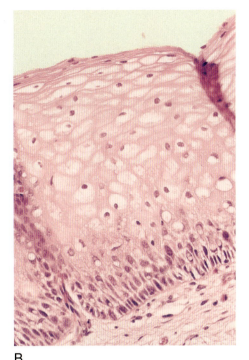

B

FIGURE 6-8 **A,** A section taken through the normal ectocervical mucosa shows the orderly progression of cells from base to surface. Under a low-power microscope, basophilic staining of the parabasal and basal cells creates a continuous thin, dark line. **B,** A high-power view shows the multilayer organization of the mature ectocervical epithelial. This epithelium is approximately 20 cell layers thick. The basal cell layer lies on the basement membrane (periodic acid-Schiff stain) that separates the epithelium from the underlying stroma. The vessels lie in the underlying stroma, and the filtration of light gives the mature ectocervix a pink-white appearance. **C,** Five cell layers are seen: 1, basal cell layer; 2, prickle cell layer; 3, clear, glycogen-containing cell layer; 4, nonvacuolated, flattened cell layer; 5, flat cells with small nuclei and keratinized cytoplasm. This layer is the stratum corneum.

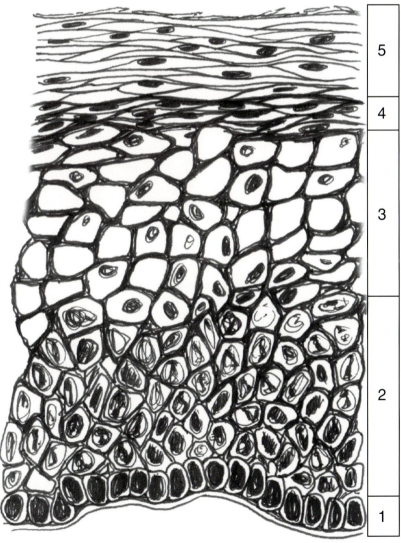

C

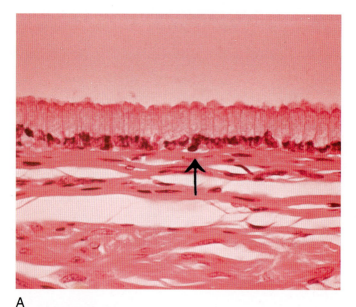

A

B

FIGURE 6-9 A, A magnified section taken through the lower one-third of the normal endocervical canal consists of a single layer of columnar mucus-secreting epithelium and shows uniform basal nuclei as well as the lack of mitotic figures. The reserve cell is seen in the underlying stroma (*arrow*). **B,** Scanning view of the endocervix shows the papillary pattern of the mucosa. Clefts between the neighboring papillae create a frond-like pattern.

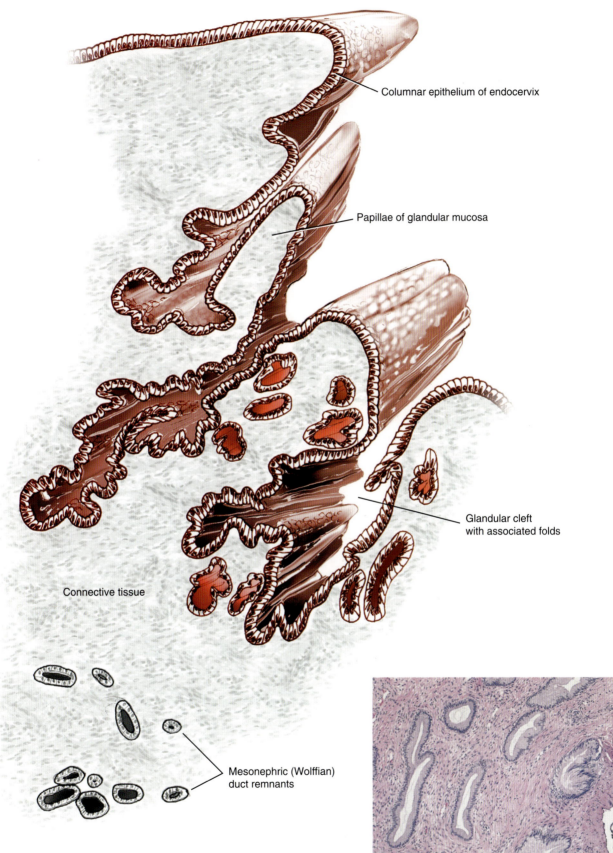

Columnar epithelium of endocervix

Papillae of glandular mucosa

Glandular cleft
with associated folds

Connective tissue

Mesonephric (Wolffian)
duct remnants

A

B

FIGURE 6-10 **A,** The macro- and microarchitecture of the endocervical canal. Mesonephric remnants are located deep in the collagenous stroma. **B,** Cross-sections of the endocervical clefts create the illusion of glands. The simple columnar mucous cell pattern seen in Figure 9A is maintained throughout the normal endocervix.

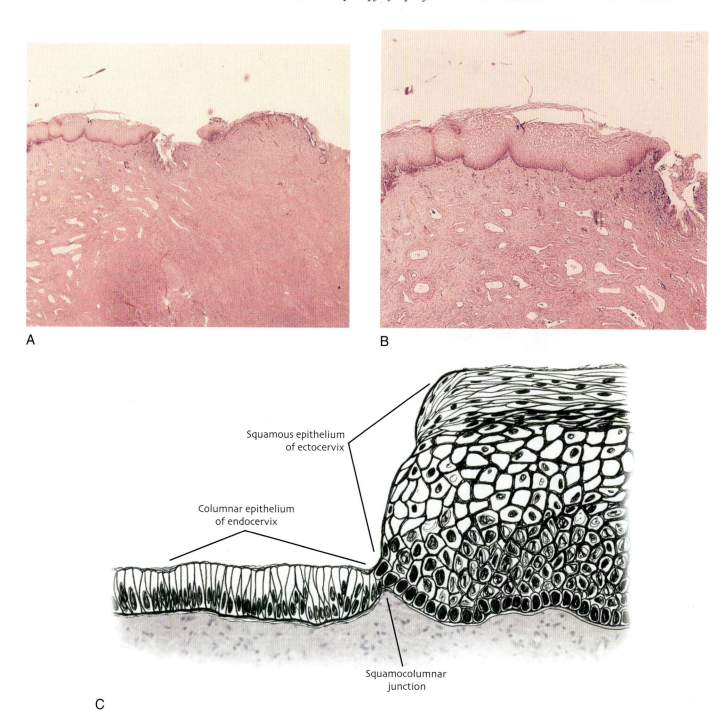

A

B

Squamous epithelium
of ectocervix

Columnar epithelium
of endocervix

Squamocolumnar
junction

C

FIGURE 6-11 **A,** Scanning photomicrograph of a normal squamocolumnar junction with a continuing view of the lower portion of the endocervical canal. **B,** Magnified view of the mature ectocervix (original squamous epithelium) and the squamocolumnar junction. **C,** An idealized squamocolumnar junction has no metaplastic cells. (continued)

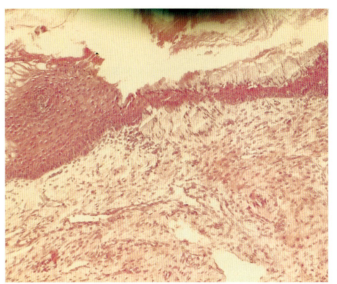

E

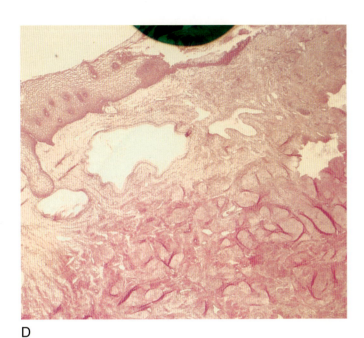

D

FIGURE 6-11 D, A low-power view of the squamocolumnar junction shows a group of red-staining cells (squamous metaplasia) that extend upward into the canal beneath the mucous endocervical epithelium. **E,** A magnified view shows multilayered maturing metaplastic cells (*left*) and less mature, three- to four-layered squamous metaplasia epithelium of the canal. Several clusters of glandular cells are pushed into the canal by the proliferating metaplastic squamous cells. **F,** An actively developing transformation zone shows extensive metaplasia in and under the endocervical canal. Several glands, or clefts, are trapped by surrounding metaplasia. Red squamous cells create the appearance of space.

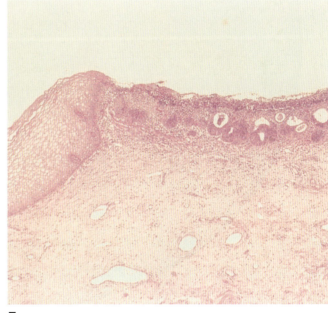

F

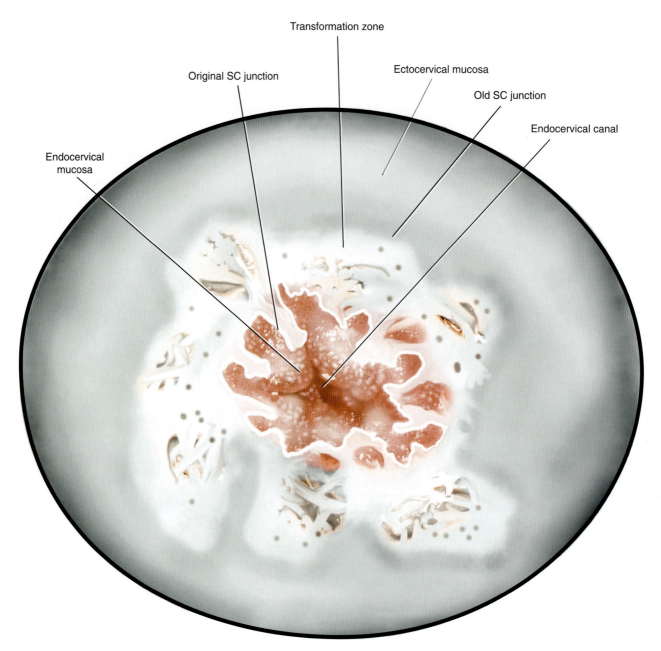

Transformation zone

Original SC junction

Ectocervical mucosa

Old SC junction

Endocervical canal

Endocervical
mucosa

FIGURE 6-12 The cervix shows evolving transformation zones. The periphery of the old transformation zone shows nearly complete metaplasia, with remnant gland openings and a few clefts. This area of advancing glandular epithelial proliferation shows outward mobilization onto the ectocervix. This change is caused by the proliferation of glandular cells as a result of pregnancy, oral contraceptive drugs, or other estrogenic stimulation.

Endocervical canal at SCJ

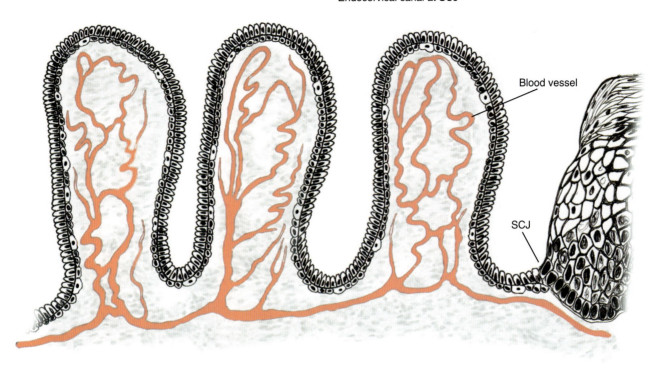

Blood vessel

SCJ

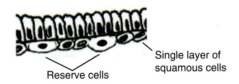

Single layer of
squamous cells

Reserve cells

A

FIGURE 6-13 **A,** The earliest phase of squamous metaplasia of the endocervical canal. The subepithelial reserve cells differentiate into a single layer of young squamous cells that sometimes are mistakenly referred to as reserve cells. The blood vessels extend high into each papillary projection. (continued)

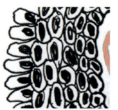

Proliferation of 4-5 layers
of squamous cells

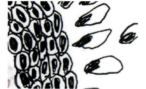

Proliferating young squamous cells
replace columnar epithelium

Endocervical cells
pushed into canal

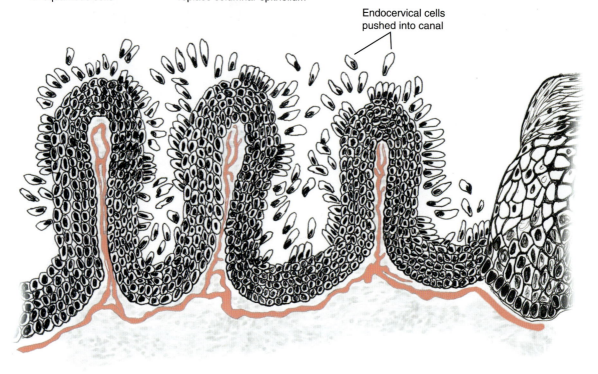

B

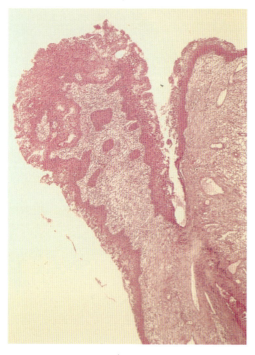

C

FIGURE 6-13 B, In stages 2 and 3 of the metaplastic
process, immature squamous cells project 5 to 12 layers
beneath the columnar epithelium. The squamous cells push
the overlying columnar, mucous cells into the endocervical
canal. As the squamous cells proliferate, the vessels are
pushed downward because the stromal vascular area recedes
as more and more squamous cells occupy the papillus core.
C, A section through the endocervical canal shows two
papillae lined by endocervical mucosa. Extensive metaplasia is
seen beneath the mucosa and within the depths of the clefts.
Red cells show stages 1 and 2 on the right and stage 3 on the
left. (continued)

FIGURE 6-13 D, High-power view of the papillus. The metaplastic (red) squamous cells surround the endocervical surface and interior cells. Several layers of metaplastic cells are seen as neighboring clefts coalesce (stage 3). **E,** Stage 4 is shown by the coalescence of papillae and the relocation of blood vessels to a basilar position. **F,** The new transformation zone is star-shaped and is located near the anatomic external os.

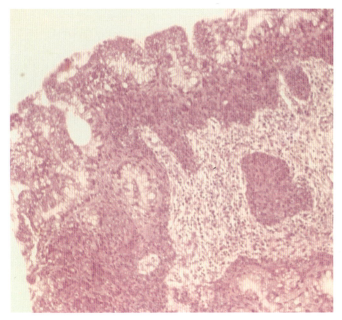

D

Papilla coalesce

Vessels pushed down

E

F

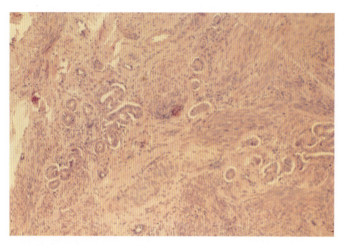

FIGURE 6-14 Tubules that are lined by cuboidal epithelium are seen deep in the underlying stroma of the upper endocervix. These tubules are remnants of the mesonephric tubules and duct (Wolffian duct). Smooth muscle cells are seen in this transition zone between the upper cervix and lower uterine corpus.

CHAPTER 7
Pathology of the Cervix

The earliest changes from normal cervical epithelium to dysplastic epithelium are seen as cellular abnormalities within squamous metaplasia (Figs. 7-1*A* to *C*). These abnormalities are referred to as cellular atypia, atypical metaplasia, atypical microglandular metaplasia, or atypical reserve cell hyperplasia (Figs. 7-2*A* to *C*). These changes are nonspecific and are not indicative of neoplasia. Inflammation causes similar atypical changes (Figs. 7-3*A* to *C*). Although most women and girls have inflammatory cells, especially plasma cells, within the stroma and in and around the transformation zone, the diagnosis of chronic cervicitis usually is based on the degree of inflammation (Figs. 7-3*D* and *E*). Inflammation, especially when associated with infection, may cause cytologic abnormalities that may be mistaken for early neoplasia (Figs. 7-4*A* to *E*). Inflammatory reactive changes usually resolve after 6 to 8 weeks of antimicrobial or antifungal therapy. In general, benign disease is reversible, whereas neoplastic disease is not; however, some benign disorders or congenital abnormalities may have enigmatic features (Figs. 7-5*A* to *H*).

Human Papillomavirus

Infection of cervical cells with human papillomavirus causes abnormalities that may be identified with a colposcope or a high-power microscope (Fig. 7-6*A*). The microscopic features seen in the squamous epithelium include acanthosis, papillomatosis, and parakeratosis (Figs. 7-6*B* and *C*). The finding of koilocytes confirms the diagnosis of human papillomavirus (Figs. 7-7*A* to *C*).

Reserve cells and cell nuclei infected by human papilloma virus follow a different developmental pathway than normal metaplastic cells. The alternate pathway leads to abnormal maturation and the formation of dysplastic cells (Fig. 7-8*A*). The proliferation of blocks of abnormal cells creates vascular abnormalities by allowing vessels to penetrate the epithelial blocks (Figs. 7-8*B* and *C*). The final products of abnormal vascular penetration are colposcopically observed punctation and mosaic patterns (Figs. 7-8*D* and *E*). Additionally, as the number of cells in a cell block increases, vessels are pushed farther apart and intervascular distance increases (Fig. 7-8*F*).

Cervical Intraepithelial Neoplasia

Grade 1

The diagnosis of cervical intraepithelial neoplasia grade 1 (CIN 1) is based on the finding of abnormal basaloid cells that show hyperchromatic nuclei, pleomorphism, an increased nuclear-to-cytoplasmic ratio, and lack of maturation that involves one-third of the thickness of the stratified squamous epithelium (Fig. 7-9*A*). Normal maturation and normal cellular forms are seen in the upper two-thirds of the cervical epithelium (Fig. 7-9*B*).

Grade 2

CIN 2 is diagnosed in patients who have abnormal cytologic changes coupled with numerous mitoses and abnormal mitotic figures that involve one-half of the epithelial thickness (Fig. 7-10*A*). Maturation progresses normally from the middle portion of the epithelium to the surface (Fig. 7-10*B*). Invasive squamous carcinoma may evolve directly from CIN 2 (moderate dysplasia) without the intervening step of progression to CIN 3 (Fig. 7-10*C*).

Grade 3

CIN 3 includes severe dysplasia of the cervix (>50% abnormality encompassing this epithelial thickness) and carcinoma in situ (full-thickness abnormality). Evidence of normal maturation and epithelial organization is absent. In severe dysplasia, a few upper layers of cells may show differentiation. Parakeratosis in the most superficial layers of epithelium does not constitute normal maturation (Figs. 7-11*A* to *D*).

Basaloid cells that have large hyperchromatic nuclei interspersed with cells that show malignant dyskeratosis and abnormal mitotic figures form a disruptive pattern of sameness from the basal to the superficial epithelial layers. Incongruous mitoses in the upper strata and individual cell keratinization within the parabasal or basal layers are seen as well (Fig. 7-12A). Typically, mitoses are abundant (Fig. 7-12B). Extension of neoplastic cells into the lining of the endocervical epithelium and the underlying endocervical clefts is more commonly seen with high-grade than with low-grade intraepithelial neoplasia. According to Fluhmann, 75% of high-grade dysplasias are associated with cleft involvement (Figs. 7-13A through C).

A serial section reconstruction study shows that the clefts are involved by direct extension of the neoplastic epithelium that arises from the squamocolumnar transformation zone and extends cranially into the endocervical canal and the clefts (Figs. 7-14A and B). This endocervical extension rarely progresses more than 1 to 1.5 cm vertically into the canal (Figs. 7-15A to C). Others studies show that dysplastic cells may penetrate the clefts to a depth of 3.8 mm into the underlying stroma.

Invasive Squamous Cell Carcinoma

Invasive disease is diagnosed when neoplastic cells or nests of cells are seen beneath the basement membrane in the cervical stroma (Figs. 7-16A and B). Involvement of the cervical glands does not constitute cleft invasion. Several patterns of invasion are seen. A tongue, or pronounced peg of epithelium, may extend into the stroma, with hypermature cells dropping off into the connective tissue (Figs. 7-17A and B). A spray of epithelial pegs may directly invade the stroma and separate from the surface epithelium. Nests of varying size are seen beneath the surface epithelium.

The cells associated with invasion are more bizarre and pleomorphic than those seen in preinvasive disease. Nuclear abnormalities also are more apparent (Fig. 7-18). Lymphatic involvement is not uncommon and is seen more often when tissue blocks are serially sectioned (Figs. 7-19A and B). A significant inflammatory response is seen around invasive foci and may suggest early invasion in sections that initially appear to be only carcinoma in situ (Fig. 7-20).

Adenocarcinoma

Although most preinvasive and invasive disease of the uterine cervix is of squamous cell origin, the incidence of adenocarcinoma is increasing. In 1970, endocervical adenocarcinoma accounted for 5% of cervical malignancies. By 1990, that figure was 20%. Adenocarcinoma in situ often coexists with squamous cell carcinoma in situ. The finding of mitotic figures within the mucus-secreting columnar cells of the endocervical canal is never normal and often accompanies early neoplasia (Fig. 7-21). The cells that line the endocervical canal and clefts also may show nuclear elongation, darkening, and multinucleation. Stratification of cells also is characteristic of neoplastic change. Budding of glands into the stroma is a sign of invasion (Fig. 7-22). The proliferation of cells associated with adenocarcinoma in situ may be difficult to differentiate from early stromal invasion that characterizes frank adenocarcinoma (Fig. 7-23). Primary adenocarcinoma of the endocervix is differentiated from secondary endometrial carcinoma by differential curettage of the endocervical canal and the endometrial cavity as well as the application of mucus stains (Figs. 7-24A and B).

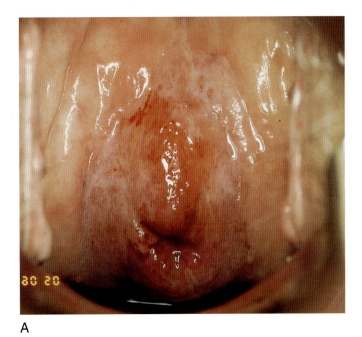

A

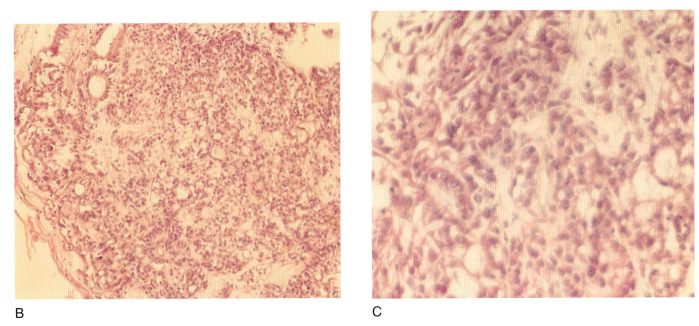

B   C

FIGURE 7-1 A, This cervix has an extensive transformation zone. Areas of immature squamous metaplasia are seen in the patient's upper left quadrant and on her right side. **B,** A biopsy specimen taken at the 1 o'clock position shows an atypical pattern of microglandular mucoid metaplasia. Small glandular spaces surrounded by solid areas of polyhedral cells may be mistaken for adenocarcinoma or adenosquamous carcinoma. In a case report published in *Obstetrics and Gynecology*, similar findings were mistaken for clear cell adenocarcinoma. **C,** A high-power view of **B** shows multiple trapped glandular spaces surrounded by immature, but benign, metaplastic squamous cells.

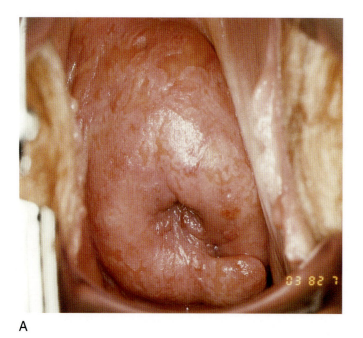

A

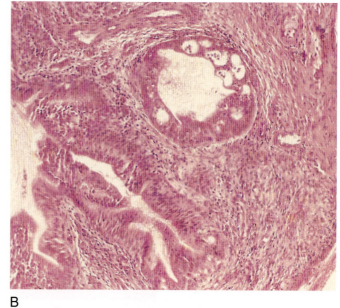

B

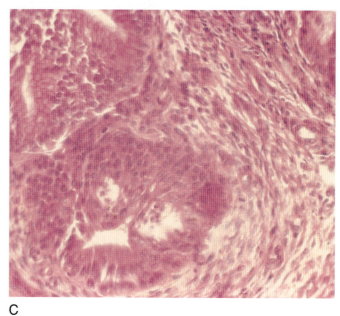

C

FIGURE 7-2 A, This cervix is nearly covered with white epithelium that extends into the vaginal fornices. The patient had no history of diethylstilbestrol exposure. The patient's mother obtained her prenatal record, which showed no exposure. **B,** Biopsy of the cervix shown in Figure 2*A* shows atypical reserve cell hyperplasia. These immature squamous metaplastic cells show mild nuclear atypia. **C,** A magnified view of **B** shows the immature squamous cells that surround definite gland structures and replace the columnar mucous cells. The structure and organization are better defined than the process seen in Figures 7-1*B* and 1*C*.

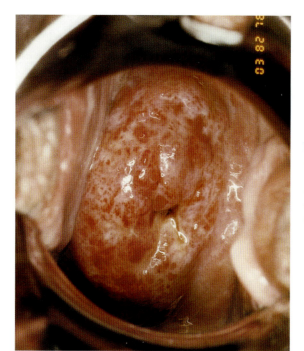

FIGURE 7-3 A, This cervix shows ectopy, squamous metaplasia, and severe inflammation. Biopsy would cause significant bleeding because of the presence of inflammatory vessels. (continued)

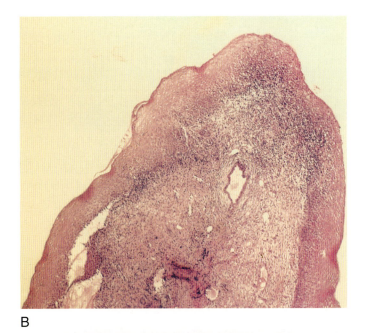

B

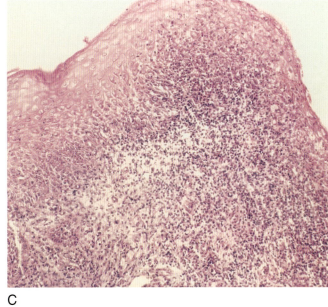

C

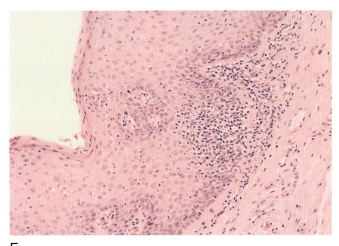

E

FIGURE 7-3 B, Ectocervical biopsy shows severe cervicitis. Many inflammatory cells are seen in the stroma and epithelium. **C,** Acute and chronic inflammatory cells have infiltrated the entire thickness of the epithelium, creating surface ulceration. **D,** This cervix has numerous red papules that are consistent with infection. **E,** Biopsy of **D** shows an epithelial reactive abnormality, parakeratosis, and mild acanthosis. Extensive chronic inflammatory cells are seen in the stroma and epithelium. Inflammation is less severe in this area than in the section seen in **C.**

D

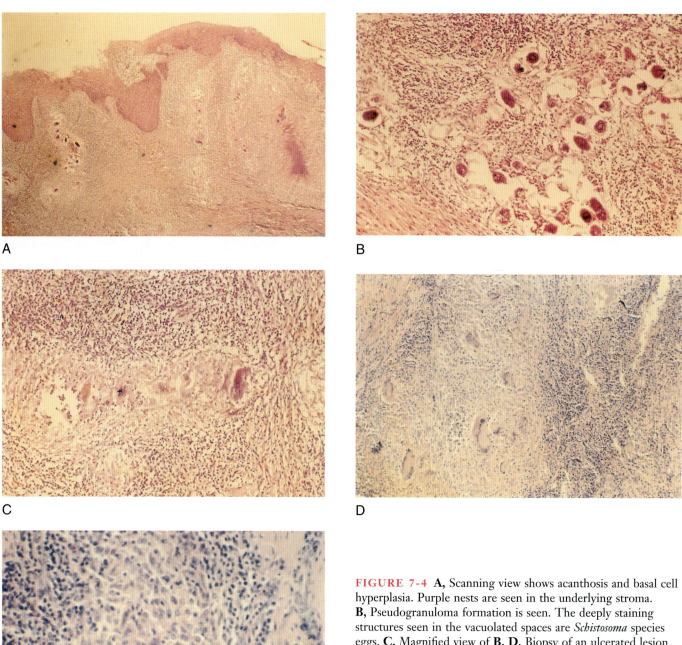

FIGURE 7-4 **A,** Scanning view shows acanthosis and basal cell hyperplasia. Purple nests are seen in the underlying stroma. **B,** Pseudogranuloma formation is seen. The deeply staining structures seen in the vacuolated spaces are *Schistosoma* species eggs. **C,** Magnified view of **B. D,** Biopsy of an ulcerated lesion on the cervix shows granuloma formation with numerous Langhans'-type giant cells. **E,** A high-power view of **D** shows giant cell and tuberculous granuloma. Acid-fast stain showed mycobacteria.

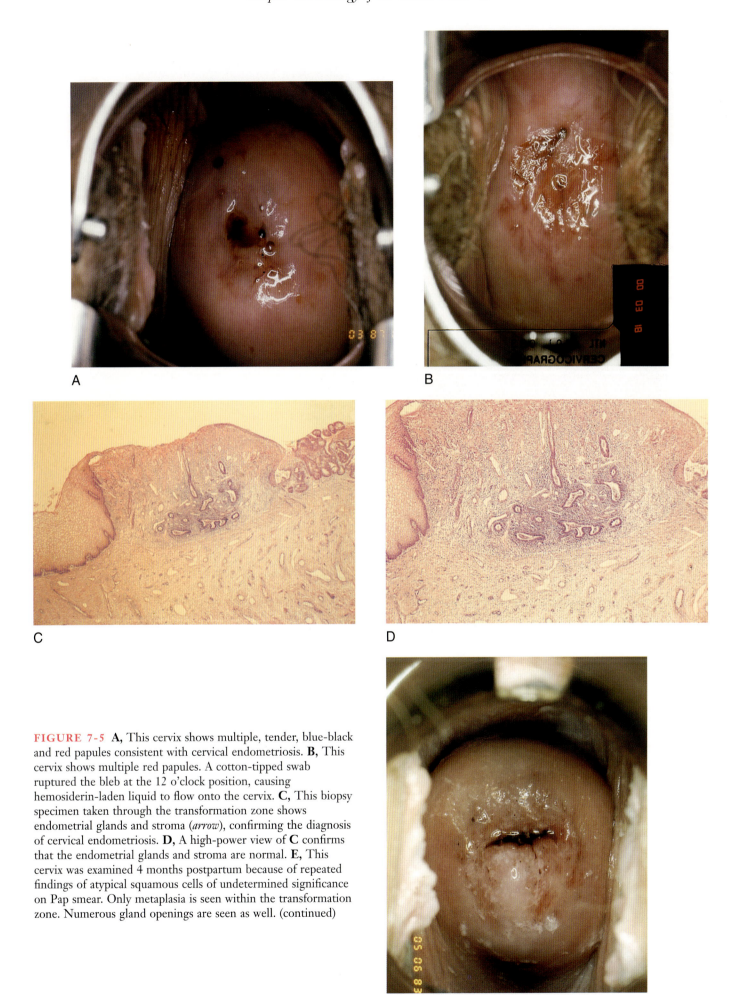

FIGURE 7-5 A, This cervix shows multiple, tender, blue-black and red papules consistent with cervical endometriosis. **B,** This cervix shows multiple red papules. A cotton-tipped swab ruptured the bleb at the 12 o'clock position, causing hemosiderin-laden liquid to flow onto the cervix. **C,** This biopsy specimen taken through the transformation zone shows endometrial glands and stroma (*arrow*), confirming the diagnosis of cervical endometriosis. **D,** A high-power view of **C** confirms that the endometrial glands and stroma are normal. **E,** This cervix was examined 4 months postpartum because of repeated findings of atypical squamous cells of undetermined significance on Pap smear. Only metaplasia is seen within the transformation zone. Numerous gland openings are seen as well. (continued)

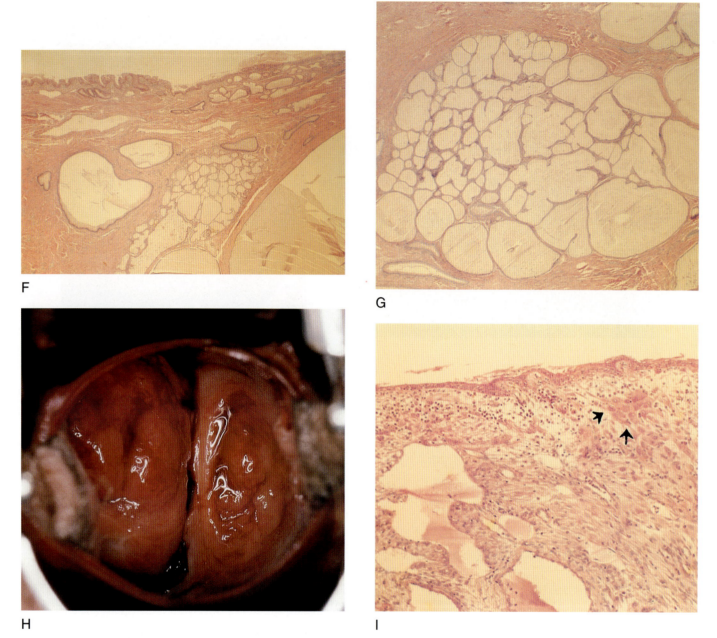

F

G

H

I

FIGURE 7-5 **F,** This biopsy taken from the transformation zone of the cervix shown in **D** shows clusters of glands and several hugely dilated spaces. **G,** This magnified view was taken through a cluster of glands lined by simple mucous columnar cells or flattened cuboid cells. Fluhmann referred to this finding as tunnel clusters, whereas others use the term endocervical glandular hyperplasia. This condition is benign and is not associated with endometrial hyperplasia. **H,** Although this cervix looks ominous, it shows a benign condition. In this photograph, taken immediately after a vaginal septum was excised, two cervices are seen. Each cervix is 2 cm high and shows extensive ectopy. **I,** This biopsy specimen was obtained from a cervix with red papules similar to those shown in Figure 7-3*D*. The large, pink cells are diagnostic of a decidual reaction (*arrows*).

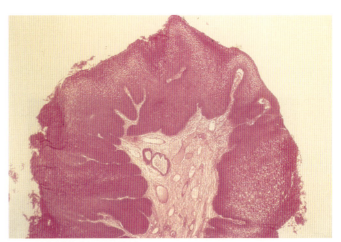

B

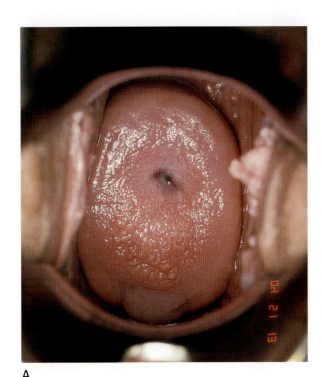

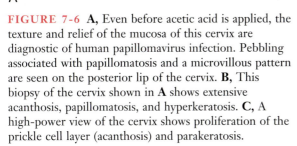

A

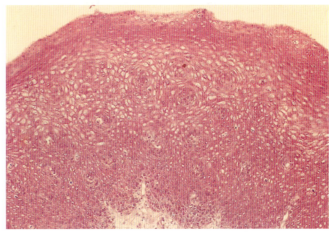

C

FIGURE 7-6 **A,** Even before acetic acid is applied, the texture and relief of the mucosa of this cervix are diagnostic of human papillomavirus infection. Pebbling associated with papillomatosis and a microvillous pattern are seen on the posterior lip of the cervix. **B,** This biopsy of the cervix shown in **A** shows extensive acanthosis, papillomatosis, and hyperkeratosis. **C,** A high-power view of the cervix shows proliferation of the prickle cell layer (acanthosis) and parakeratosis.

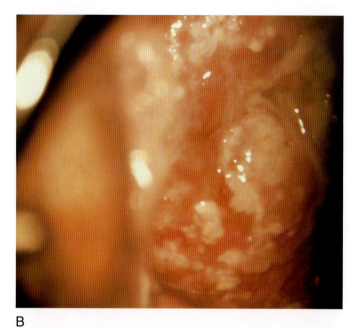

B

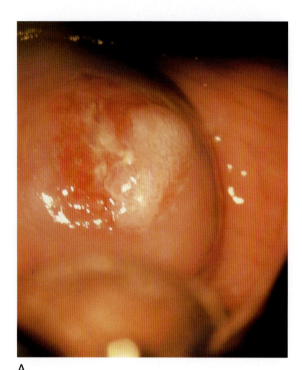

A

FIGURE 7-7 A, This white lesion occupies the patient's left half of the abnormal transformation zone and is diagnostic of a flat wart. **B,** This patient is approximately 10 weeks pregnant. An extensive abnormal transformation zone and multiple areas of white epithelium show a pattern typical of flat warts. **C,** This fragment of tissue shows atypical condylomatous change with many koilocytes.

C

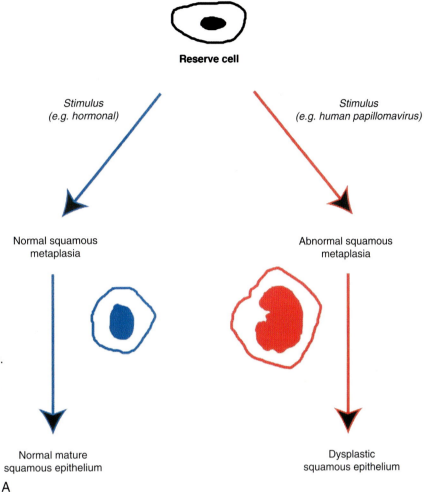

FIGURE 7-8 **A,** The two metaplastic developmental pathways taken by reserve cells. **B,** The reserve cells that underlie the columnar mucous cells in the endocervical canal are infected with human papillomavirus. The progeny of the infected reserve cells are abnormal metaplastic cells. As these cells proliferate, they create more atypical cells. The native mature glandular cells are cast off into the canal, and the endocervical papillae are composed of blocks of atypical, or dysplastic, squamous metaplastic cells. (continued)

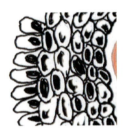

Nuclei abnormal

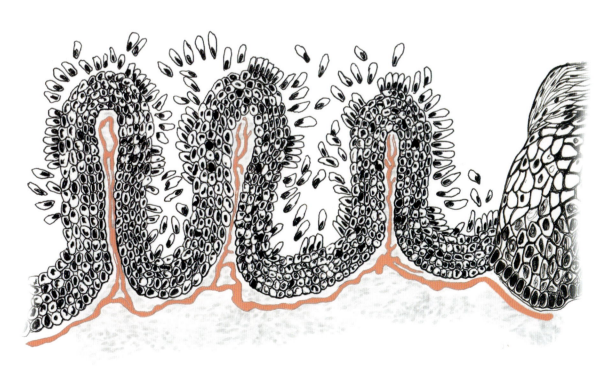

B

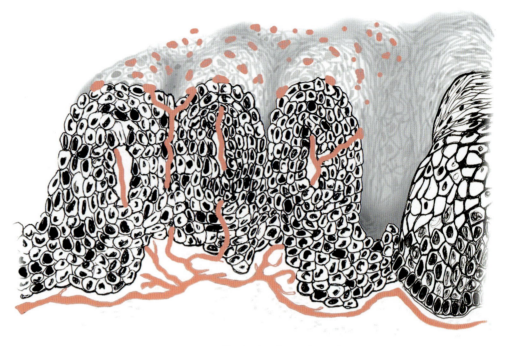

Penetrating abnormal vessels
(punctate)

C

Blocks of tissue proliferating

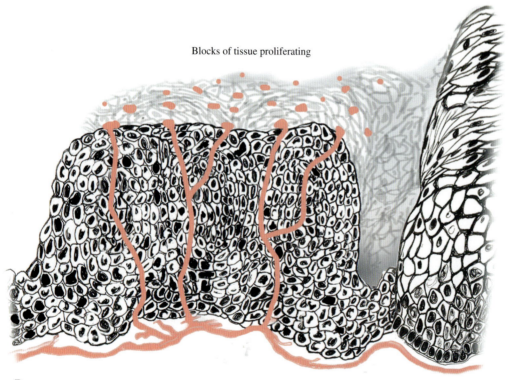

D

FIGURE 7-8 C, As the blocks of cells expand and coalesce, the original vessels are incorporated into the epithelial blocks and the vessels proliferate within the atypical epithelium. **D,** Compression of the terminal vessels creates punctation patterns. As the dysplastic process increases in volume and severity, the intraepithelial vessels are pushed farther apart. The intercapillary distance mirrors the grade of dysplasia. (continued)

Mosaic

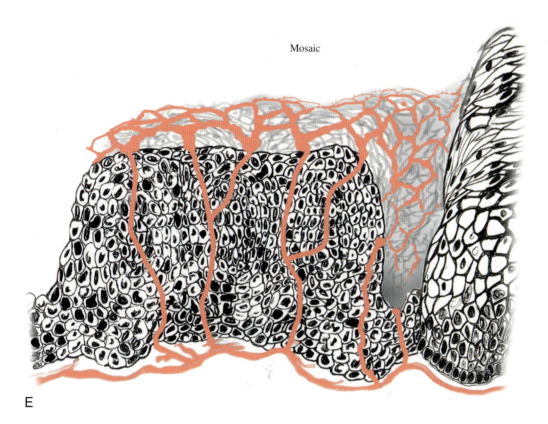

E

Mosaic

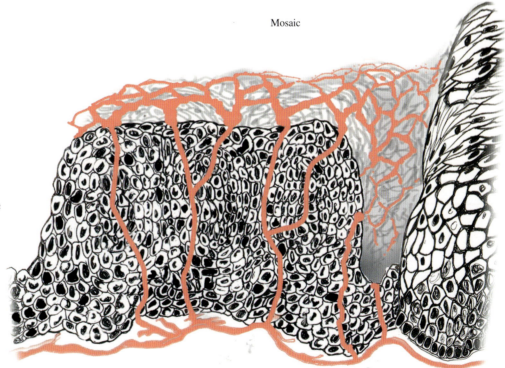

F

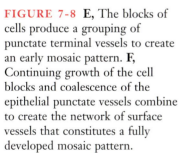

FIGURE 7-8 E, The blocks of cells produce a grouping of punctate terminal vessels to create an early mosaic pattern. **F,** Continuing growth of the cell blocks and coalescence of the epithelial punctate vessels combine to create the network of surface vessels that constitutes a fully developed mosaic pattern.

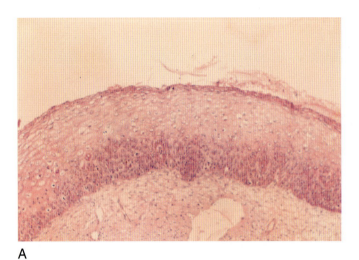

A

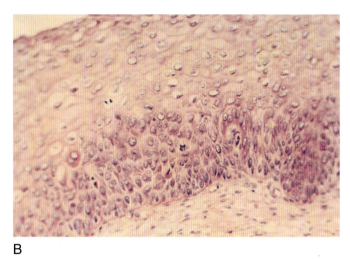

B

FIGURE 7-9 **A,** A low-power view of this section is diagnostic of mild dysplasia. The sharp, well-defined basal layer has been obliterated by the proliferation of basaloid cells to approximately one-third the thickness of the epithelial layer. **B,** A high-power view of **A** shows abnormal cells and mitotic figures occupying 33% of the epithelial thickness. At the one-third internal point, the epithelium abruptly begins the normal maturation process. This section shows mild dysplasia.

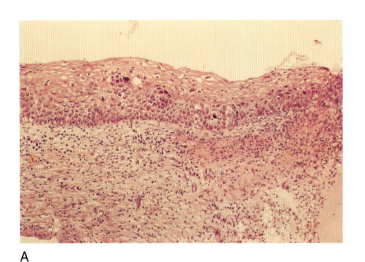

A

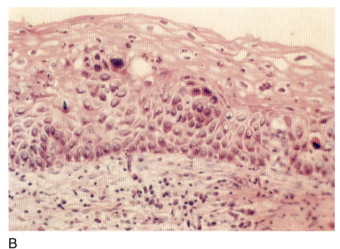

B

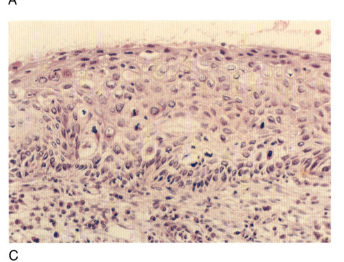

C

FIGURE 7-10 **A,** Compared with Figure 7-9*A* and *B*, definite progression is seen relative to the grade of dysplasia. Cellular abnormalities occupy 50% of the epithelial strata before normal maturation begins. **B,** A magnified view of **A** shows neoplastic cells that range from a single keratinized cell in the prickle cell layer, where it clearly does not belong, to hyperchromatic pleomorphic cells that border the zone of normal maturation. This section shows moderate dysplasia. **C,** This section shows moderate to severe dysplasia. Several mitotic figures are seen, even at the midepithelial level. Although maturation is evident in the upper third, it is atypical, with parakeratosis.

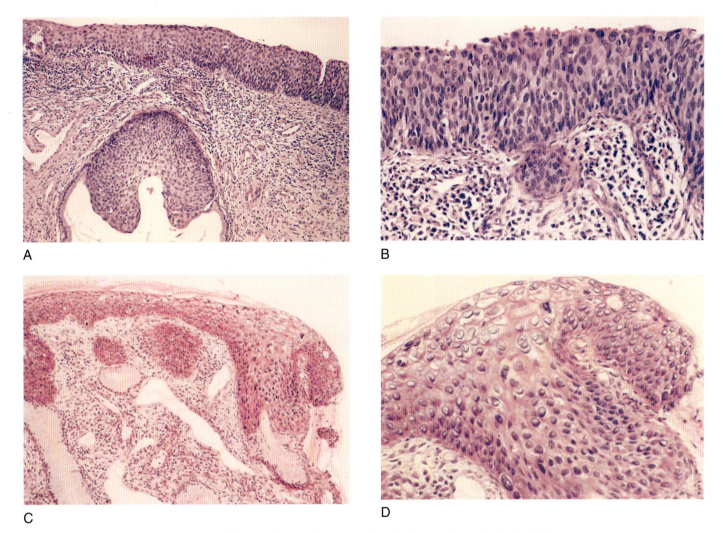

A

B

C

D

FIGURE 7-11 A, Carcinoma in situ of the cervix is involvement of neoplastic cells through the full thickness of the epithelium. No normal maturation is present, as in mild or moderate dysplasia. Severe dysplasia of the endocervical clefts is clearly seen. **B,** A high-power view of Figure 7-11*A* shows hyperchromatic basaloid cells that extend through the epithelium, from top to bottom. The layers show no organization, and the entire thickness of the epithelium is homogeneously configured by neoplastic cells. Serial sections must be examined to exclude microscopic invasion in the area of the small, circular clump of cells below the basement membrane. **C,** This section shows severe dysplasia. Severe dysplasia and carcinoma in situ are equally severe. **D,** A high-power view of **C** shows a marginal cluster of cells that extends into an endocervical cleft. Although this process clearly shows upward extension into the endocervical canal, it does not alter the prognosis.

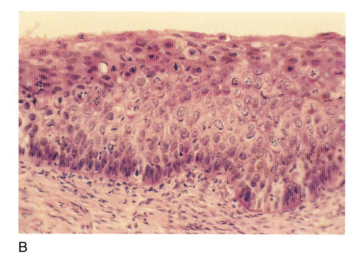

B

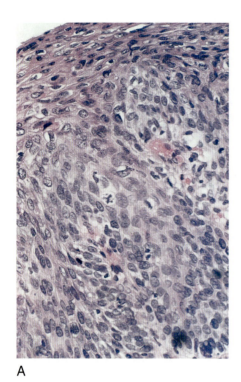

A

FIGURE 7-12 **A,** Dilated blood vessels penetrate deeply into the upper layers of the epithelium and cause the colposcopic findings of mosaic and punctation. **B,** This section of severe dysplasia shows individual cellular anaplasia. Many abnormal mitotic figures are seen in the upper third of the epithelium (*right*).

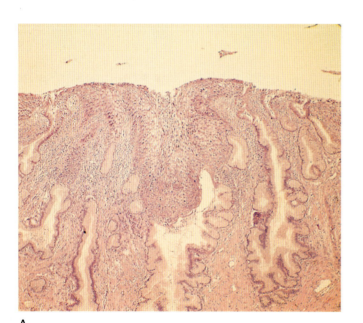

A

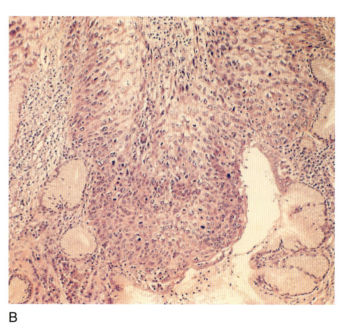

B

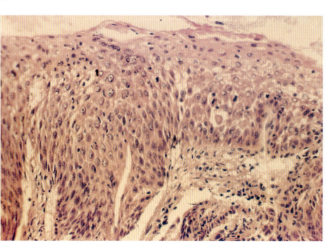

C

FIGURE 7-13 **A,** At least 50% of lesions that show severe dysplasia or carcinoma in situ extend into the endocervical canal through direct extension from the transformation zone. **B,** A high-power view of **A** shows neoplastic tissue intruding into a cleft that is lined by normal columnar mucous cells. **C,** Another section shows neoplastic cells extending into underlying clefts.

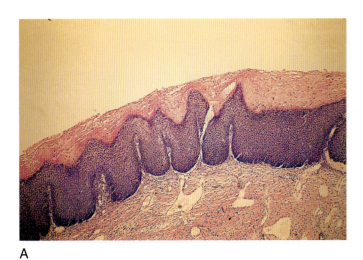

A

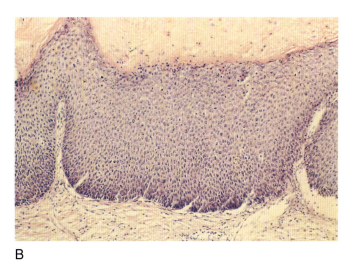

B

FIGURE 7-14 A, This type of carcinoma in situ is associated with more mature cells and hyperkeratosis than similar lesions; however, its behavior is the same. The colposcopic appearance is thick, white epithelium with no vascular abnormalities. These cellular changes are referred to as Bowenoid. **B,** A high-power view of **A** shows round cells with clear cytoplasm and round hyperchromatic nuclei. These cells are known as corps ronds.

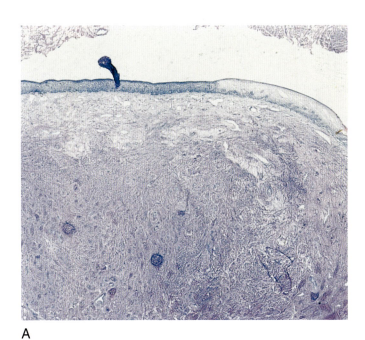

A

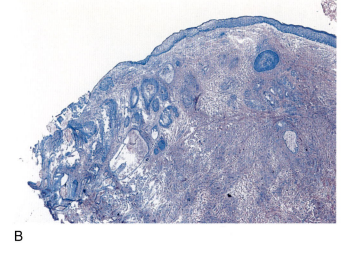

B

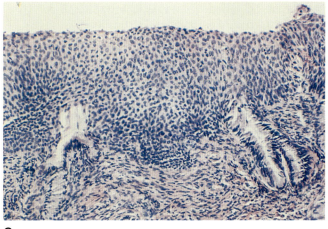

C

FIGURE 7-15 A, A cryostat cone section (scanning power) shows extension of carcinoma in situ into the endocervical canal. **B,** A section of the case shows extension to the 1-cm margin of the endocervical canal. A 1.5-cm margin is recommended. **C,** High-power view of **B**.

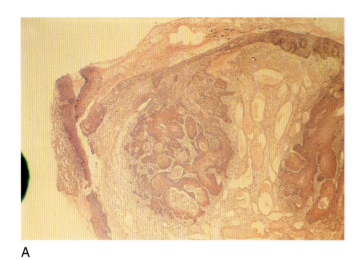

A

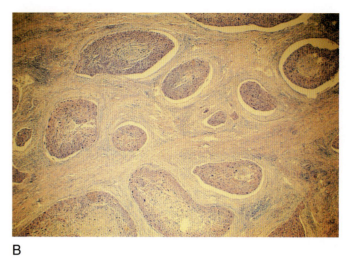

B

FIGURE 7-16 **A,** A scanning view shows early stromal invasion. **B,** Plugs of squamous carcinoma fill the endothelial lined spaces, i.e., lymphatic vessels.

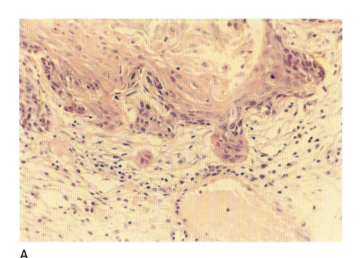

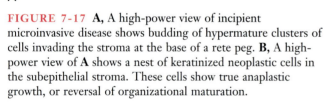

A

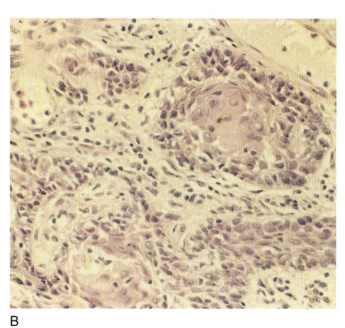

B

FIGURE 7-17 **A,** A high-power view of incipient microinvasive disease shows budding of hypermature clusters of cells invading the stroma at the base of a rete peg. **B,** A high-power view of **A** shows a nest of keratinized neoplastic cells in the subepithelial stroma. These cells show true anaplastic growth, or reversal of organizational maturation.

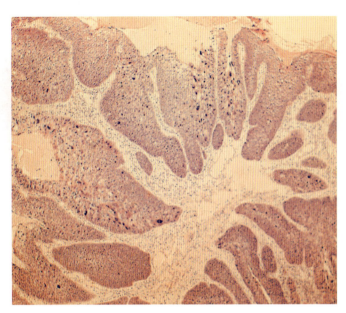

FIGURE 7-18 Biopsy of a papillomatous cervical lesion shows extreme individual cell anaplasia associated with invasive cancer.

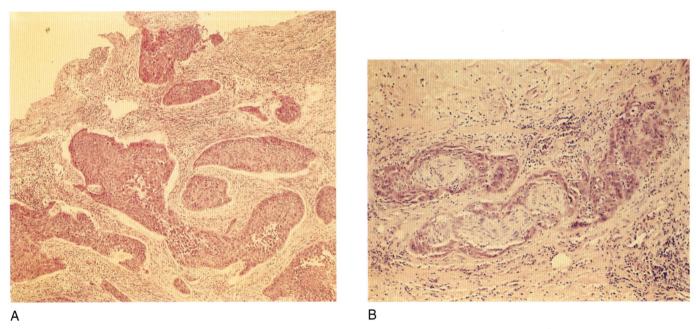

A

B

FIGURE 7-19 **A,** Invasive fingers of squamous carcinoma extend through the cervical stroma and invade the base of the bladder. **B,** Squamous cell carcinoma invades the perineural lymphatic spaces.

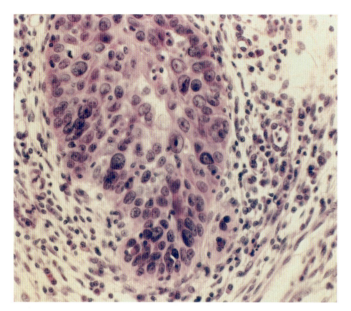

FIGURE 7-20 An inflammatory response surrounds this tongue of neoplastic tissue within the cervical stroma. A line of plasma cells is seen.

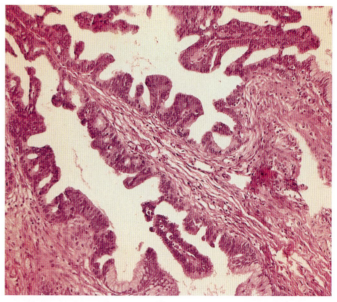

FIGURE 7-21 This section shows adenocarcinoma in situ. Compared with normal mucous cells, the neoplastic cells show stratification, the nuclei are hyperchromatic, and mitoses are present. A sharp transition is seen between normal mucous cells on the right and neoplastic epithelium on the left.

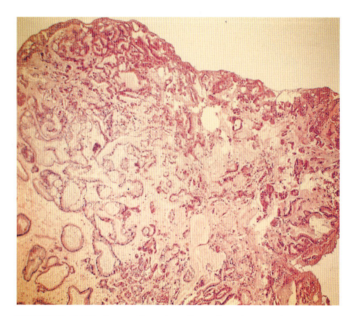

FIGURE 7-22 A scanning view shows invasive mucinous adenocarcinoma in the endocervical canal.

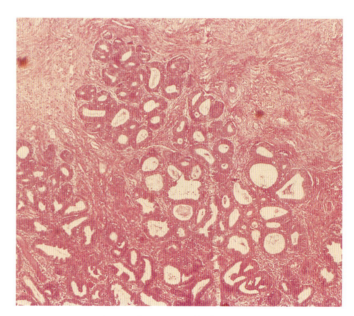

FIGURE 7-23 Stromal invasion of adenocarcinoma of questionable origin is seen. An endometrial primary lesion is suspected.

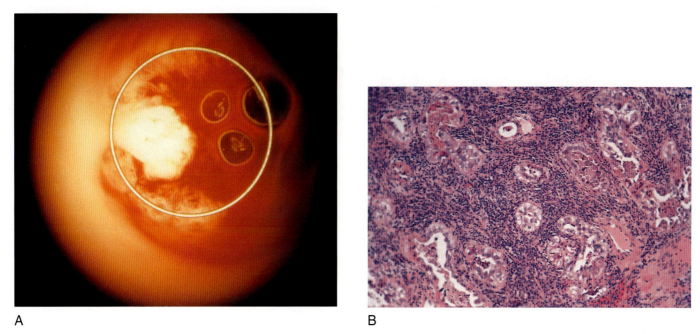

A

B

FIGURE 7-24 A, Contact hysteroscopic examination of the endocervix shows a 3-mm focus of neoplastic tissue at the 9 o'clock position. **B,** Microscopic sections of the lesion shown in **A** show invasive adenocarcinoma.

CHAPTER 8
Terminology

To communicate with each other, colposcopists need a uniform descriptive terminology. Over the last 60 to 70 years, although the semantics have changed, the features being described have remained consistent.

Basic Terminology

Atypical transformation zone: Diagnosis is based on the following findings on colposcopy: white appearance of the epithelium after the application of 3% acetic acid solution; red appearance of the endocervical epithelium, with some raised areas; abnormal vascular patterns, including mosaic or punctation patterns; and no staining after the application of Lugol's iodine solution.

Leukoplakia (white plaque): This term leukoplakia has been replaced by the term white epithelium. Ground leukoplakia is the white background that sets off the abnormal red vascular patterns. Plaque formation describes hyperkeratosis sometimes combined with flat papillomatosis.

White epithelium: The former term for this change is ground leukoplakia. White epithelium is graded according to the degree of whiteness, the focality of the area, and the degree of relief, or extension above the surrounding normal epithelium. Grade 1 is cloudy or veiled whitish-pink (Fig. 8-1). Grade 3 is densely chalky white and often shows greater relief than grade 1 (Fig. 8-2). Grade 2 is intermediate between grades 1 and 3. White epithelium may be present before 3% acetic acid is applied and always is seen in an abnormal transformation zone after 3% acetic acid is applied.

Condylomatous pattern: White epithelium forms islands on the ectocervix and may be located well away from the transformation zone (Fig. 8-5). The wavy papillomatosis creates a golf ball–like surface (Figs. 8-3 and 8-4). Another pattern has a microvillous or micropapillomatous appearance that is characterized by fine white spicules with red punctation at the tip of each projection. This pattern is associated with human papillomavirus infection.

Vascular Patterns

The cervix has a rich vascular supply. The vascular pattern seen in a normal cervix depends on the thickness of the stratified squamous epithelium. Most cervices show no distinctive vascular pattern; however, atrophy thins the epithelium sufficiently to allow a clear view of the architecture of the blood vessels. The two most common patterns are branching and network patterns. Branching is often seen over nabothian cysts (Fig. 8-6). Network patterns are diffuse and often involve the entire ectocervix.

Punctation pattern: Grades of punctation range from fine to coarse (Figs. 8-7 to 8-9). This pattern consists of dots that are created by the upward course of blood vessels that are squeezed by proliferating blocks of neoplastic cells. As the neoplastic disorder progresses, intercapillary distances increase. Greater intercapillary distance indicates more significant underlying pathology. The normal intercapillary distance is 100 µm. Early dysplasia is associated with intercapillary distances of 250 µm, and advanced dysplasia is associated with intercapillary distances of 350 to 450 µm (Fig. 8-10). Typically, large, coarse punctation is associated with high-grade dysplasia, whereas fine, closely spaced dots indicate a benign condition. Typically, dysplastic lesions have a clear focus. Diffuse lesions usually indicate inflammation of normal tissue. Inflammatory disorders are associated with single vessels, double hairpin vessels, or network punctation (Figs. 8-11 and 8-12).

Mosaic pattern: Early mosaic patterns are groupings of punctation that initially form the outline of a mosaic. As the lesion develops, the dots connect to form a solid vascular boundary (Figs. 8-13 to 8-15). A sharp, clear mosaic pattern suggests a severe lesion, whereas a diffuse mosaic pattern usually is associated with diethylstilbestrol-related disease or another benign disorder. A focal mosaic pattern seen in white epithelium that has an intercapillary distance of greater than 250 μm suggests high-grade disease (cervical intraepithelial neoplasia grade 2 or 3).

Unsatisfactory Colposcopy

In an unsatisfactory colposcopic examination, the squamocolumnar transformation zone cannot be seen (Fig. 8-16). Several causes are possible. First, cervical stenosis may prevent colposcopic assessment of the endocervical canal. Second, in some elderly women, the squamocolumnar junction is relocated high in the endocervical canal as a result of estrogen deprivation. Finally, radiation therapy or cervical surgery may lead to the formation of scars that may shorten and distort the cervix.

Atypical (Abnormal) Vessels

Atypical vessels include bizarre branching and horizontal types (Fig. 8-17). The branches are not tree-like, but are short and irregular, with abrupt terminations. No regular branching pattern is seen. The caliber of the branching vessels is bizarre, with distended surface vessels that have bulbous terminations. The horizontal vessels have no precise starting source and simply appear in a more or less haphazard fashion traversing short distances. In contrast to the punctation and mosaic patterns, these vessels are neither uniform nor even. A cerebral pattern, suggestive of the gyri of the brain, strongly suggests underlying malignancy. Irregular vessels typically suggest invasive carcinoma (Fig. 8-18*A* and *B*).

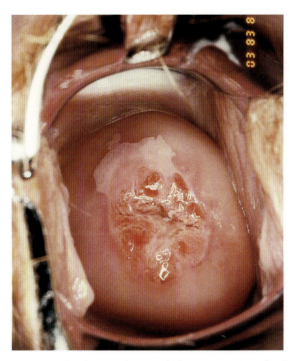

FIGURE 8-1 Grade 1-2 white epithelium is seen in a focal lesion that extends at the perimeter of the transformation zone from the 11 o'clock position to the 1 o'clock position.

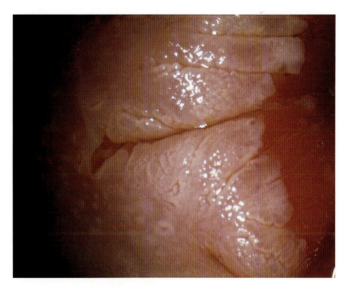

FIGURE 8-2 Grade 3 white epithelium occupies most of the abnormal transformation zone. Large clefts and smaller peripheral cleft openings are seen.

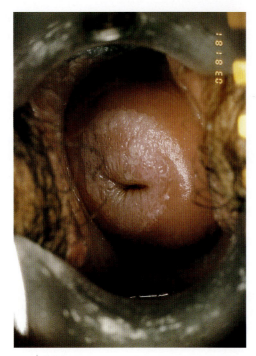

FIGURE 8-3 This extensive white epithelium shows papillomatosis, or pebbling, and microvillous formation. This appearance is diagnostic of condylomatous atypia.

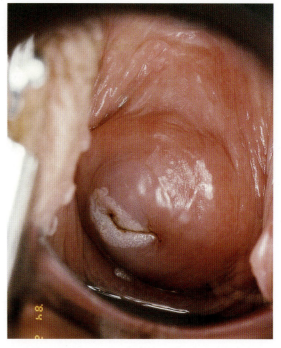

FIGURE 8-4 Dense white epithelium shows a geographic microvillous pattern and a focalized abnormal transformation zone. This pattern is typical of human papillomavirus infection and dysplasia.

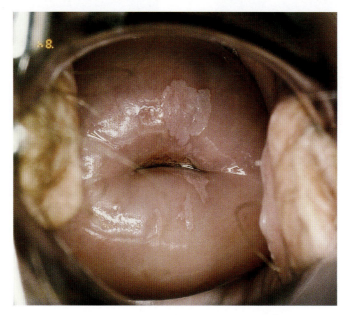

FIGURE 8-5 Isolated islands of grade 1 white epithelium seen at the 12 o'clock and 6 o'clock positions suggest human papillomavirus infection.

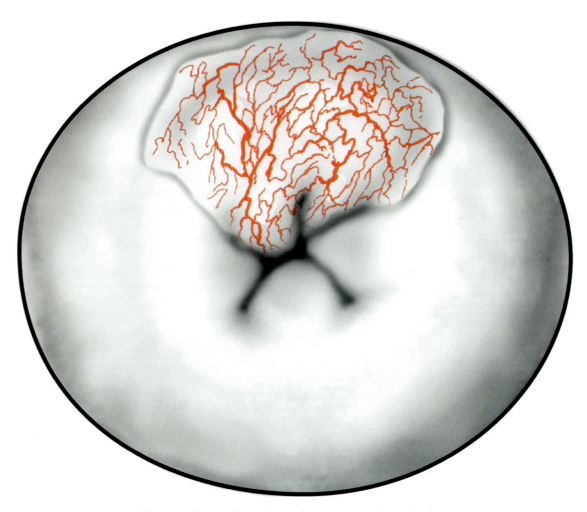

FIGURE 8-6 The normal cervical vasculature shows organized, tree-like branching.

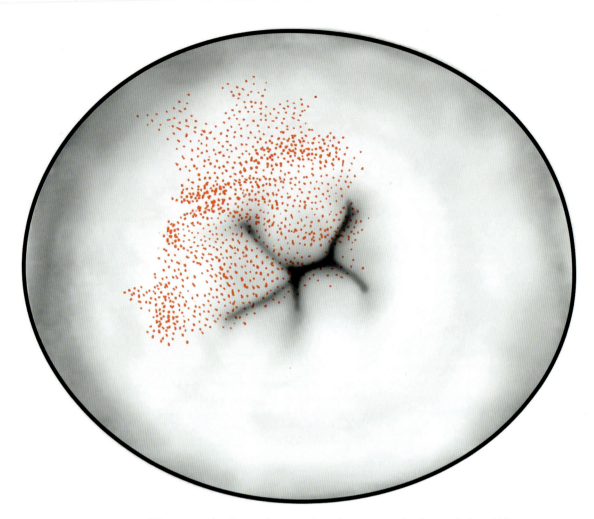

FIGURE 8-7 Fine punctation is seen in normal cervices as a result of metaplasia, within atrophic cervices, and within inflamed cervices. Fine punctation usually is not associated with white epithelium.

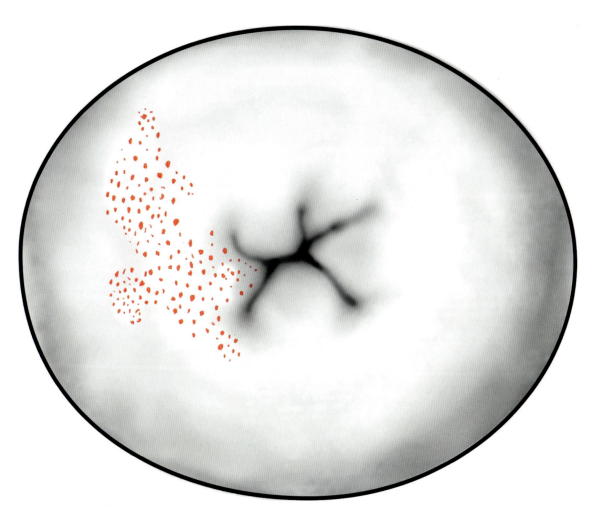

FIGURE 8-8 Early intermediate papillary punctation with an intercapillary distance of greater than 250 μm. The pattern is set off by white epithelium. The contrast of red on white enhances the view of the abnormal transformation zone.

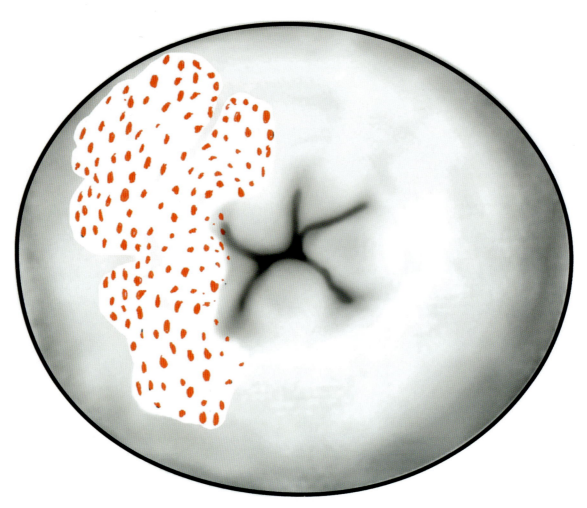

FIGURE 8-9 True papillary punctation. The terminal portion of the capillaries is compressed by proliferating blocks of neoplastic cells. These blocks increase intercapillary distance and create large, bulbous spots. The terminal capillaries usually are focal and are set against a background of white epithelium.

Intercapillary Distance

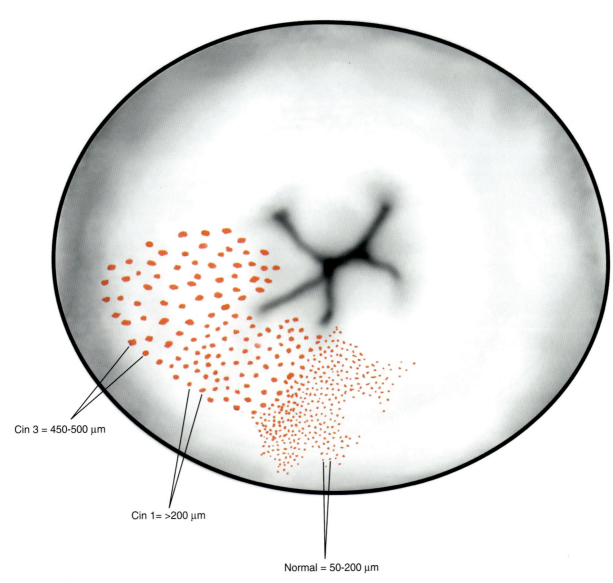

Cin 3 = 450-500 µm

Cin 1= >200 µm

Normal = 50-200 µm

FIGURE 8-10 Normal versus abnormal intercapillary distance and the relative size of punctate terminal capillaries.

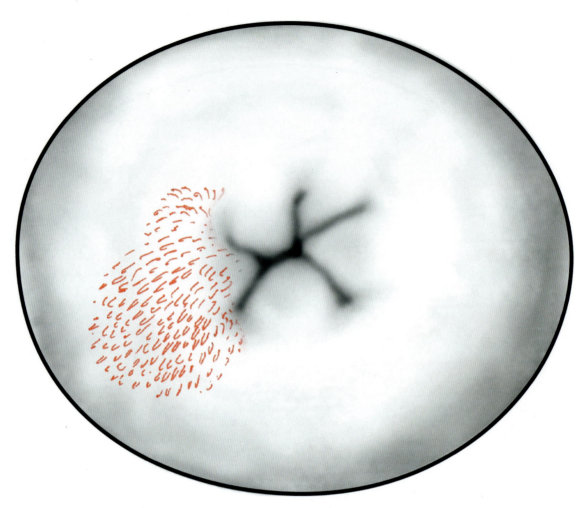

FIGURE 8-11 Hairpin capillaries are associated with inflammatory conditions that range from bacterial to parasitic infestations.

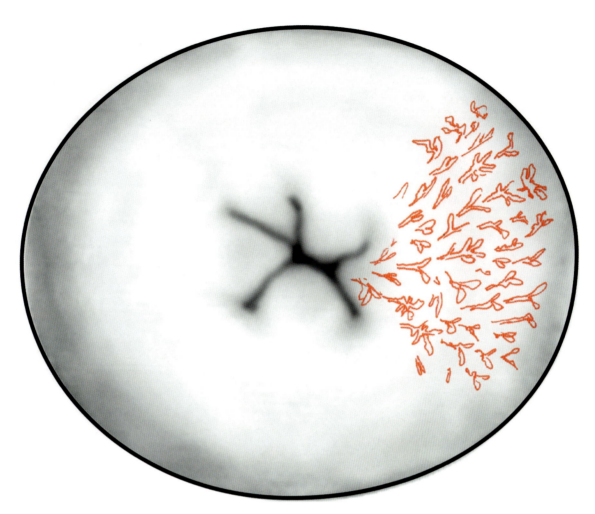

FIGURE 8-12 Double hairpin capillaries and network capillaries are seen in atrophic and inflammatory conditions.

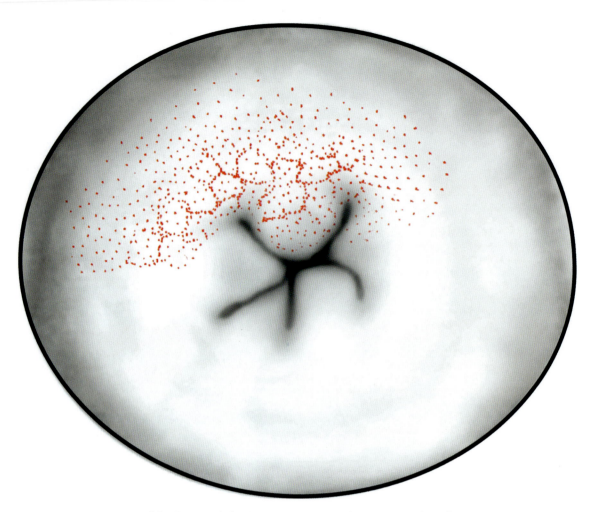

FIGURE 8-13 Mosaic patterns begin as punctation, with groupings of capillaries that outline proliferating blocks of tissues. Early mosaic patterns typically show this pattern. Although mosaic patterns usually are seen in association with neoplasia, they also are seen in association with metaplastic processes, especially in women exposed to diethylstilbestrol.

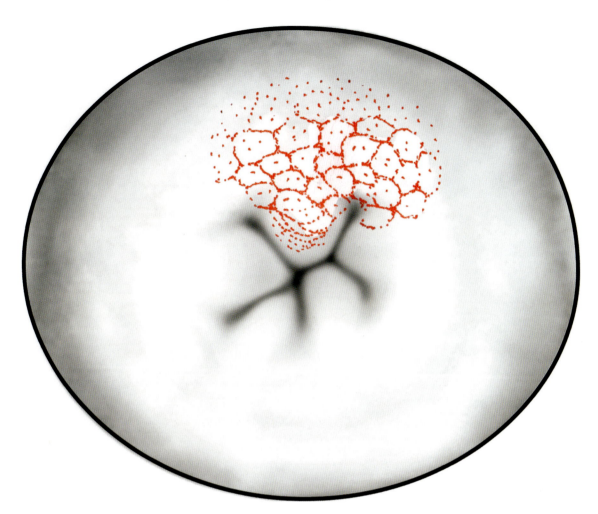

FIGURE 8-14 Intermediate mosaic formation is associated with white epithelium and a high-grade squamous intraepithelial lesion.

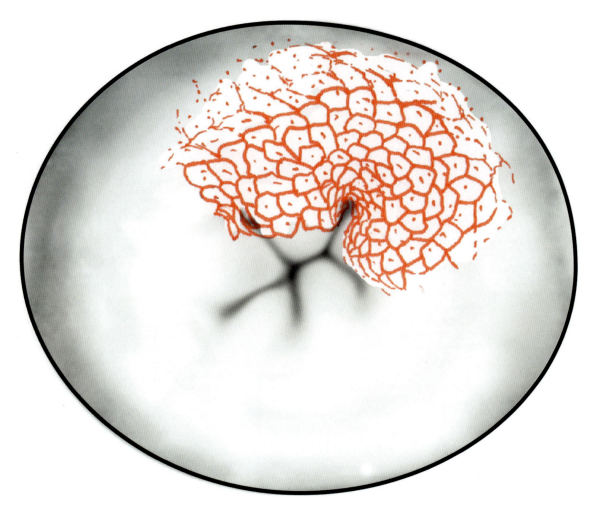

FIGURE 8-15 A severe mosaic pattern suggests carcinoma in situ or severe dysplasia. These lesions usually are focal, but may occupy all or most of extensive abnormal transformation zones. The vascular pattern is seen against white epithelium, the outlines of the vessel are sharp and thick, and the intercapillary distances are great (>350 μm).

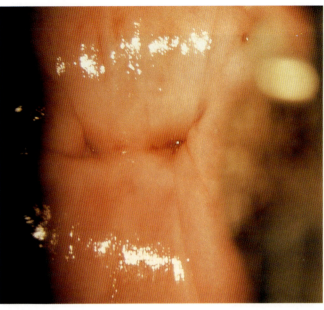

FIGURE 8-16 In an unsatisfactory colposcopic examination, the squamocolumnar transformation zone cannot be seen. The transformation zone is not seen here because the patient has iatrogenic scarring as a result of cone biopsy. The anterior and posterior lips of the cervix are joined as a result of bilateral stenosis.

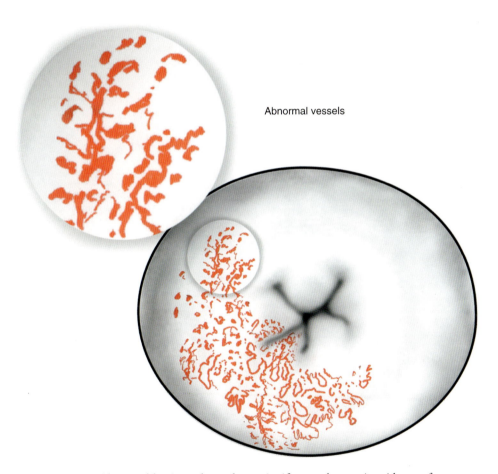

Abnormal vessels

FIGURE 8-17 Abnormal horizontal vessels are significant colposcopic evidence of stromal invasion. The vascular patterns are bizarre and follow no logical branching pattern.

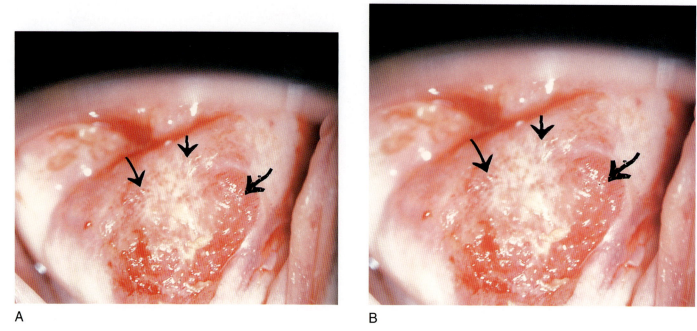

A

B

FIGURE 8-18 **A,** This cervix has abnormal vessels within the abnormal transformation zone, from the 11 o'clock position to the 1 o'clock position. Biopsy showed invasive squamous cell carcinoma (*arrows*). **B,** A magnified view of **A** shows horizontal and bulbous abnormal vessels.

CHAPTER 9
Colposcopic Technique

The patient is placed in the lithotomy position on a motorized gynecologic examination table. The patient's legs are abducted as widely as is comfortable. The colposcope is swung into position, and the table is raised to a height that is comfortable for the examiner. If a video camera is attached to the beam splitter, the monitor is adjusted to allow the patient to view the examination. The magnification is set on scanning power (×4) (Fig. 9-1).

The external genitalia, perianal skin, and vestibule are examined. Next, a Pederson speculum is inserted into the vagina and the cervix is located (Fig. 9-2). The speculum is opened carefully to fully expose the cervix midway between the anterior and posterior blades of the speculum. A Pap smear is performed, and ectocervical and endocervical cells are obtained, first with a spatula and then with a cytobrush. Care is taken to limit bleeding (Figs. 9-3A to C).

The examiner focuses the colposcope onto the cervix and inspects the ectocervix, transformation zone, and surrounding vaginal fornices. A portion of the endocervical canal may be seen by manipulating the cervix with a cotton-tipped applicator or a long-handled, fine hook (Figs. 9-4A and B). This examination is most conveniently performed at ×6 magnification.

Next, a 3% acetic acid solution is applied to the cervix. The transformation zone and surrounding ectocervix are doused with the solution while the examiner views the field at ×4 to ×6 magnification (Fig. 9-5A). This process is repeated two to three times with large, cotton-tipped proctoscopic swabs (Scopettes) (Fig. 9-5B). After 30 to 40 seconds, the magnification is increased to ×10 and the transformation zone is studied systematically, beginning at the 12 o'clock position and working clockwise around the cervix (Fig. 9-6).

The examiner notes the size and location of the transformation zone, indicates whether this zone is normal or abnormal, and describes the disposition and extent of the endocervical canal. In addition, the examiner notes the presence of white epithelium, mosaic or punctation patterns, or atypical vessels. If necessary, the examiner increases the magnification to ×16 to ×25 to perform a more detailed examination and to grade colposcopic abnormalities. The examiner may supplement written documentation by obtaining a colposcopic or cervicoscopic photograph.

To determine whether the abnormal transformation zone extends into the endocervical canal, differential pressure is applied to the anterior or posterior lips of the cervix with a small, dry, cotton-tipped applicator or a fine cervical hook (Figs. 9-7A and B). Some practitioners use an endocervical speculum to examine the canal, but others find this instrument unwieldy. During the examination, additional 3% acetic acid may be applied to the cervix to enhance the view of abnormalities and to identify the abnormal transformation zone. The boundaries of this zone fade as the effects of the initial application of acetic acid subside (Fig. 9-8A). In response to the application of acetic acid, the color of the endocervical mucosa changes from red-orange to pink and the mucosa appears grape-like (Fig. 9-8B), i.e., the mucosal papillae coalesce.

True directed biopsy always is performed while the examiner views the field with a colposcope. Usually, the magnification is decreased to ×4 to allow the examiner to view a wider field than that obtained with higher magnification.

As with directed punch biopsy, endocervical curettage is performed under colposcopic magnification (see "Sampling Techniques"). After the cervical examination is completed, the examiner views the vagina while manipulating and withdrawing the speculum.

Most colposcopes are equipped with a green filter that filters red wavelengths and sharpens the contrast when the examiner views vascular changes. Because vessels appear black when the filter is used, its utility is limited, and it should be used only for the relevant portion of the examination.

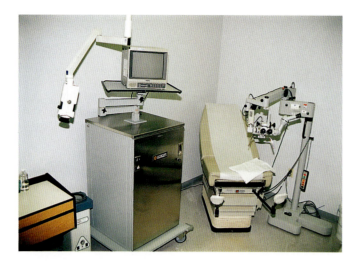

FIGURE 9-1 An ideal arrangement for an examination room in a private office. The examination table is motorized. To the left of the table is a console that contains a video system that is coupled to the colposcope. The colposcope is located to the right of the table and is mounted on an S-2 stand. A halogen examination light is mounted on the ceiling.

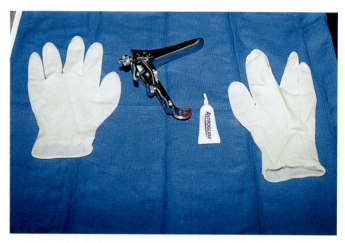

FIGURE 9-2 A Pederson speculum has narrow blades and provides greater comfort for the patient than the standard Graves speculum. As a lubricant, Astroglide is preferred over K-Y jelly because it is less irritating to the vestibular skin and glands. Lubricant is used for the bimanual examination that is performed after colposcopy is completed.

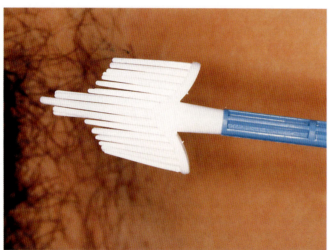

A

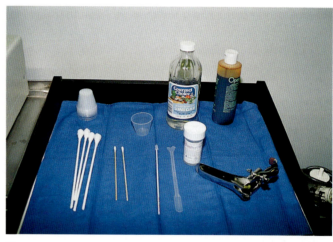

B

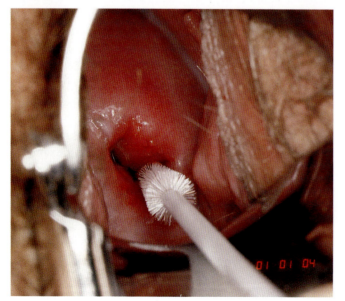

C

FIGURE 9-3 A, A broom-like cytology brush is used to obtain ectocervical and endocervical specimens with a single stroke. **B,** The equipment stand contains the devices needed for thin prep cytology, including a plastic spatula, a cytobrush, and a bottle of fixative. **C,** The cytobrush is inserted into the endocervical canal to obtain a sample of cells.

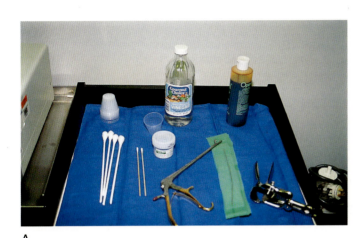
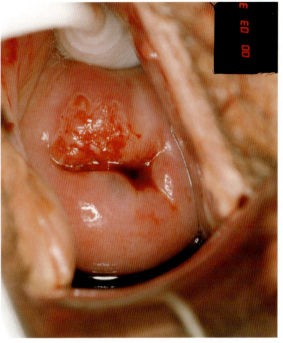

A   B

FIGURE 9-4 A, Equipment for colposcopy includes 3% or 4% acetic acid, large cotton swabs (Scopettes), small cotton swabs, a baby Hegar dilator, a biopsy clamp, and a formalin fixation jar. **B,** Before the acetic acid is applied, the cervix is observed with a colposcope. A dry cotton-tipped applicator is used to manipulate the cervix to permit an unobstructed view.

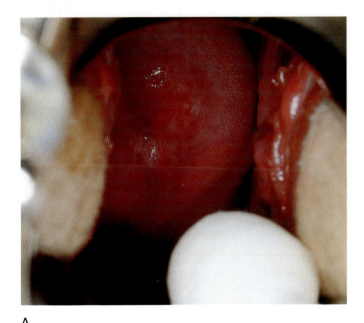
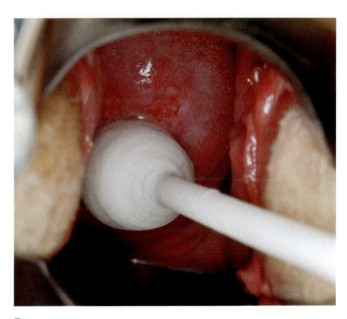

A   B

FIGURE 9-5 A, A cotton-tipped swab is soaked in acetic acid and introduced into the vagina. **B,** The examiner douses the cervix lightly, taking care to avoid rubbing the tissue.

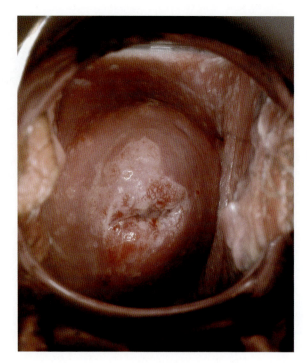

FIGURE 9-6 Thirty seconds after acetic acid is applied, the cervix shows a startling change as the white epithelium highlights the mosaic vascular pattern.

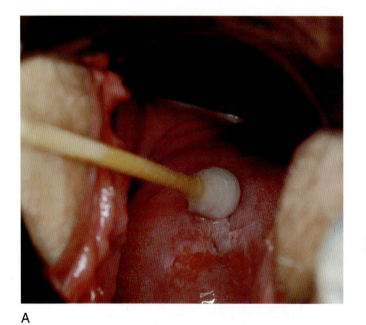

A

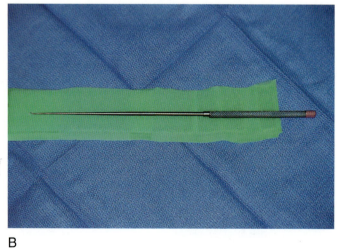

B

FIGURE 9-7 A, A small cotton-tipped swab is used to manipulate the cervix without causing trauma or bleeding. **B,** Alternatively, the cervix may be manipulated gently with a long titanium hook.

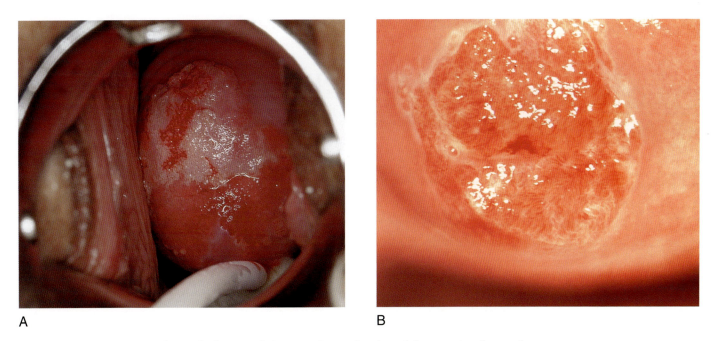

A

B

FIGURE 9-8 A, Acetic acid is applied a second time to enhance the view of the extensive abnormal transformation zone on the anterior lip of the cervix. **B,** Application of 3% acetic acid enhances the orange-red, grape-like appearance of the endocervical mucosa.

CHAPTER 10
Sampling Techniques

Directed Biopsy

Directed cervical biopsy is the primary technique used to obtain a tissue sample for pathologic evaluation. The tissue sample is fixed, embedded in paraffin, and cut into thin slices that are placed on glass slides. A series of chemicals are applied, and the section is stained and studied under the lens of a microscope (Fig. 10-1A).

The most common histopathologic stain consists of hematoxylin and eosin (H&E stain). Hematoxylin gives the cells a blue appearance, and eosin causes the cells to appear pink. Typically, three or four cuts are made at different levels of the paraffin block, resulting in three or four slides (Fig. 10-1B). However, when precise information about the tissue is needed, step serial sections are cut and 50 to 100 slides are produced.

A variety of cervical biopsy clamps are used. Although some hospitals continue to use outdated types, such as cup biopsy forceps, a contemporary biopsy forceps offers many advantages over cup devices and Witner forceps (Fig. 10-2A).

Modern biopsy forceps have three main parts: jaws, shaft, and handle (Fig. 10-2B). The jaws of the clamp are the chief area of difference between instruments. Sharp articulating jaws are necessary to obtain a good biopsy specimen. Because the cervix has a hemispherical shape as seen through the vagina, the jaws must be able to open widely to grasp and remove a portion of the cervix (Figs. 10-2C and D). Typically, the posterior jaw is fixed and the anterior jaw articulates. As the jaw closes, the upper (anterior) jaw fits tightly inside the lower jaw (Figs. 10-2E and F). The serrated cutting surface of the jaws is similar to the teeth of a shark, which slice as they bite into soft tissue (Fig. 10-2G).

The shank of the biopsy forceps is 8 inches long and provides easy access to the entire vagina and the cervix. Because the shank is narrow, it provides both an unobstructed view of the field through the colposcope and access to hard-to-reach areas of the cervix. The principal

function of the shank is to transmit the force created in the handle to the jaws of the clamp through a mechanical spring-like action (Fig. 10-2H).

Whereas older forceps used a modified scissors action, the handle of the modern forceps consists of a pistol-like grip that efficiently transfers force from the handle to the jaw. An extension of the rear grip rests on the skin fold between the thumb and the index finger to provide stability as the handle rests on the thenar eminence and palm. The remaining four fingers are used to grasp the front grip. High-quality biopsy forceps are constructed of heavy-gauge stainless steel, and some have gold-plated handles (Fig. 10-2I).

After the biopsy specimen is obtained, a small, cotton-tipped applicator is dipped in Monsel solution (ferric substrate) and applied to the biopsy site to stop the bleeding (Figs. 10-3A to D).

Alternate Techniques

An electrosurgical loop also may be used to obtain a biopsy specimen. The only disadvantage of this device is the thermal artifact produced by the heating of tissue. The advantage of the technique is that a relatively bloodless biopsy can be performed as a result of coagulation of the blood vessels. The 5-mm square or rounded loop is best suited for a single excisional biopsy (Fig. 10-4A). Power should be set at 35 to 50 W, with the pure cut setting selected on the electrosurgical generator. A superficial tissue sample is adequate (Fig. 10-4B). Monsel solution is applied to control residual bleeding.

Endocervical curettage has been used for more than 30 years to assess the endocervical canal for neoplastic tissue. Although this method of sampling has drawbacks, it is direct and simple to perform, and has minimal complications. Endocervical curettage is appropriate in the following cases: a squamous intraepithelial neoplastic lesion extends from the transformation zone into the canal; cytologic screening shows atypical glandular cells; the squamocolumnar transformation zone cannot be seen colposcopically; colposcopy shows an abnormal transformation zone that requires an ectocervical biopsy, but the examiner is not an expert colposcopist. Only an expert colposcopist is qualified to decide to delete the endocervical curettage, which should be otherwise performed in conjunction with ectocervical biopsy (Figs. 10-5*A* to *D*).

A single-tooth tenaculum may be used to stabilize the anterior aspect of the cervix (Fig. 10-6*A*). A sharp Kevorkian-type curette is inserted through the endocervical canal until the operator meets the resistance of the internal cervical os (Fig. 10-6*B*). A nonadherent sponge is placed in the posterior vaginal fornix and led out below the posterior lip of the cervix. Curettage is performed by pulling the curette down toward the external os, but not out of the canal (Fig. 10-6*C* and *D*). The curette is swept in successive motions, clockwise or counterclockwise, through the 3 o'clock, 6 o'clock, and 9 o'clock positions or through the 9 o'clock, 6 o'clock, and 3 o'clock positions until it returns to the 12 o'clock position. Typically, a long strand of mucus that contains bits of endocervical tissue extends from the external os to the inserted blade of the speculum (Figure 10-6*E*). A Kelly clamp is used to twist the strand of mucus like a long piece of spaghetti and deposit it on a dry paper towel (Figs. 10-6*F* and *G*). The towel is placed in a jar of formalin and sent for pathologic evaluation (Fig. 10-6*G*). Endocervical curettage rarely allows orientation of epithelium and stroma; therefore, grading of neoplastic tissue obtained with this technique is difficult and may be accurate. Even though the sample is obtained blindly, however, the technique successfully shows abnormal epithelium within the canal.

Several devices allow the examiner to see into the depths of the canal through the colposcope. The best known is the endocervical speculum (Figs. 10-7*A* and *B*). However, this device is unwieldy to use, traumatizes the canal, and is undependable when used in conjunction with colposcopy to track the extension of neoplastic epithelium that originates at the transformation zone (Fig. 10-7*C*).

A long, fine titanium hook is used to lift and manipulate the cervix to permit the examiner to peer into the endocervical canal for a short distance. The hook is essential for vaginal colposcopy (Figs. 10-8*A* and *B*).

A dry cotton-tipped applicator can be used to manipulate the anterior and posterior lips of the cervix to expose the distal endocervical canal. Because this tool and the associated technique are simple to use, the practitioner should use a cotton-tipped applicator before resorting to a hook or an endocervical speculum to gain a better view into the endocervical canal. The baby Hegar dilator is used to probe stenotic cervices (Fig. 10-9).

Several instruments can be used to view the endocervical canal directly and facilitate directed biopsy within the canal. These include small endoscopes, e.g. a 3-mm–diameter hysteroscope, and a contact-type hysteroscope. Hyskon is the ideal medium to use when distension of the endocervical canal is required, as for panoramic hysteroscopy. Carcinoma has a characteristic appearance and often produces abnormal vascular patterns. When direct-view endocervical endoscopy is combined with endocervical curettage, endocervical neoplasia can be diagnosed with a high degree of accuracy (Fig. 10-10).

When a larger tissue sample is required, cervical conization is performed with a knife, an electrosurgical loop electrode, or a CO_2 laser (see Chapter 23).

Loop electrical excision of the transformation zone is a quick, office-based technique that is used to perform shallow cone biopsy. Colposcopy is performed immediately before the loop excision is done and the margins of the abnormal transformation zone are identified. A 1:100 mixture of vasopressin and local anesthetic (1 mL vasopressin in 99 mL 1% lidocaine [Xylocaine]) is injected into the cervix, outside the margins of the abnormal transformation zone (Fig. 10-11*A*). The mixture causes concurrent vasoconstriction and local anesthesia. A loop electrode is attached to a handheld receptacle that is connected by a wire to an electrosurgical generator (Figs. 10-11*B* and *C*). Cutting current vaporizes cells and allows an 8- to 10-mm section of cervix to be excised within a few seconds (Figs. 10-11*D* to *F*). Additional hemostasis may be obtained by substituting a ball electrode for the cutting loop. The coagulation mode can be used to shower the cone bed with current, causing superficial coagulation of bleeding vessels (Fig. 10-11*G*). The specimen is sent for pathologic evaluation.

Knife or laser conization usually is performed in the operating room. After colposcopic examination is performed, the cervix is injected with a vasopressin solution. A sharp scalpel (no. 15 blade) or a superpulsed laser beam is used to cut around the periphery of the abnormal transformation zone. The incision is deepened and beveled toward the endocervical canal. The ideal height of the cone is 1 cm. A cone-shaped cylinder of tissue is removed. The specimen is wrapped in a saline-soaked sponge and sent for pathologic evaluation. Additional hemostasis is obtained by the placement of 3-0 Vicryl sutures.

Although most cervical biopsies are performed without anesthesia, anesthesia is indicated in patients who are anxious or especially sensitive to pain. Local anesthesia (1% Xylocaine, with or without epinephrine) may be obtained by injection directly into the cervix through a triple-ring, 10-mL syringe attached to a 1.5-inch, 25- to 26-gauge needle. The injection should be made superficially, i.e. just beneath the mucosa, and should encompass the entire biopsy region.

Cone biopsy or electrical loop excision biopsy always requires anesthesia. The technique is similar to that described earlier, but a vasoconstrictor is added to the 1% Xylocaine solution. A 1:100 vasopressin solution is recommended. Additionally, the entire circumference of the cervix must be infiltrated to provide adequate anesthesia.

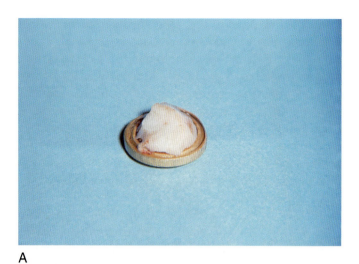

A

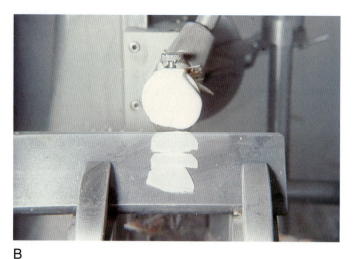

B

FIGURE 10-1 A, A cervical biopsy specimen is mounted on a disk with collodian and frozen before it is sectioned on a dermatome. **B,** Sections of the specimen are cut on a dermatome and placed on a microscopic slide. Then the slide is stained.

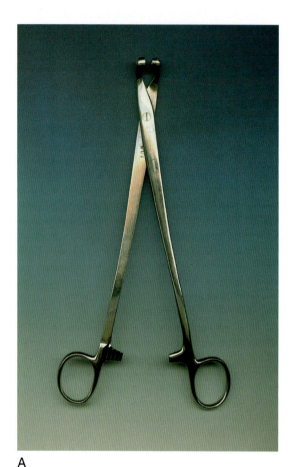

A

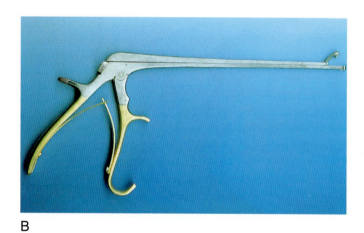

B

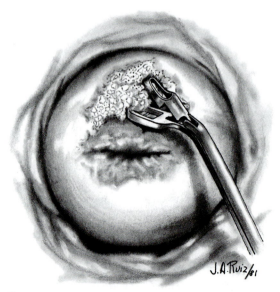

C

FIGURE 10-2 A, This antiquated biopsy forceps was commonly utitized in the 1960s. It is too large and cumbersome for precise colposcopically directed biopsies. **B,** A contemporary biopsy clamp has three essential components: jaws, shaft, and handle. **C,** Because the cervix is rounded, the teeth of the clamp, which usually are prominently located on the posterior jaw, dig into the cervical tissue to stabilize it during the biopsy procedure. (continued)

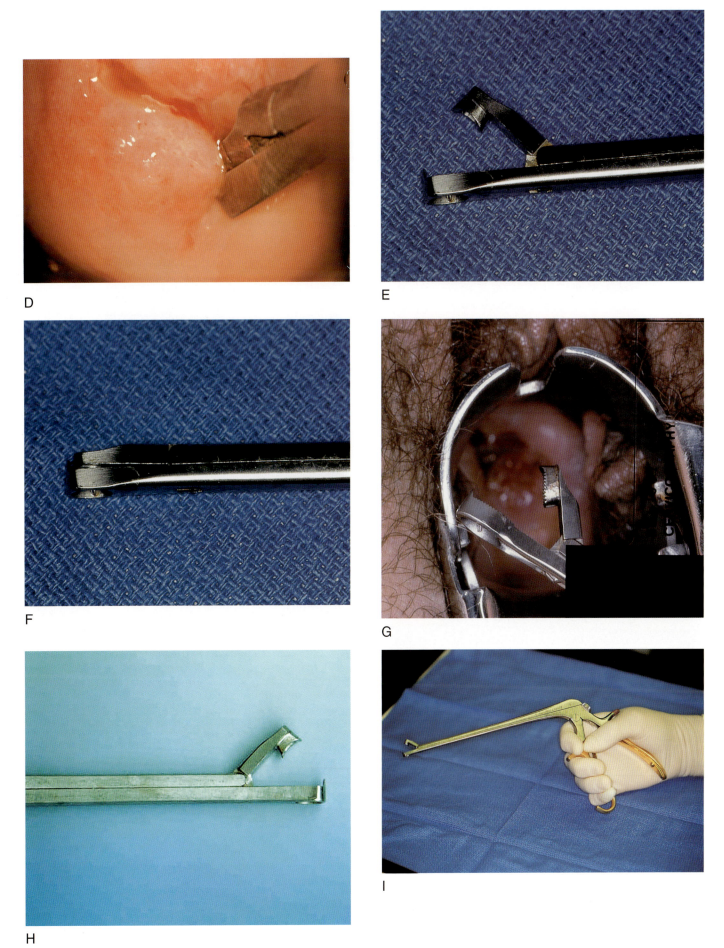

FIGURE 10-2 D, The anterior jaw cuts the tissue as it closes into the posterior jaw of the clamp during directed biopsy. In true directed biopsy, the details of the procedure are seen accurately through the colposcope. **E,** The anterior jaw articulates upward to fully open the jaws of the biopsy clamp. The toothed posterior jaw is fixed. **F,** The anterior jaw is closed and fits tightly into the posterior jaw. The sharp edges of the jaw cut through the tissue and separate the specimen from the surrounding tissue. **G,** The jaws of the biopsy clamp have serrated edges that cleave through tissue. For optimal performance, the instrument must be sharpened regularly. **H,** In its resting state, the upper component of the shaft retracts and opens the anterior jaw of the clamp. As the direction of the shaft is reversed by the spring action of the handle grip, the jaw closes firmly. **I,** The pistol grip efficiently transfers force to the jaws of the clamp.

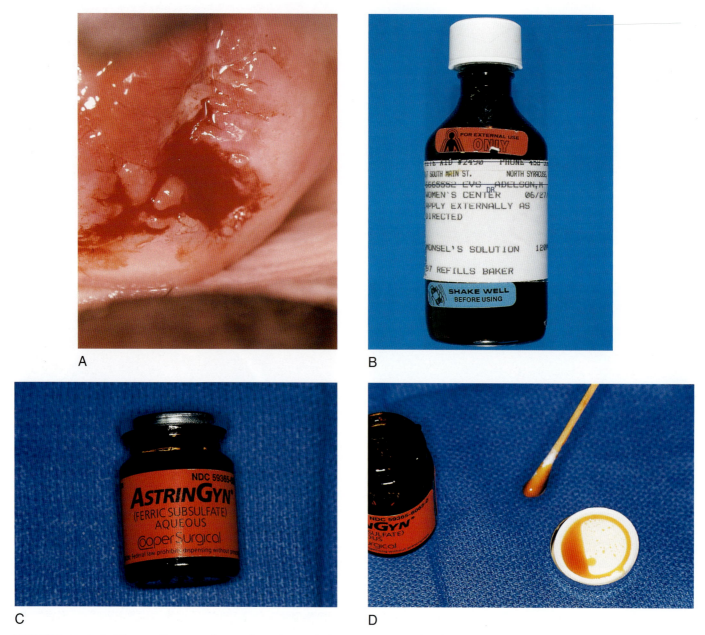

FIGURE 10-3 A, The excellent vascular supply to the cervix is seen as soon as the clamp is withdrawn from the biopsy site. **B,** The most rapid and convenient method to control bleeding is through the application of ferric subsulfate (Monsel solution) to the biopsy crater. **C,** Another hemostatic preparation is concentrated Monsel paste. **D,** Monsel solution or paste is caustic and must be applied sparingly with a small, cotton-tipped applicator to reduce tissue necrosis.

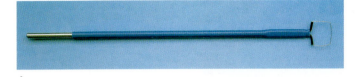

A

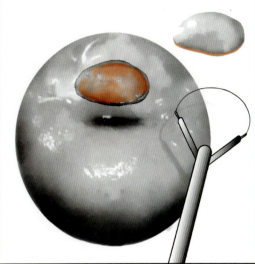

FIGURE 10-4 **A,** A small electrosurgical loop electrode may be used to obtain a blood-free biopsy specimen. To reduce thermal artifact, the pure cut setting is used. **B,** The key to successful loop electrosurgical cervical biopsy is a superficial loop excision. This technique provides both a generous tissue sample and hemostasis.

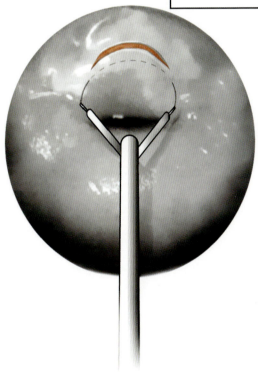

B

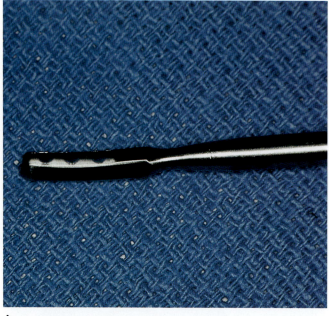

A

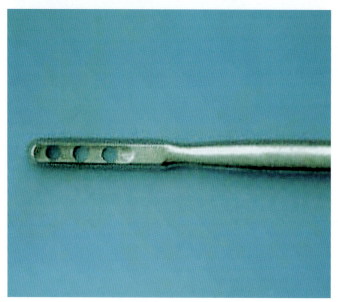

B

FIGURE 10-5 **A,** Because a colposcope does not allow the operator to observe lesions in the endocervical canal, this blind spot is routinely sampled when directed biopsy for cervical intraepithelial neoplasia is performed. The Kevorkian curette can be used to perform this sampling because of its low profile and sharp edges. **B,** The closed back wall of the curette is perforated to permit drainage of fluid that accumulates while endocervical fragments are obtained. (continued)

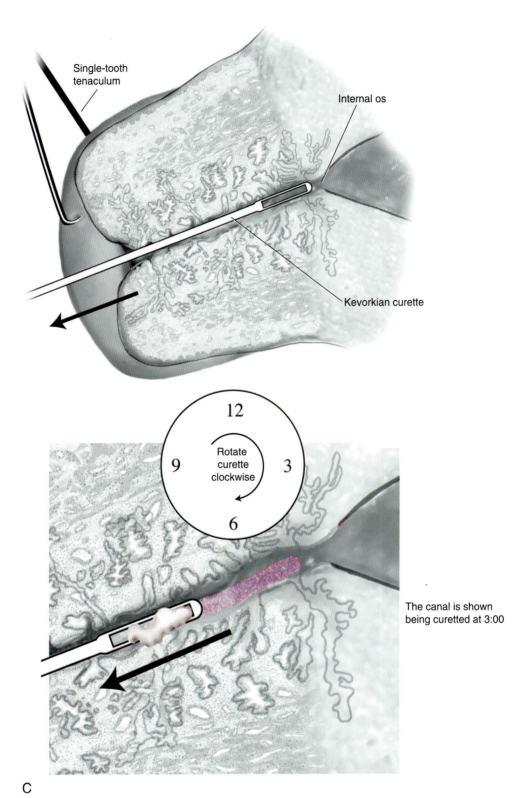

C

FIGURE 10-5 **C,** During endocervical curettage, the curette is positioned in the endocervical canal, at the level of the internal os. As the curette is drawn down to the external os, the curette scrapes away endocervical mucosa. The curette is rotated 10 to 15 degrees clockwise, and the process is repeated until the curette has rotated 360 degrees. (continued)

FIGURE 10-5 D, The tissue, which is encased in mucus, is collected on a piece of nonadherent sponge that is tucked partly into the posterior vaginal fornix. The strands of mucus and endocervical tissue are twisted free with a long Kelly clamp. The specimens and sponge are placed in formalin.

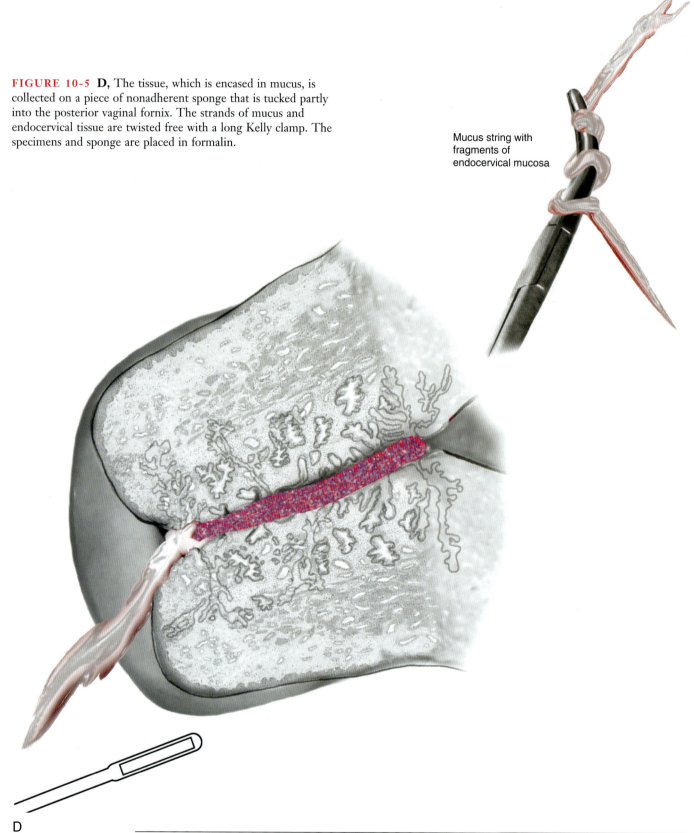

Mucus string with fragments of endocervical mucosa

D

FIGURE 10-6 A, Endocervical curettage may be performed either before or after ectocervical biopsy. In this case, the cervix is swabbed with acetic acid and curettage will be done immediately. **B,** A Kevorkian curette is inserted into the vagina and readied for entry into the cervical canal. **C,** Endocervical curettage is performed by scraping the canal downward in a clockwise or counterclockwise direction. **D,** The curette is drawn towards the external os (different patient). **E,** The curette together with endocervical fragments exits the external os (different patient). **F,** The specimen, which is encased in mucus, is placed on a nonadherent dressing pad, rolled, and placed into a bottle of fixative. **G,** An additional specimen is placed on a nonadherent dressing pad and sent for pathologica evaluation.

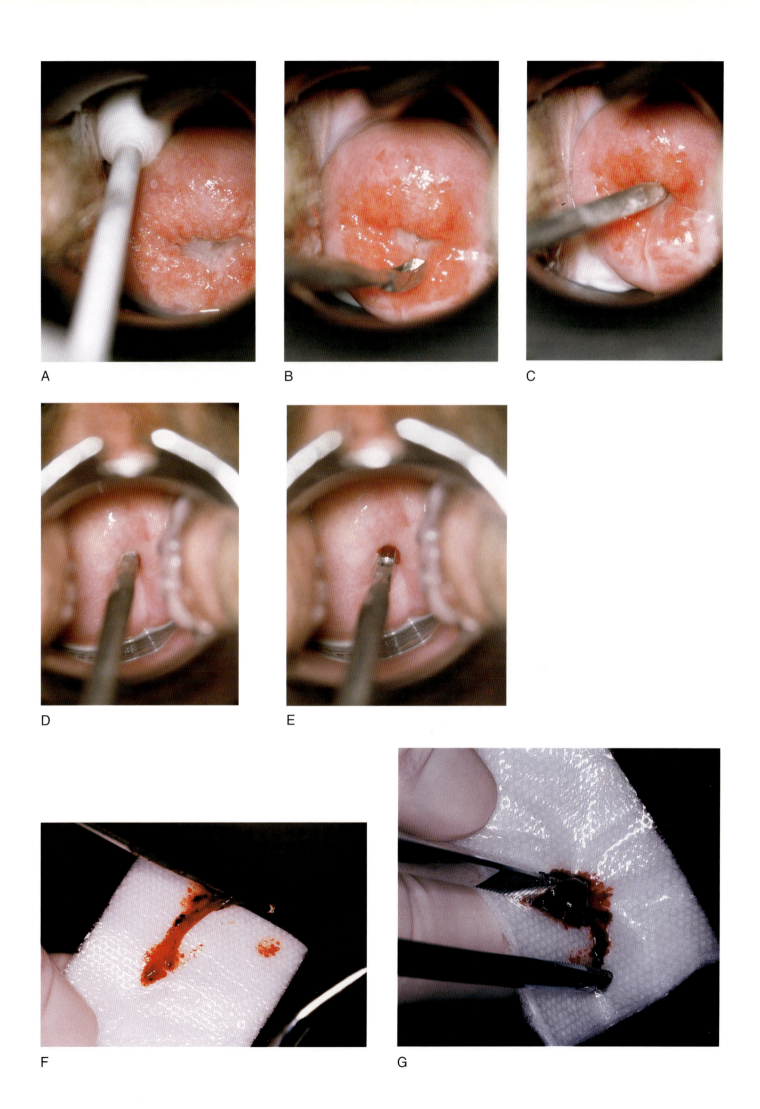

A

B

C

D

E

F

G

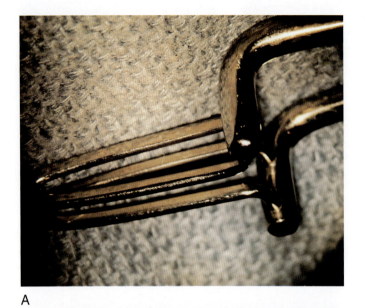

A

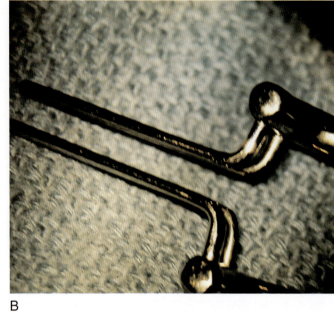

B

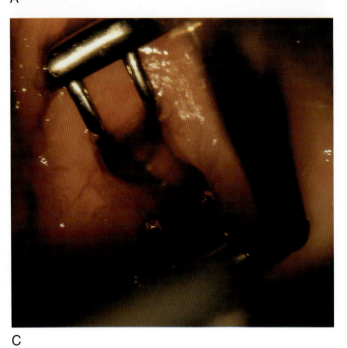

C

FIGURE 10-7 A, The endocervical speculum was designed to spread the lower cervical canal open to allow colposcopic examination. **B,** A ratchet device permits the jaws to separate. **C,** The endocervical speculum does not permit satisfactory colposcopic examination of the endocervical canal. This instrument may traumatize the endocervical mucosa and initiate bleeding.

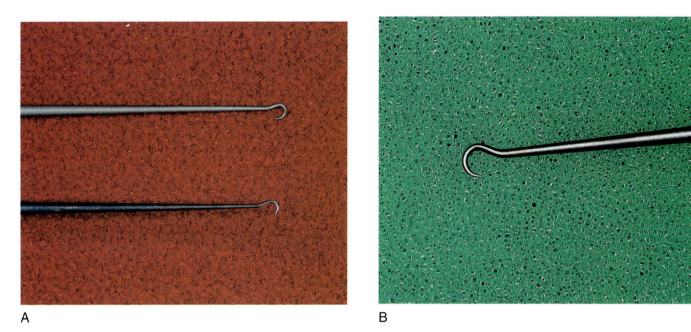

A   B

FIGURE 10-8 **A,** A long-handled, fine titanium hook is used to manipulate the cervix and retract the endocervical canal. **B,** The operator can place the hook into small spaces to facilitate colposcopic examination of hard-to-see areas.

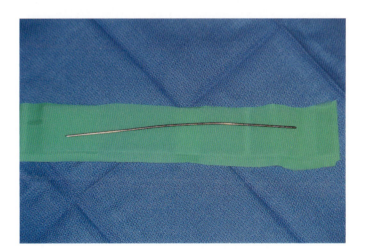

FIGURE 10-9 The diameter of the narrow end of a baby Hegar dilator is 1.5 mm. The diameter of the wide end is 2.0 mm. The instrument is ideal for probing stenotic cervices to determine the axis of the endocervical canal and enter the corpal portion of the uterine cavity.

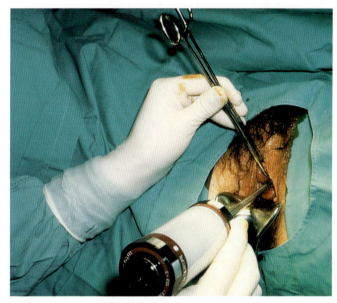

FIGURE 10-10 A small-caliber endoscope is ideal for viewing the endocervical canal. No anesthesia is required. A 6-mm–diameter contact hysteroscope requires no medium and no sheath.

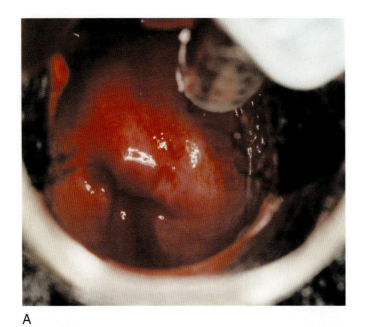

A

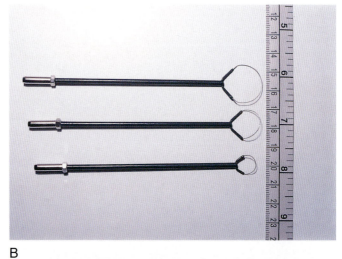

B

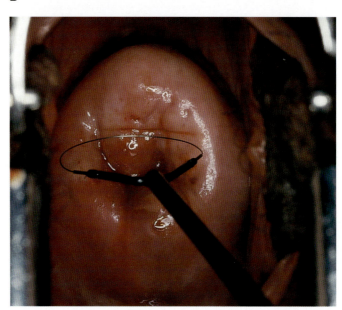

C

D

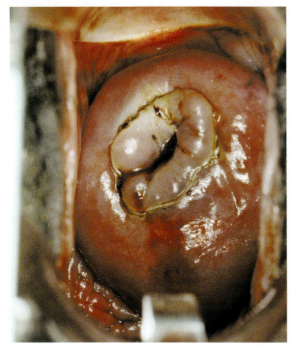

E

FIGURE 10-11 **A,** A syringe and a needle are seen in the upper right corner. The 26-gauge needle has superficially penetrated the anterior lip of the cervix. No vasopressin has been injected. **B,** Loop electrodes are available in a variety of sizes. The size of the abnormal transformation zone and the height and diameter of the cervix must be considered before a loop is selected. **C,** The D-shaped loop has an insulated (Teflon-coated) base. The height of the bar is fixed at 8 to 10 mm. Ball electrodes are used for postexcision coagulation. **D,** The cutting loop is placed perpendicular to the cervix, beyond the peripheral boundary of the abnormal transformation zone. As the electric current flows, the 0.2-mm wire vaporizes cells and is pressed lightly into the cervix to a depth of 8 to 10 mm. **E,** The loop travels through the cervical tissue and exits on the opposite end of the abnormal transformation zone. A white area of thermal coagulation is seen. No bleeding is seen. (continued)

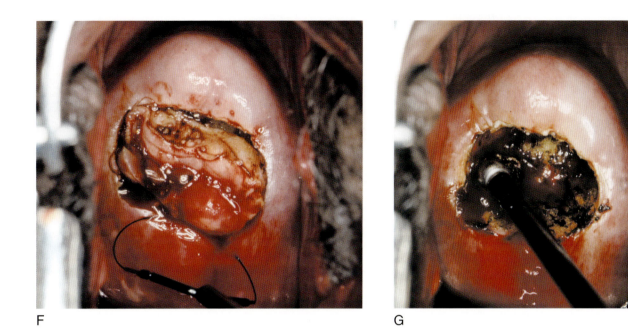

F

G

FIGURE 10-11 **F,** The excised tissue is removed, placed in fixative, and sent for pathologic examination. The excisional bed shows light bleeding. **G,** The loop electrode is discarded. A ball electrode is substituted, and the current is switched to coagulation mode. Bleeding vessels are fulgurated circumferentially with spray coagulation.

CHAPTER 11
Case Examples

Mosaic Patterns

Case 1

A 42-year-old woman underwent colposcopic examination after a Pap smear suggested a severe squamous intraepithelial lesion, or severe dysplasia. Two years earlier, a Pap test showed atypical squamous cells of undetermined significance (ASCUS) and a subsequent Pap smear was normal (Figs. 11-1 and 11-2).

Case 2

A 20-year-old woman was referred for colposcopy because of prenatal exposure to diethylstilbestrol. Previous cervical cytologic findings were normal (Fig. 11-3).

Case 3

A 23-year-old woman underwent colposcopy after Pap smear showed a low-grade squamous intraepithelial lesion (Fig. 11-4).

Case 4

A 19-year-old woman underwent colposcopy after she had abnormal cytologic findings over a period of 2 years. Four Pap smears showed ASCUS, a low-grade squamous intraepithelial lesion, ASCUS, and ASCUS (Fig. 11-5).

Case 5

A 31-year-old woman was referred for colposcopy by a family planning agency. She was taking oral contraceptives and had a history of two chlamydia infections as well as genital herpes infection that was suppressed by med-

ication. Routine Pap test showed high-grade squamous intraepithelial lesion (Fig. 11-6).

Case 6

A 30-year-old woman had a Pap smear that showed a high-grade squamous intraepithelial lesion initial. Colposcopy was performed when she was 28 weeks' pregnant, but no biopsy was performed. She was referred for repeat colposcopy 6 weeks postpartum (Fig. 11-7).

Case 7

A 45-year-old women underwent cryosurgery for CIN grade 2 six years earlier. Two consecutive Pap smears were abnormal and showed ASCUS and a high-grade squamous intraepithelial lesion. The patient underwent colposcopic examination and directed biopsy (Fig. 11-8).

Case 8

An 18-year-old woman underwent colposcopy because of prenatal exposure to diethylstilbestrol (Fig. 11-9).

Punctation Patterns

Case 9

A 29-year-old woman underwent colposcopy because a Pap smear showed a high-grade squamous intraepithelial lesion. The patient had not had a Pap smear for 5 years before the current Pap smear. The patient stated that she had moved out of town and had no gynecologist or primary care provider. When she became ill (on one occasion), she went to an emergency room. She was referred from there to a clinic where the Pap smear was done (Fig. 11-10).

Case 10

A 50-year-old woman underwent colposcopy because a Pap smear showed carcinoma in situ (Figs. 11-11 and 11-12).

Case 11

A 24-year-old woman underwent colposcopic examination after two consecutive Pap smears showed ASCUS (Fig. 11-13).

Case 12

A 22-year-old woman underwent colposcopy because of prenatal exposure to diethylstilbestrol. The congenital hood, or rim, at the cervicovaginal junction is a common site of vascular abnormalities (Fig. 11-14).

Case 13

A 30-year-old woman who had prenatal exposure to diethylstilbestrol underwent colposcopic examination because of structural changes and a Pap smear that showed a low-grade squamous intraepithelial lesion as well as condylomatous cellular changes that suggested human papillomavirus infection (Figs. 11-15 and 11-16).

Case 14

A 38-year-old woman underwent colposcopic examination because three consecutive Pap smears showed ASCUS. The last Pap smear showed human papillomavirus infection as well (Fig. 11-17).

Case 15

A 42-year-old woman had two Pap smears that showed ASCUS with reactive changes. She underwent 6 months of antimicrobial therapy for chlamydia, mycoplasma, and *Candida* species. Repeat Pap smear showed ASCUS favoring a low-grade squamous intraepithelial lesion (Fig. 11-18).

White Epithelium and Condylomata

Cases 16 and 17

These patients underwent colposcopic examination as part of a routine mapping survey of the lower genital tract. The survey was performed because of the finding of condylomata acuminata. Typically, genital warts are first detected on the vulva or perianal skin. Gross warts such as these usually are associated with infection with human papillomavirus types 6 and 11 (Figs. 11-19 and 11-20).

Case 18

An 18-year-old woman underwent colposcopy because of recurrent low-grade squamous intraepithelial (condylomatous) cervical cytology. She had undergone loop electrical excision of the transformation zone 1 year earlier (Figs. 11-21 and 11–22).

Case 19

A 22-year-old woman was seen twice during her pregnancy with vaginal and vulvar warts and condylomatous changes of the cervix. No therapy was administered during the pregnancy. At the 4-week postpartum visit, the vaginal and vulvar warts were gone. Because a Pap smear showed cells consistent with human papillomavirus infection, or a low-grade squamous intraepithelial lesion, she was referred for colposcopy (Fig. 11-23).

Case 20

A 29-year-old woman underwent colposcopy after a Pap smear showed a high-grade squamous intraepithelial lesion. The patient was taking oral contraceptives. One year earlier, Pap smear showed a low-grade squamous intraepithelial lesion. No therapy was administered for the low-grade squamous intraepithelial lesion; the patient elected observation and follow-up every 6 months. Unfortunately, she did not keep her appointment at 6 months and returned instead at 1 year, after a certified reminder letter (Fig. 11-24).

Case 21

A 49-year-old woman had a past history of undergoing sharp conization of the cervix for carcinoma in situ. For 5 years, annual Pap smears showed no abnormality, but when the most recent Pap smear showed a low-grade squamous intraepithelial lesion, she was referred for colposcopic examination (Fig. 11-25).

Case 22

A 20-year-old woman underwent colposcopy after pregnancy termination. The family planning clinic initially performed cervicography and referred the patient to the colposcopy clinic for colposcopy and possible directed biopsy (Fig. 11-26).

Case 23

A 21-year-old woman who was 13 to 14 weeks' pregnant with her first child underwent colposcopy because a Pap smear showed high-grade cytologic abnormalities. Findings on a previous Pap smear were abnormal, but no medical record was available to document the severity of the findings (Fig. 11-27).

Case 24

A 19-year-old woman underwent colposcopy after two Pap smears showed ASCUS that suggested a low-grade squamous intraepithelial lesion rather than reactive atypia (Fig. 11-28).

Case 25

A 28-year-old pregnant woman had CIN grade 2 that was diagnosed by Pap smear and biopsy. No therapy was administered during pregnancy, and she was referred for repeat colposcopy and biopsy 6 weeks postpartum (Fig. 11-29).

Case 26

A 23-year-old woman who had prenatal exposure to diethylstilbestrol was evaluated as part of a routine annual examination. Over 4 years of follow-up visits, extensive squamous metaplasia was seen. Pap smear showed atypical squamous cells and atypical glandular cells (Fig. 11-30).

Case 27

A 31-year-old nulliparous woman was referred for colposcopy by a continuity clinic. Pap smear showed changes that suggested human papillomavirus infection. Previously, the results of annual Pap smears were normal (Fig. 11-31).

Case 28

A 21-year-old woman was referred for colposcopy by a family planning clinic. Over a period of 1 year, three Pap smears showed ASCUS. The patient has taken oral contraceptives since the age of 17 years (Fig. 11-32).

Case 29

An 18-year-old woman delivered her third child and returned for a 6-week postpartum examination. During the examination, a Pap smear was obtained and showed a low-grade squamous intraepithelial lesion. The patient was referred for colposcopy and sampling. The patient missed two appointments and returned to the colposcopy clinic approximately 6 months after the first scheduled appointment (Fig. 11-33).

Case 30

A 16-year-old girl was referred for colposcopy by social services. She had been sexually active since the age of 12 years. She had no pregnancies because she began to use oral contraceptives at the age of 13 years. She had previ-

ous episodes of vulvar genital warts and had positive antibodies for herpes simplex virus type 2 (Fig. 11-34).

Case 31

A 50-year-old woman was referred for colposcopy by her primary care physician because she had a cauliflower-like cervical lesion, a malodorous discharge, and dyspareunia. She had not undergone a Pap smear for more than 3 years. She used no contraception and had had no pregnancies for 15 years (Fig. 11-35).

Case 32

A 43-year-old woman underwent laser vaporization for CIN 1 with condylomatous atypia. Pap smear obtained 1 year later showed ASCUS favoring a low-grade squamous intraepithelial lesion. She was referred for colposcopic examination (Fig. 11-36).

Case 33

A 32-year-old woman had vaginal discharge and itching. She was diagnosed as having a yeast infection and treated with fluconazole (Diflucan). Her symptoms continued, and because of the unusual epithelial pattern seen on her cervix, she was referred for colposcopic evaluation (Fig. 11-37).

Case 34

A 27-year-old woman was referred for colposcopy after two consecutive Pap smears showed a low-grade squamous intraepithelial lesion. The patient took oral contraceptives (Fig. 11-38).

Case 35

A 25-year-old woman had Pap smears that showed a low-grade squamous intraepithelial lesion. She underwent colposcopy and biopsy, but received no treatment for 2 years (Fig. 11-39).

Case 36

A 29-year-old woman had very heavy mucous discharge and an extensive transformation zone after the birth of her last child. Pap smear showed ASCUS (Fig. 11-40).

Ectopy and Metaplasia

Case 37

A 38-year-old woman who underwent laser vaporization of the cervix for CIN grade 2 returned for a 6-month follow-up colposcopic examination (Fig. 11-41).

Case 38

A 32-year-old woman was referred for colposcopy because of a heavy vaginal discharge. When acetic acid was applied, papillary lesions were seen in the cervix (Fig. 11-42).

Case 39

A 41-year-old woman was concerned because she and her sexual partner felt a "bump" on her cervix. Results of Pap smears were normal (Fig. 11-43).

Case 40

A 33-year-old pregnant woman had extensive ectopy that was attributed to pregnancy. A Pap smear obtained at 10 weeks' gestation showed high-grade squamous intraepithelial lesion (Fig. 11-44).

Case 41

A 21-year-old woman was referred for colposcopy postpartum because several Pap smears showed ASCUS with reactive changes (Fig. 11-45).

Case 42

A woman had postcoital bleeding and a persistent foul-smelling, green-yellow vaginal discharge. Because of the alarming appearance of the cervix, the patient was referred for colposcopy (Fig. 11-46).

Abnormal Vessels

Case 43

A 49-year-old woman had a Pap smear that showed ASCUS. A repeat Pap smear showed a high-grade squamous intraepithelial lesion. Results of previous Pap smears were normal (Fig. 11-47).

Case 44

A 50-year-old woman had an annual Pap smear that showed cells that suggested invasive squamous cell carcinoma (Figs. 11-48*A* and *B*).

Case 45

A 38-year-old woman had persistent postcoital bleeding. No gross abnormality of the cervix was seen. Pap smear showed a high-grade squamous lesion that suggested carcinoma in situ (Fig. 11-49).

Infections

Case 46

A 32-year-old woman underwent colposcopic examination as part of the follow-up after loop excision of the cervix. A nurse practitioner was concerned about the colposcopic findings and referred the patient to the dysplasia clinic (Figs. 11-50*A* and *B*).

Case 47

A 28-year-old woman had intense itching and a watery, greenish discharge. A wet saline preparation showed *Trichomonas vaginalis* infection of the vagina and cervix (Fig. 11-51).

Case 48

A 25-year-old woman underwent vaginal examination because of initial infection of the vulva with herpes simplex virus. The cervix and vagina were swabbed for herpes culture (Figs. 11-52*A* and *B*).

Diethylstilbestrol-Related Lesions

Cases 49 to 59

These patients, ranging in age from 16 to 30 years, underwent colposcopic examination because they had prenatal exposure to diethylstilbestrol that initially occurred within the first trimester and early second trimester (<16 weeks). Because these patients were at risk for adenocarcinoma and squamous intraepithelial neoplasia, follow-up included colposcopic examination and directed biopsy (Figs. 11-54 through 11-63*A* and *B*).

Adenocarcinoma

Case 60

A 46-year-old woman had postcoital bleeding. Examination showed extensive cervical erosion. No biopsy was performed, but the patient underwent cryosurgery. Ten weeks after cryosurgery, the patient returned for an examination, and the endocervical tissue appeared more exuberant than before surgery. The patient was referred for colposcopy and biopsy (Figs. 11-64 and 11-65).

Other Cervical Lesions

Case 61

A 34-year-old woman had a history of vaginal bleeding. Examination showed a deformity of the cervix that was identified as a diethylstilbestrol-related abnormality (Figs. 11-66 through 11-68*A* and *B*).

Case 62

A 52-year-old woman presented with a large mass occupying the position of her cervix. She related a history of one month of heavy vaginal bleeding (Fig. 11-69).

Case 63

Polypoid masses are seen at the external os. These masses may cause no symptoms or may cause intermittent contact bleeding and spotting (Figs. 11-70*A* and *B*, 11-71).

Case 64

A 23-year-old secundigravida was referred for colposcopic examination because a Pap smear showed a low-grade squamous intraepithelial lesion. The patient was approximately 22 weeks' pregnant (Fig. 11-72).

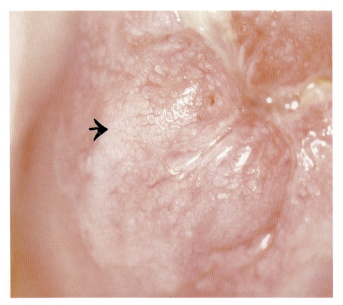

FIGURE 11-1 In this colposcopic view (×10), the patient's right half of this hypertrophied, lacerated cervix (old) is enveloped in a large abnormal transformation zone (*arrow*). A well-developed mosaic pattern is seen against the white epithelium, or ground leukoplakia. The widely spaced capillaries (*center*) are diagnostic of cervical intraepithelial neoplasia (CIN) grade 3.

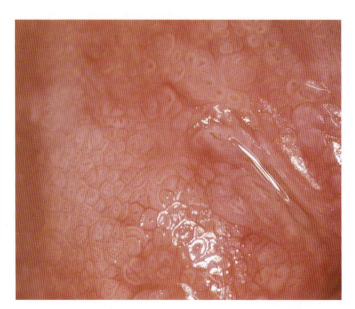

FIGURE 11-2 Thirty seconds after the reapplication of 3% acetic acid, the cervix seen in Figure 11-1 was examined at higher magnification (×16 and ×25). Even before a biopsy specimen was obtained, the mosaic pattern interspersed with small areas of punctation (patient's *middle right* and patient's *lower right*) confirmed the diagnosis of CIN grade 3.

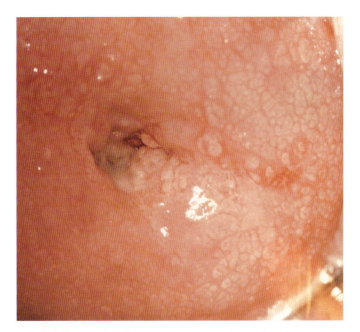

FIGURE 11-3 A colposcopic view (×6) shows that the entire cervix, from the squamocolumnar junction to the vaginal fornices, is covered with a diffuse, intermediate mosaic pattern. The lesion has no apparent focus. Although the mosaic vasculature is well developed, the capillaries are not as widely spaced as in Figures 11-1 and 11-2. Biopsy showed extensive squamous metaplasia.

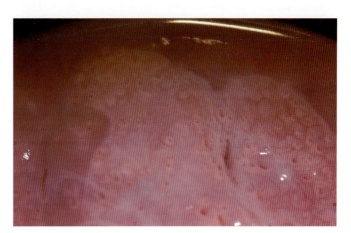

FIGURE 11-4 The abnormal transformation zone occupies the anterior lip of the cervix, extending from the 11 o'clock position to the 1 o'clock position within an area of squamous metaplasia. The findings of several gland openings and cloudy white epithelium suggest metaplasia. An early (fine) mosaic pattern at the periphery of the abnormal transformation zone suggests a low-grade intraepithelial lesion, or CIN grade 1.

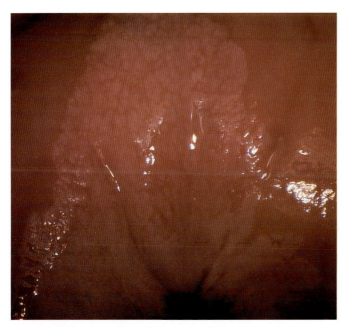

FIGURE 11-5 A colposcopic view (×16) shows white epithelium at the 12 o'clock position in the abnormal transformation zone. The white epithelium drifts off at the 11 o'clock position and extends onto the ectocervix at the 1 o'clock position. A fine mosaic pattern shows a short intercapillary distance. This lesion is compatible with condylomatous atypia, or CIN grade 1.

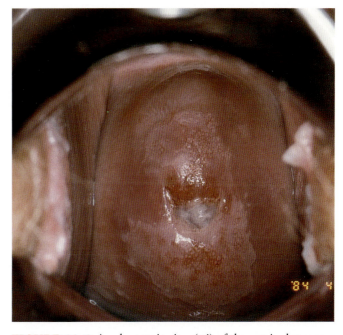

FIGURE 11-6 A colposcopic view (×4) of the cervix shows an extensive abnormal transformation zone that extends well out onto the portio on both the anterior and posterior aspects of the cervix. Unlike the rest of the cervix, the area from the 9 o'clock position to the 11 o'clock position appears normal. Even under low power, a well-developed mosaic pattern is clearly seen, particularly on the posterior lip. Directed biopsy specimens were obtained through the abnormal transformation zone at the 6 o'clock and 12 o'clock positions. The specimen obtained at the 6 o'clock position showed carcinoma in situ, and the specimen obtained at the 12 o'clock position showed CIN grade 2.

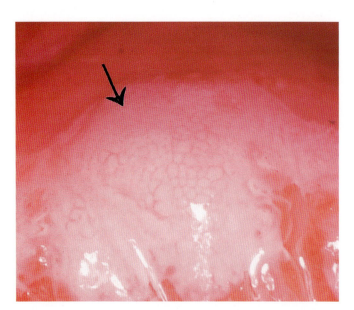

FIGURE 11-7 An extensive abnormal transformation zone is seen extending from the 9 o'clock position to the 3 o'clock position (×10). The white epithelium is fairly dense, grade 2. An early mosaic pattern is seen where punctate areas coalesce (*arrows*). Colposcopic examination suggested CIN grade 1 to CIN grade 2; however, directed biopsy showed CIN grade 1. The patient underwent loop excision of the entire transformation zone, and the specimen showed CIN grade 1.

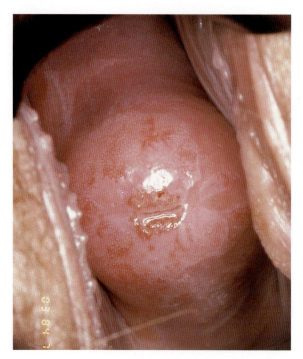

FIGURE 11-8 An abnormal transformation covers 80% of the epithelial surface of the cervix and extends into the posterior fornix of the vagina. Even at low power (×4), a mosaic pattern is seen (red zones). Biopsy specimens obtained at the 7 o'clock and 11 o'clock positions and in the posterior vaginal fornix showed CIN 3.

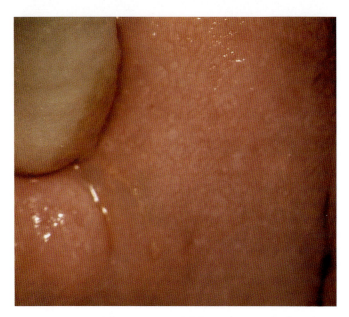

FIGURE 11-9 A large cotton swab is used to manipulate the cervix. The hooded rim of the cervix shows an early, diffuse mosaic pattern (×25). No white epithelium, or ground leukoplakia, is seen. Biopsy showed squamous metaplasia.

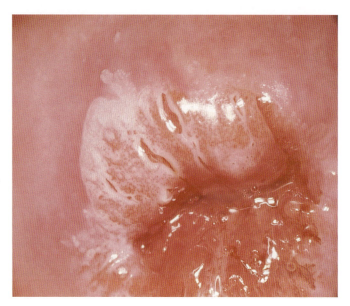

FIGURE 11-10 A colposcopic view (×10) shows an abnormal transformation zone that extends from the 7 o'clock position to the 1 o'clock position and consists of white epithelium and punctation. The punctation is focalized, and the intercapillary distance varies from intermediate to wide. Directed biopsy at the 11 o'clock position, just below the endocervical cleft, showed CIN grade 2 to 3 with glandular involvement. Endocervical curettage showed dysplasia.

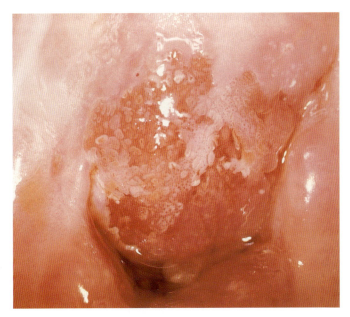

FIGURE 11-11 An abnormal transformation zone is seen in a peninsula-like area that begins near the external os, within everted endocervical mucosa. The area broadens as it extends upward onto the ectocervix. The lower areas show papillary punctation and wide intercapillary distances. The portio contains largely dense white epithelium. An early mosaic pattern is seen at the 1 o'clock position. Biopsy confirmed carcinoma in situ with glandular involvement.

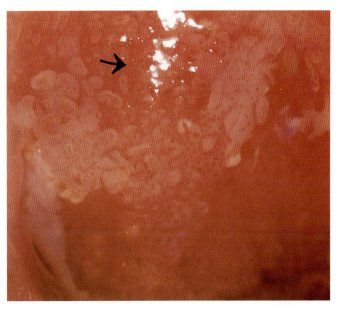

FIGURE 11-12 A high-power colposcopic view (×16) of case 11 shows papillary (large) punctation (*center*). The intercapillary distance is more than 350 μm. The white epithelium, or ground leukoplakia, shows both fine punctation (patient's *left*) and intermediate punctation with mosaic formation (patient's *right* and *above*). An early mosaic pattern is seen as well (*top, arrow*).

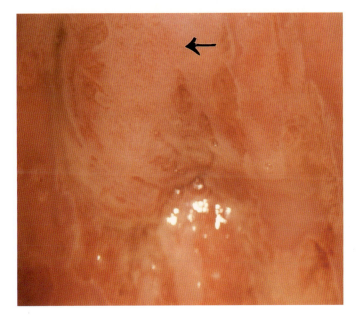

FIGURE 11-13 Colposcopic examination (×10) shows extensive squamous metaplasia. Endocervical clefts and mucosa are surrounded by thin, white tissue that corresponds to immature squamous epithelium. A fine punctation pattern with normal intercapillary distance is seen (*arrow*). Directed biopsy at the 12 o'clock position showed atypical squamous metaplasia.

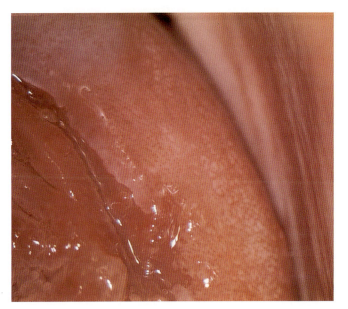

FIGURE 11-14 After the application of 4% acetic acid, the rim at the cervicovaginal junction shows extensive punctation and a mosaic pattern. Cervical biopsy at the 3 o'clock position showed CIN grade 1.

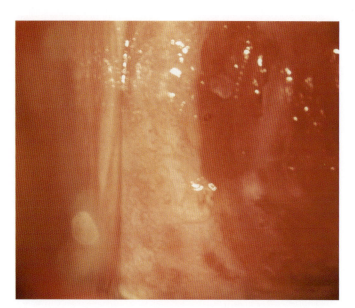

FIGURE 11-15 The cervicovaginal junction on the patient's right shows dense white epithelium. A close-up colposcopic view (×10) shows punctation that is particularly well seen at the 9 o'clock position. The pattern is compatible with the cytologic findings.

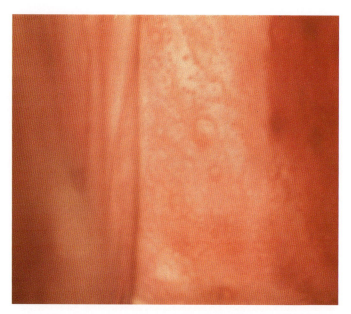

FIGURE 11-16 A magnified view (×16) of Figure 11-15 shows punctation with intermediate intercapillary distance (*center*) at the cervicovaginal junction. The upper half of this area shows punctation, and the lower half shows an early mosaic pattern.

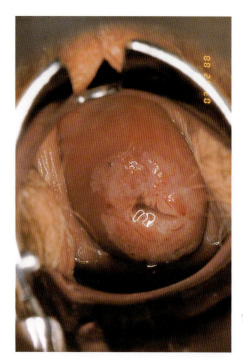

FIGURE 11-17 A low-power view (×4) of the cervix shows squamous metaplasia of the entire transformation zone. Endocervical clefts, or glands, are surrounded by a veil of cloudy metaplastic epithelium. At the 11 o'clock and 1 o'clock positions, fine, focal areas of punctation are seen within white epithelium, or ground leukoplakia. Cervical biopsy showed CIN 1, or condylomatous atypia. Endocervical curettage did not show dysplastic (CIN) cells.

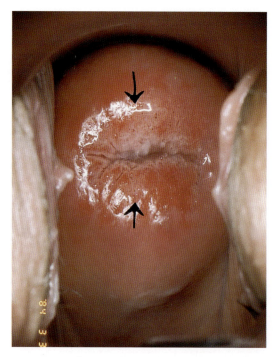

FIGURE 11-18 The transformation zone is extensive, with multiple areas of metaplasia. Ectopy is seen on the glandular epithelium on the portio. Two small foci of punctation are seen, the larger on the anterior lip (*arrow*) and the smaller on the posterior lip (*arrow*). Biopsy at the 12 o'clock position showed CIN grade 1. Results of endocervical curettage were negative for dysplasia.

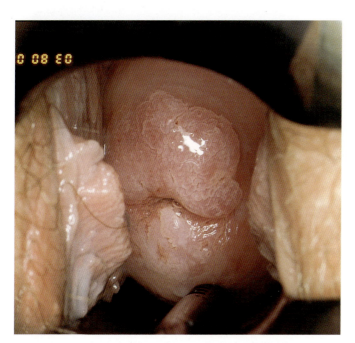

FIGURE 11-19 Colposcopic examination (×6) shows a large wart that occupies the entire anterior lip of the cervix.

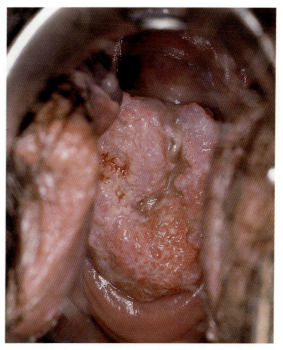

FIGURE 11-20 Two to three confluent warts virtually encompass the cervix. A small piece of the posterior cervix is seen (*bottom*). Biopsy is indicated when this type of warty lesion is seen. Biopsy of this lesion showed a benign condyloma.

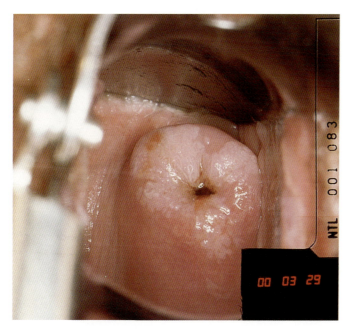

FIGURE 11-21 The transformation zone is abnormal and has been replaced by a dense, white, flat, papillomatous lesion that is consistent with flat, warty (condylomatous) epithelium (×4).

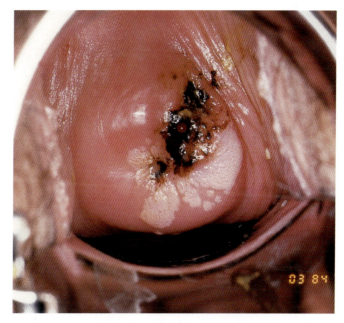

FIGURE 11-22 This condylomatous lesion is similar to the lesion seen in Figure 11-21 (×4). A generous biopsy specimen was taken through the transformation zone at the area from 1 o'clock to 2 o'clock. Monsel solution was applied for hemostasis. Biopsy showed condylomatous atypia and a flat condyloma, i.e. CIN grade 1. The pebbly appearance of the warty epithelium is pathognomonic of human papillomavirus infection.

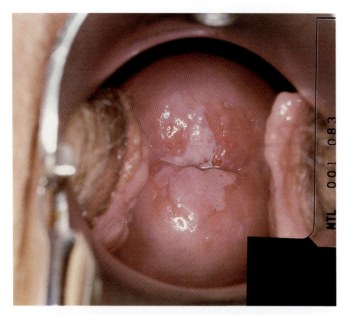

FIGURE 11-23 An abnormal transformation zone is seen, with white epithelium extending onto the portio, both anteriorly and posteriorly, as well as into the endocervical canal. Fine punctation is seen. Directed biopsy showed CIN grade 1; endocervical curettage showed CIN.

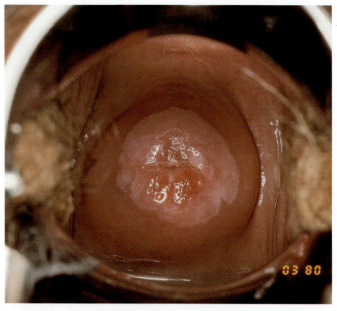

FIGURE 11-24 A colposcopic view (×4) shows a circumferential abnormal transformation zone that consists of white epithelium that extends halfway onto the portio as well as into the endocervical canal. The patient underwent endocervical curettage and a 10-mm-deep loop excision of the entire abnormal transformation zone. The endocervical margin was positive. Pathologic examination showed CIN grade 2 with glandular involvement. Endocervical curettage showed no dysplasia.

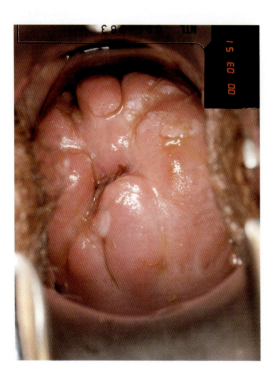

FIGURE 11-25 The cervix is deformed as a result of the prior sharp cone biopsy. The squamocolumnar junction is not well seen. Plaques of pebbly white epithelium are seen at the 6 o'clock, 11 o'clock, 12 o'clock, 1 o'clock, 2 o'clock, and 3 o'clock positions. The epithelium varies in whiteness and contains condylomatous patches.

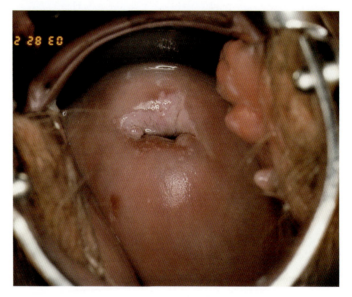

FIGURE 11-26 The abnormal transformation zone is small, occupying the anterior lip of the cervix. A small island of white epithelium is seen on the ectocervix at the 12 o'clock position. Biopsy showed CIN grade 1, or condylomatous changes. Endocervical curettage showed no dysplasia.

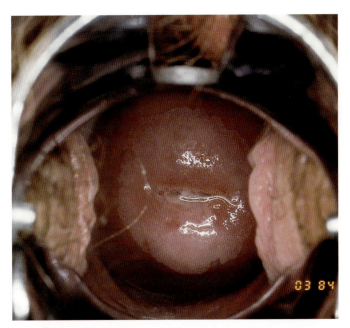

FIGURE 11-27 The cervix is dusky because of the pregnancy. An extensive, circumferential abnormal transformation zone shows white epithelium and a peripheral mosaic pattern (from the 12 o'clock position to the 2 o'clock position) that suggests high-grade dysplasia. Directed biopsy was performed without excessive bleeding at the 1 o'clock position and showed CIN grade 3.

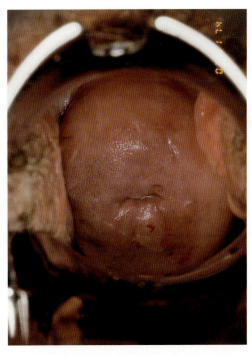

FIGURE 11-28 An excellent example of reverse mosaic. A pattern of red endocervical papillae tips surrounded by white metaplastic epithelium is seen on the anterior aspect of the cervix, extending from the 10 o'clock position to the 12 o'clock position. To a lesser extent, this pattern is seen at the 1 o'clock position. The lesion corresponds to atypical metaplasia and typically evolves into obvious dysplasia. This incipient dysplastic lesion is not commonly seen.

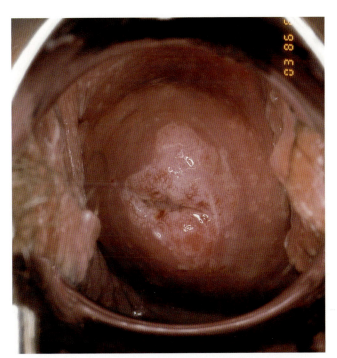

FIGURE 11-29 Colposcopic examination (×6) shows an abnormal transformation zone that is characterized by white epithelium that circumferentially surrounds the external os and extends onto the ectocervix at the 12 o'clock, 6 o'clock, and 3 o'clock positions. A well-developed severe mosaic pattern is seen at the 11 o'clock and 12 o'clock positions. Islands of white epithelium are seen on the ectocervix at the 3 o'clock position. Biopsy at the 10 o'clock position showed carcinoma in situ, and biopsy at the 5 o'clock position showed CIN grade 2. Biopsy of the ectocervix at the 3 o'clock position showed condylomatous atypia.

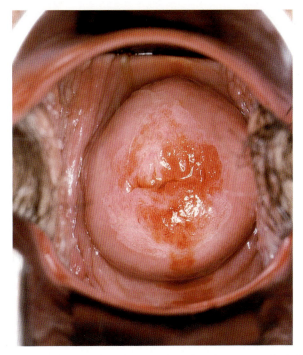

FIGURE 11-30 Colposcopic examination shows metaplasia in the central portion of the abundant glandular epithelium of the ectocervix. This finding is characteristic of prenatal exposure to diethylstilbestrol. Additionally, far out on the portio, white epithelium characteristic of atypical metaplasia is seen at the margins of the transformation zone. Multiple biopsies confirmed atypical metaplasia.

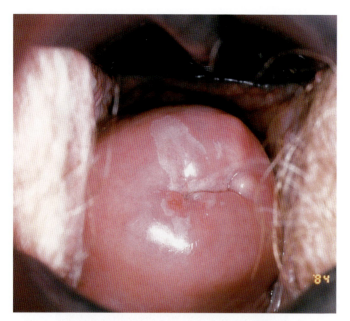

FIGURE 11-31 The cervix shows two areas of white epithelium jutting out from the transformation zone onto the ectocervix. The anterior projection extends far out onto the portio at the 11 o'clock position. Two small islands of white epithelium are seen between the 5 o'clock and 6 o'clock positions. Smaller islands are seen on the ectocervix and on the anterior and posterior lips of the cervix. These lesions show no vascular changes and are typical of human papillomavirus infection. Multiple biopsies confirmed condylomatous changes.

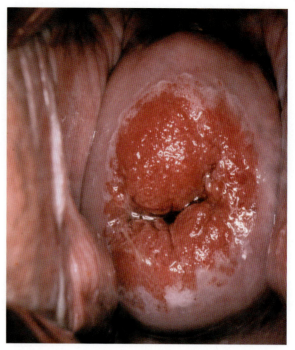

FIGURE 11-32 The cervix shows extensive ectopy as a result of oral contraceptive use. An abnormal transformation zone is seen along the periphery of the endocervical epithelium. Fingers of white epithelium extend outward onto the ectocervix. The largest projection of white epithelium, at the 12 o'clock position, extends to the anterior vaginal fornix. Directed biopsy at three projections showed condylomatous atypia, or CIN grade 1.

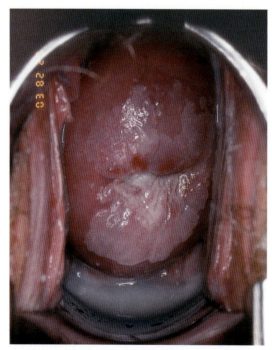

FIGURE 11-33 The cervix shows an extensive abnormal transformation zone that encompasses more than 50% of the anterior and posterior portions of the cervix. The major abnormality is marked by extensive white epithelium. A minimal mosaic pattern is seen in the upper right quadrant of the cervix (patient orientation), from the 9 o'clock position to the 12 o'clock position. An even less remarkable minimal mosaic pattern is seen along the outer posterior margin of the transformation zone. Cervical sampling of the more severe lesion (from the 9 o'clock position to the 12 o'clock position) showed CIN grade 2.

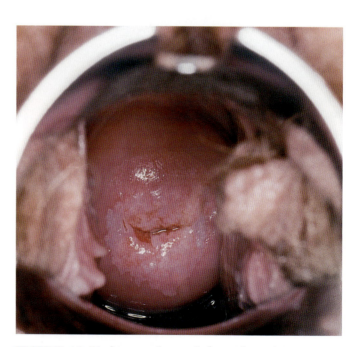

FIGURE 11-34 An extensive atypical transformation zone shows white epithelium with light and intermediate density. Biopsies at the 6 o'clock and 12 o'clock positions showed CIN 1, or condylomatous atypia.

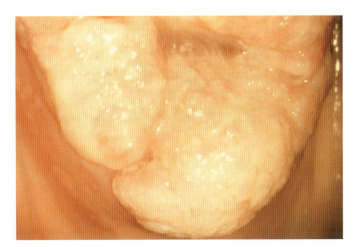

FIGURE 11-35 A colposcopic view (×10) shows a dense, stark white lesion that covers the entire cervix. No normal cervical tissue and no abnormal vessels are seen. Four biopsy specimens obtained randomly showed invasive keratinizing squamous cell carcinoma.

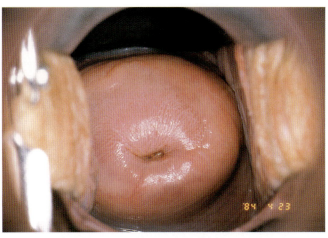

FIGURE 11-36 Streak-like tracts of raised, pebbly white epithelium are seen, particularly on the anterior portion. This pattern suggests human papillomavirus infection. Cervical biopsy showed a flat, warty lesion.

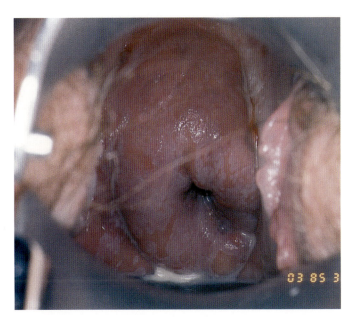

FIGURE 11-37 The cervix shows diffuse areas of white epithelium. This appearance suggests recent severe fungal infection rather than a neoplastic process. Biopsy of hyperkeratotic areas showed hyphae on fungal staining.

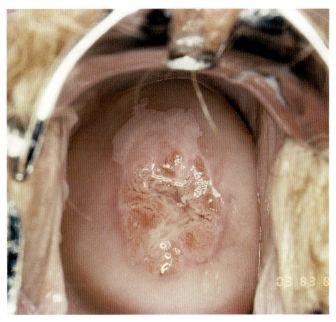

FIGURE 11-38 Dense white epithelium is seen within the transformation zone at the 12 o'clock position. The relief, even in this two-dimensional view, suggests papillomatosis. Biopsy confirmed a flat, warty lesion that suggested CIN grade 1, or condylomatous atypia.

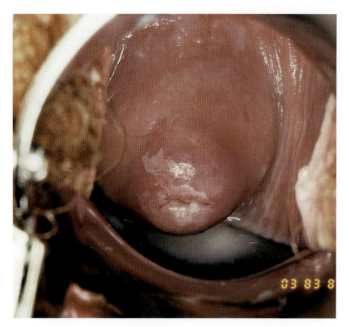

FIGURE 11-39 A colposcopic view (×6) shows little change from the findings 6 months earlier. The atypical transformation zone involves both a small area of the posterior lip at the 5 o'clock position and a larger site at the anterior lip, where the white epithelium juts upward, at the 11 o'clock position. The lesion was excised in toto by loop electrical excision to a depth of 10 mm. All margins were clear. The diagnosis was CIN grade 1.

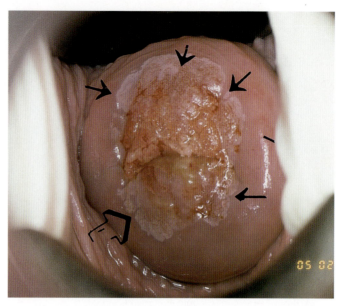

FIGURE 11-40 An abnormal transformation zone at the periphery of the transformation zone is characterized by white epithelium (*arrows*). Punctation is seen in the white epithelium at the 7 o'clock position (*open arrow*). Biopsy at the 11 o'clock and 1 o'clock positions showed condylomatous changes. Biopsy at the 7 o'clock position showed CIN grade 2.

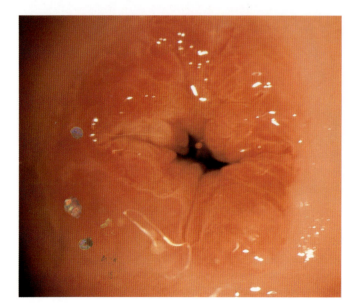

FIGURE 11-41 The ectocervix is pink. The squamocolumnar transformation zone is normal. The endocervical mucosa has migrated a short distance beyond the external os (buttoning). The entire transformation zone is normal.

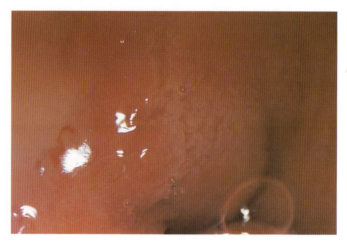

FIGURE 11-42 After the application of acetic acid, the grape-like pattern of the migrated, or ectopic, endocervical tissue is seen. This change is caused by the action of oral contraceptives on the cervix. No warts are seen, and colposcopic findings are normal (×25).

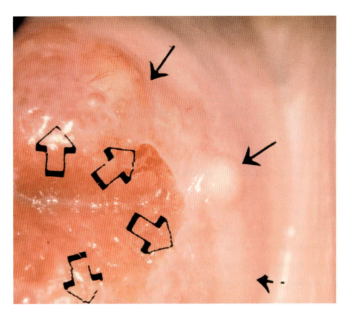

FIGURE 11-43 Colposcopic examination (×10) shows a normal transformation zone. Both an old transformation zone (*arrows*) and a new transformation zone (*open arrows*) are seen. The bump is a nabothian cyst at the 3 o'clock position.

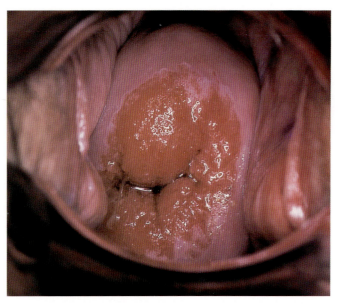

FIGURE 11-44 Colposcopic examination (×6) shows a bluish cervix with extensive ectopy. At the 12 o'clock periphery, a small zone of white epithelium contains intermediate to coarse punctation. White epithelium and punctation also are seen at the 6 o'clock periphery. Biopsy at the 12 o'clock position showed CIN 2.

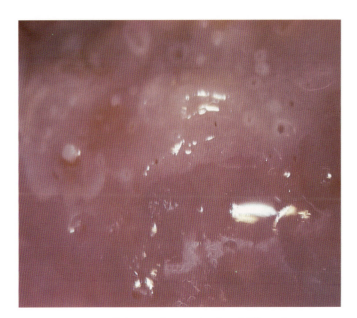

FIGURE 11-45 Colposcopic examination (×25) at the transformation zone shows the pink, mature squamous epithelium of the ectocervix. Many gland openings are seen and are surrounded by a cloudy veil of white epithelium. This veil contains young metaplastic cells and shows squamous metaplasia.

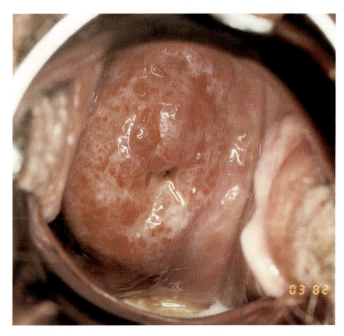

FIGURE 11-46 The cervix has several large, punctate areas as well as large, coalescing red spots. It also shows extensive ectopy and metaplasia. Several cultures were obtained, and directed biopsy was performed through the 9 o'clock position. Bacteriologic examination showed heavy growth of β-hemolytic streptococci. The patient received 1.2 million units of penicillin G and was treated with ampicillin for 7 days. Biopsy showed severe acute and chronic cervicitis.

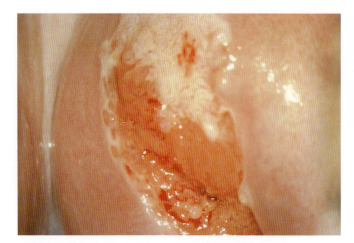

FIGURE 11-47 Colposcopic examination (×10) shows that a sharply focal abnormal transformation zone at the 12 o'clock position, which extends from the endocervix upward onto the portio. The white epithelium is dense and contains abnormal nonbranching vessels as well as horizontal and bizarre vessels. Directed biopsy showed CIN grade 3 with microscopic invasion.

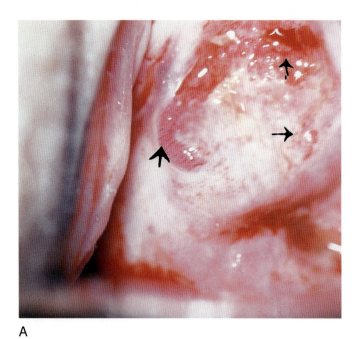

A

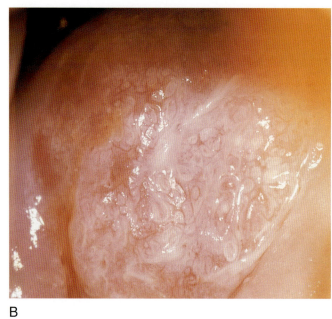

B

FIGURE 11-48 **A,** Raised white and red cervical tissue contains many abnormal vessels (*arrows*). **B,** Directed biopsy showed invasive squamous cell carcinoma with vascular involvement.

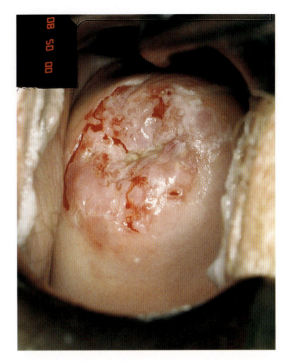

FIGURE 11-49 Colposcopic examination (×6) shows enlargement of the cervix. The white epithelium is condylomatous and shows many bizarre, transverse abnormal vessels. Cervical biopsy showed microscopic invasion and carcinoma in situ.

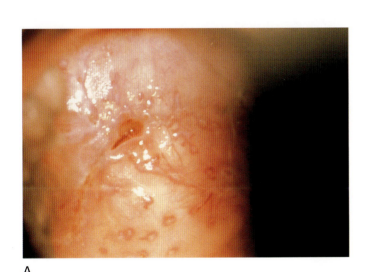

A

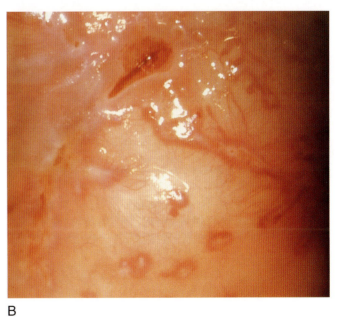

B

FIGURE 11-50 A, A colposcopic view (×16) shows squamous metaplasia. The looped, branching vessels do not involve neoplasia. **B,** Magnified view of **A.**

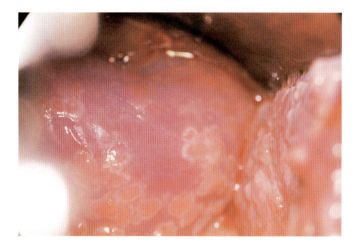

FIGURE 11-51 The cervix is pushed to the patient's right with a large cotton swab (*far left*). Large, shallow ulcers outlined by white borders cover the cervix and are seen on the lateral vaginal wall. Directed cervical biopsy of an ulcer showed *T. vaginalis.*

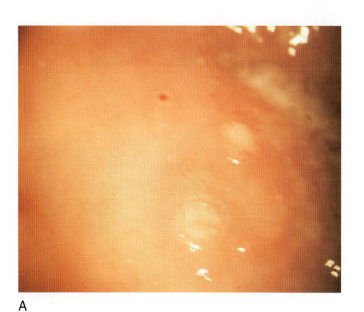

A

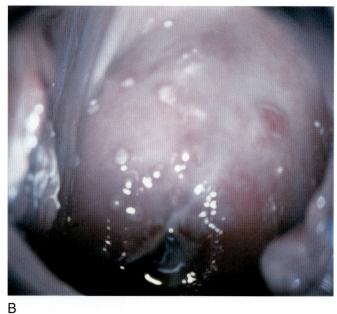

B

FIGURE 11-52 A, An oblique colposcopic view of the cervix (×16) shows white craters, which are herpes ulcers that are filled with fibrin. Culture and biopsy confirmed the presence of herpes simplex virus, type 2. **B,** Multiple herpetic vesicles and ulcers are seen on the portio of this cervix.

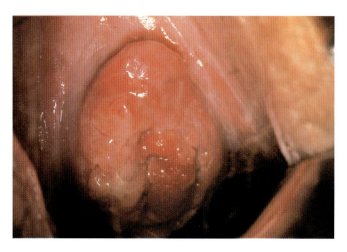

FIGURE 11-53. The cervix is deformed. The entire cervix appears to consist of endocervical columnar (red) mucous epithelium. The cleft formation is consistent with the structure of the endocervical canal in non-diethylstilbestrol-exposed women.

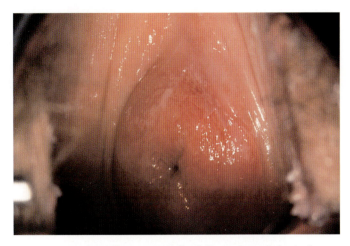

FIGURE 11-54 The congenitally deformed cervix is similar to that shown in Figure 11-53. The ectocervix is attenuated and forms a hood, or comb, at the base of the main glandular component of the cervix. The hood is the boundary between the cervix and the vagina. This iatrogenic anomaly creates a large transformation zone.

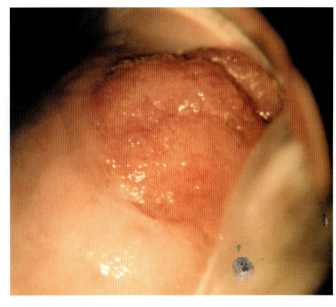

FIGURE 11-55 The squamous portion of the cervix is better developed than those seen in Figures 11-53 and 11-54. It is likely that diethylstilbestrol exposure began later in the gestation. The hood of the cervix is approximately 1 cm high and joins the protruding glandular element in an area of squamous metaplasia.

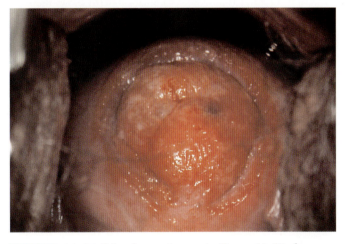

FIGURE 11-56 Like the cervix seen in Figure 11-55, the squamous rim is better developed than in Figures 11-53 and 11-54; however, the metaplastic zone is much wider.

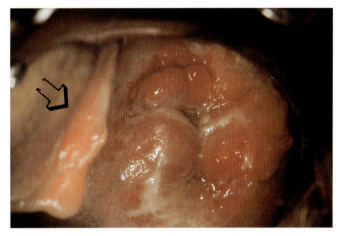

FIGURE 11-57 This cervix consists of endocervical elements, including the tiny remnant of a rim (*arrow*). Another common defect is a relaxed or poorly developed internal os that increases the risk of cervical insufficiency during pregnancy.

FIGURE 11-58 This cervix shows several stigmata of prenatal DES exposure. The main ectocervix is composed of glandular epithelium. A hood is present at 12 o'clock. Extensive squamous metaplasia is present. Adenosis is seen in the fornices.

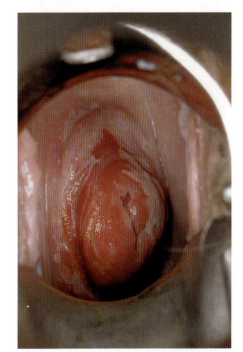

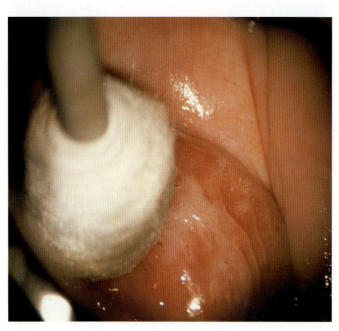

FIGURE 11-59 A large cotton swab is used to push the cervix downward. A central area of white epithelium is seen. Biopsy showed squamous metaplasia.

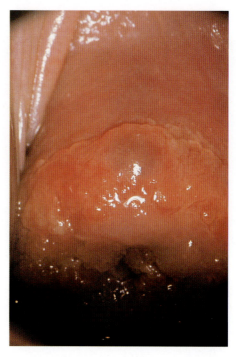

FIGURE 11-60 Colposcopic examination (×16) shows the grape-like consistency of the cervix in a patient with prenatal exposure to diethylstilbestrol. Early central squamous metaplasia is seen as well.

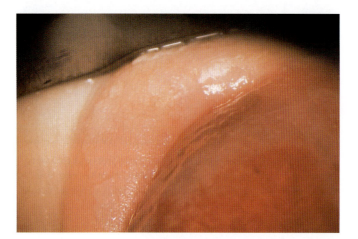

FIGURE 11-61 Atypical condylomatous metaplasia caused by human papillomavirus infection is seen in the hood at the base of the glandular cervix. A recessed area is seen between the squamous and glandular components of the cervix.

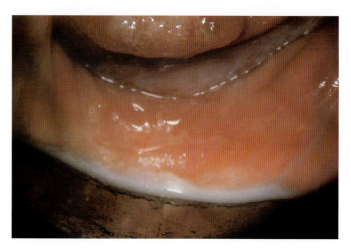

FIGURE 11-62 A colposcopic view obtained at the junction of the posterior rim of the squamous component of the cervix, where it joins the main glandular component. Areas of active and normal squamous metaplasia are seen.

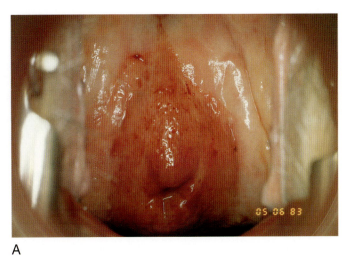

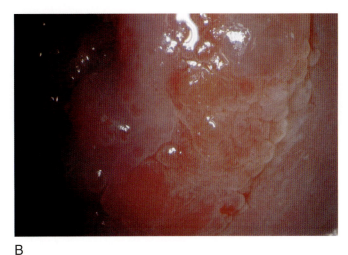

A

B

FIGURE 11-63 A, Atypical metaplasia, as evidenced by ground leukoplakia and mosaic, is seen within the lateral portion of the cervical hood. The diffuse mosaic seen within the glandular epithelium is not atypical. **B,** A high-power colposcopic view (×25) of the glandular tissue in **A.**

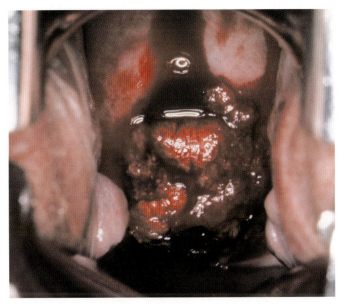

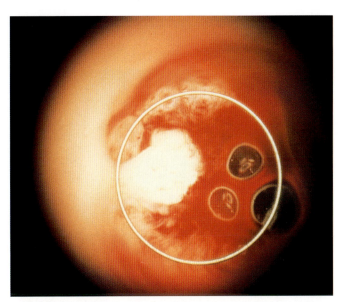

FIGURE 11-64 Reddish glandular tissue fills the cervix and spills out into the posterior fornix of the vagina. This tissue bled at the lightest touch. Cervical biopsy was performed and showed adenocarcinoma. Bimanual rectal and vaginal examination showed a small uterus, normal adnexa, and no parametrical thickening.

FIGURE 11-65 Contact hysteroscopy was performed in the endocervical canal. This stark white lesion was seen at the junction of the lower corpus and the internal cervical os. Biopsy showed adenocarcinoma.

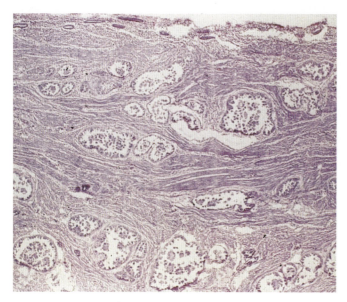

FIGURE 11-66 A biopsy specimen from the patient seen in Figure 11-67 shows adenocarcinoma.

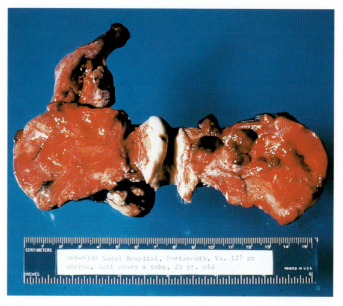

FIGURE 11-67 The uterus and vagina of a young woman show clear cell adenocarcinoma of the upper vagina and cervical rim. The patient had early, prolonged prenatal exposure to large doses of diethylstilbestrol.

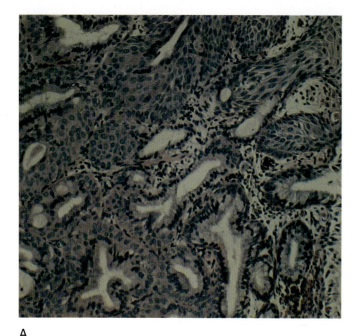

A

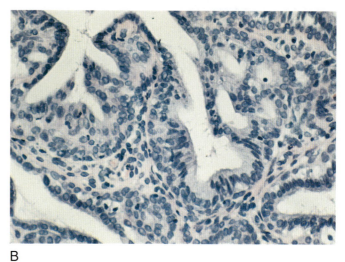

B

FIGURE 11-68 **A,** An area of the vagina that is adjacent to the tumor shown in Figure 11-67 shows benign adenosis, or glandular tissue with surrounding squamous metaplasia. **B,** A high-power view shows metaplasia at the base of the endocervical epithelium. These findings are characteristic of adenosis.

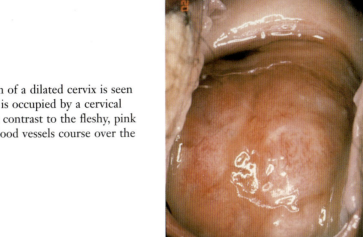

FIGURE 11-69 The rim of a dilated cervix is seen (*top*). The rest of the field is occupied by a cervical myoma that is pink-red in contrast to the fleshy, pink cervix. Many branching blood vessels course over the surface of the myoma.

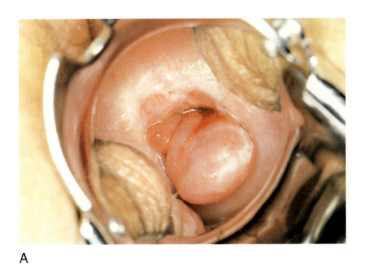

A

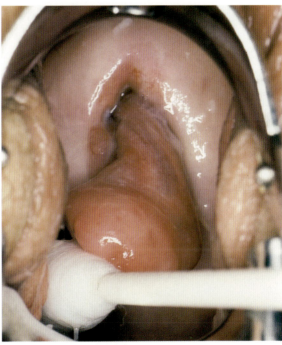

B

FIGURE 11-70 **A,** A polyp emerges from the endocervix. A clamp was placed on the polyp and its base was clamped. The polyp was excised and a 3-0 vicryl ligature was placed around the base. **B,** A large polyp extends from high in the cervical canal or from the lower uterine (corpus) segment. The polyp was excised. Pathologic examination showed a benign endometrial polyp.

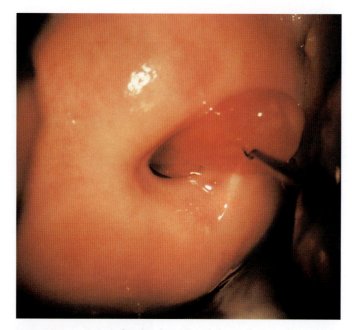

FIGURE 11-71 A fine hook is placed through a small cervical polyp, and the lesion is placed on traction. The base of the polyp arises from the endocervical canal. The polyp is twisted and removed. Pathologic examination showed a benign endocervical polyp.

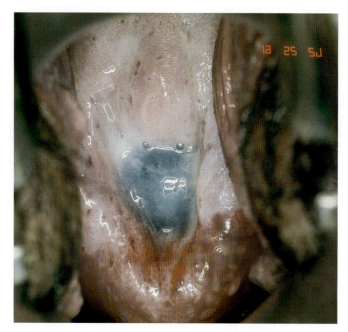

FIGURE 11-72 Obvious cervical dilation with exposure of the membranes within the cervical canal. The cervix has an abnormal transformation zone, with white, condylomatous epithelium that is especially notable at the 9 o'clock and 3 o'clock positions.

B
Colposcopy of the Vagina

CHAPTER 12
Anatomy and Microanatomy of the Vagina

The vagina is a potential space that extends between its attachments to the cervix, cardinal, and uterosacral ligaments (upper vagina) to the vestibule at the level of the hymenal ring (lower vagina) (Figs. 12-1*A* to *C*). Anteriorly, the vagina is intimately attached to the urethra and bladder (Fig. 12-2). Posteriorly, the vagina is attached to the anus and rectum. Laterally, the vagina is supported by the levator ani muscles. The lower third of the vagina is closely apposed to the bulbocavernosus muscle, Bartholin's gland, the bulb of the vestibule, and the corpora cavernosa of the clitoris (Figs. 12-3*A* to *F*). In the dorsal lithotomy position, the anterior and posterior walls of the vagina droop so that they touch each other. In the knee-chest position, the walls are pushed open by in-flowing air (Figs. 12-4*A* and *B*). The anterolateral and posterolateral walls are attached to the levator ani muscles and paravaginal connective tissue, creating sulci, or furrows (Figs. 12-5*A* and *B*). The lateral walls of the vagina are located between the anterolateral sulcus and the posterolateral sulcus (Fig. 12-6).

There is some controversy about the embryonic origin of the vagina. Most studies support a combined derivation from the müllerian ducts and the urogenital sinus (Fig. 12-7).

Based on observations of women who had exposure to diethylstilbestrol during the first 12 to 14 weeks of gestation, the role of the müllerian ducts is conclusive. The presence of müllerian mucus epithelium in the vagina, or adenosis, confirms this role (Figs. 12-8*A* and *B*). Additionally, the formation of a septum, with uterine and cervical duplication, is further evidence of the key role played by the müllerian ducts in the formation of the vagina (Figs. 12-9*A* through *C*). In a mature woman (20 to 40 years of age), the vagina is 8.0 to 9.5-cm long from the hymenal ring to the top of the anterior or posterior fornix. The anterior wall consists of smooth muscle and collagen that is shared with the bladder and urethra. The distance between the anterior vaginal mucosa and the bladder mucosa is approximately 3 mm (Fig. 12-10). The distance between the urethra and the vagina is 2 to 3 mm. Posteriorly, the rectovaginal septum shares smooth muscle and collagen with the posterior vagina and anterior rectal wall. The thickness of the septum ranges from 2 to 3 mm (see Fig. 12-10).

In a mature woman, the vaginal mucosa has a rich, pink color and has pleats or ridges known as rugae that increase the surface area (Fig. 12-11). The vagina is pliable and stretches to accommodate the penis and, during delivery, the fetus. Vaginal capacity is increased with slow, gradual stretching. Acute stretching tears the mucosa and underlying stroma, leading to laceration.

In most cases, the vaginal epithelium consists only of nonkeratinized stratified squamous epithelium (Figs. 12-12*A* and *B*). A well-developed stratum corneum is seen when significant vaginal prolapse occurs and the vaginal mucosa is exposed to the outside environment (Fig. 12-13). The multilayered squamous mucosa is identical to that of the ectocervix. In proliferative phase of the normal menstrual cycle, the squamous mucosa is 20 to 30 cell layers thick (Fig. 12-14). In contrast, in a postmenopausal woman who does not receive estrogen replacement, the vagina is thin and smooth and the epithelial layer is only five to ten layers deep (Fig. 12-15). Under normal circumstances, no mucus, or glandular epithelium, is seen in the vagina (Fig. 12-16). The underlying stroma has many vascular channels within a loose matrix that consists of collagen, elastic tissue, and smooth muscle (Figs. 12-17*A* to *C*). Compared with the cervix, the characteristics of the vaginal stroma reflect its potential for expansion. The vaginal stroma contains both elastic tissue and smooth muscle (Fig. 12-18). Most importantly, the vagina is a passive conduit between the external environment and the uterus.

Remnants of the mesonephric system found in the stroma of the vagina include the vestigial Wolffian duct and occasionally mesonephric tubules (Fig. 12-19).

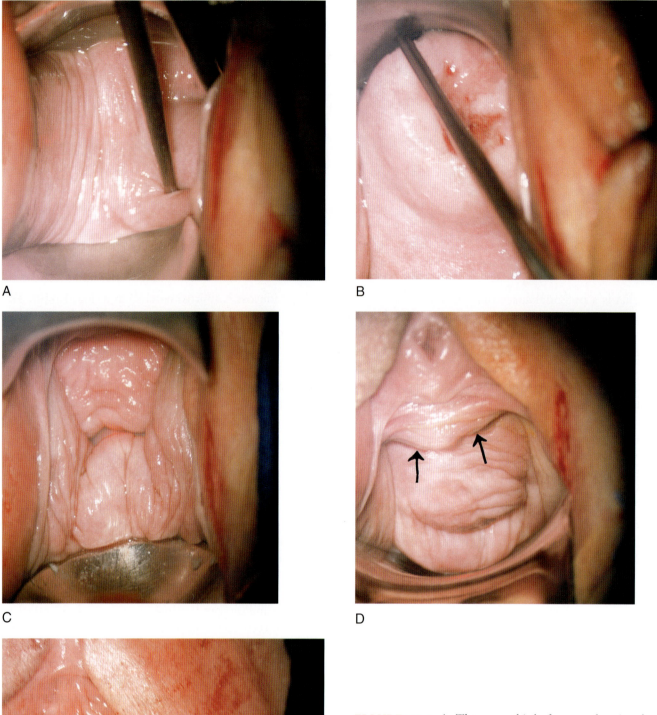

FIGURE 12-1 A, The upper third of a normal vagina shows the attachment of the vagina to the cervix and paracervial connective tissue. A tenaculum pushed the cervix to the left exposing the right vaginal fornix. **B,** The patient increases intraabdominal pressure, which causes the posterior fornix to bulge. **C,** The middle is seen. The anterior and posterior walls are in close apposition. **D,** Observing through the introitus, the urethro-vesical junction is seen (*arrows*). **E,** The lower third of the vagina is seen just above the hymenal ring, which separates the vagina from the vestibule. A band-like rugal pattern is seen on the posterior wall.

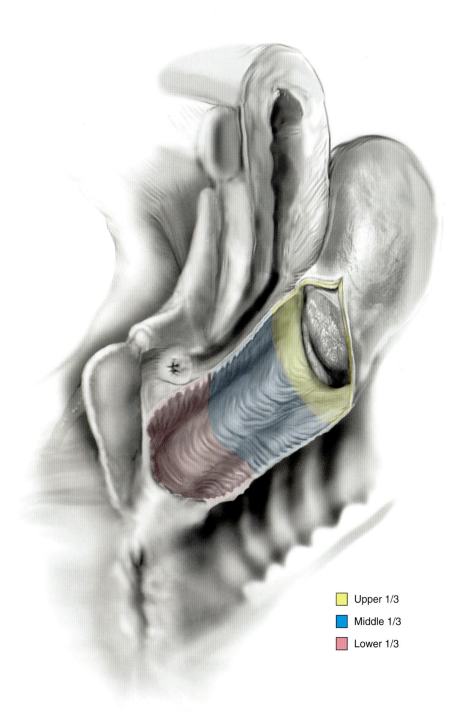

FIGURE 12-2 A three-dimensional view of the vagina shows the close relationships between the vagina and its neighboring structures. The vagina is divided into thirds for purposes of description.

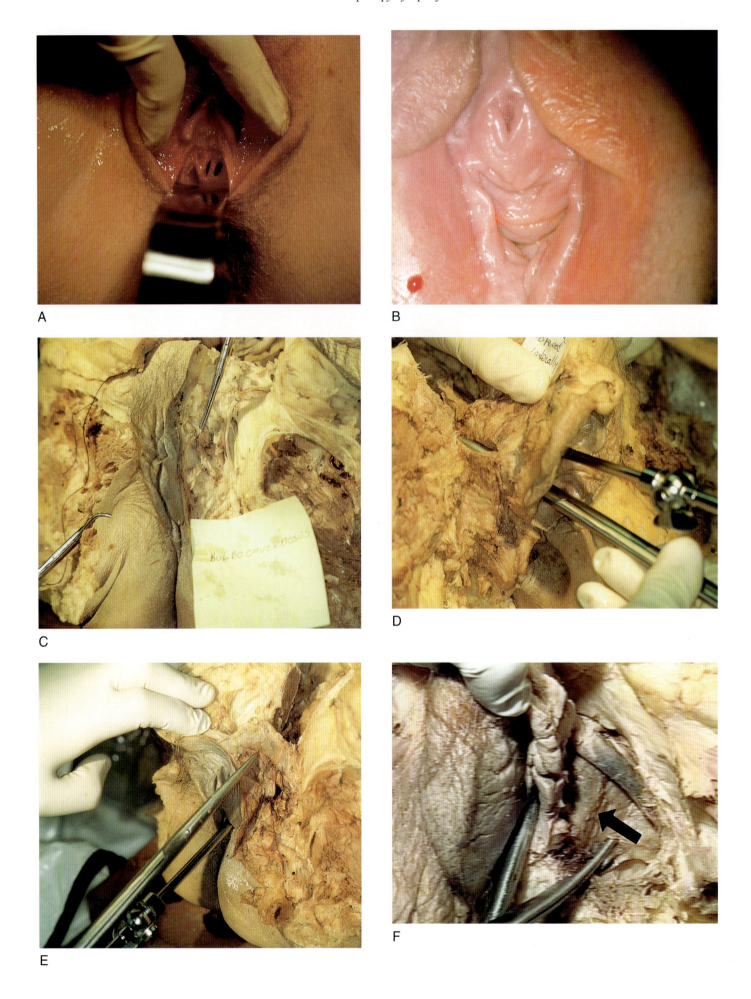

A

B

C

D

E

F

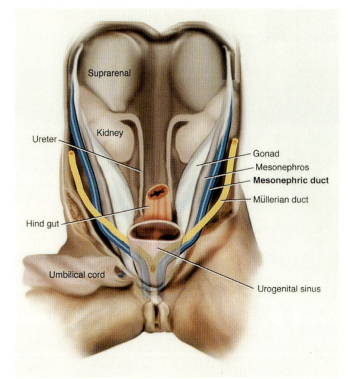

FIGURE 12-7 The vagina is formed by fusion of the müllerian ducts (yellow) and the urogenital sinus epithelium. Remnants of the once prominent mesonephric ducts (blue) are vestigial structures buried deeply within the lateral vaginal walls.

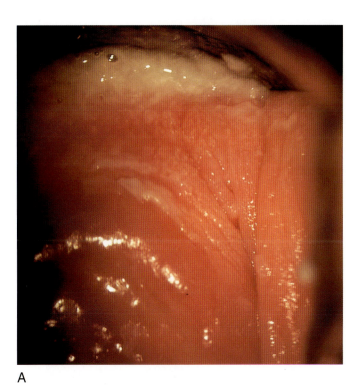

A

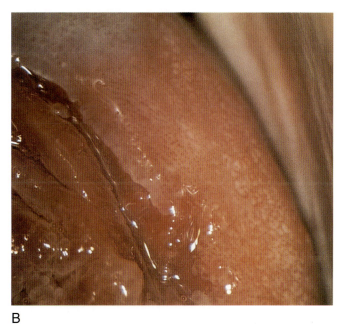

B

FIGURE 12-8 A, Vaginal adenosis in the anterior vaginal fornix is characterized by reddish, mucus-secreting glandular tissue. This tissue provides evidence of the müllerian contribution to the formation of the vagina. **B,** Cervical-vaginal hood or rim anomaly secondary to DES exposure is shown here. The red areas represent vaginal adenosis. Note the presence of mosaic and punctation vascular patterns.

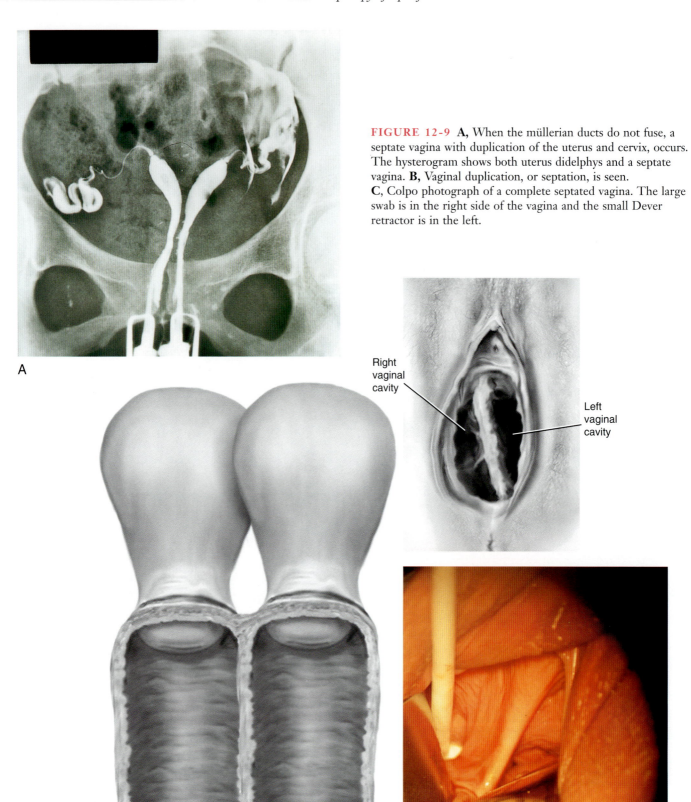

FIGURE 12-9 A, When the müllerian ducts do not fuse, a septate vagina with duplication of the uterus and cervix, occurs. The hysterogram shows both uterus didelphys and a septate vagina. **B,** Vaginal duplication, or septation, is seen. **C,** Colpo photograph of a complete septated vagina. The large swab is in the right side of the vagina and the small Dever retractor is in the left.

Right vaginal cavity

Left vaginal cavity

A

B

C

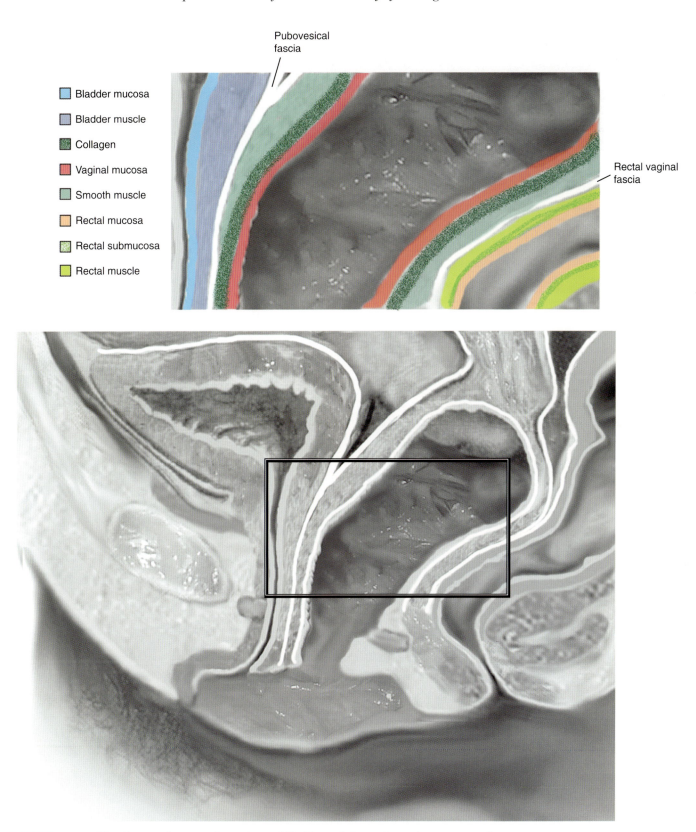

Bladder mucosa

Bladder muscle

Collagen

Vaginal mucosa

Smooth muscle

Rectal mucosa

Rectal submucosa

Rectal muscle

Pubovesical
fascia

Rectal vaginal
fascia

FIGURE 12-10 The distances between the vagina and bladder and the vagina and rectum are a few millimeters. The color codes identify the vaginal epithelium, anterior rectal wall, and posterior bladder epithelium (*inset*). The stromal walls are shared with the vaginal wall.

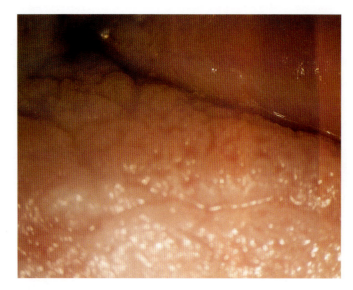

FIGURE 12-11 A magnified view (×16) of the normal vaginal wall shows many small mucosal fissures and folds.

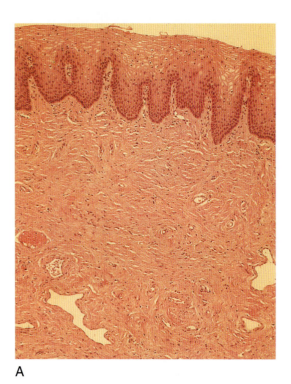

A

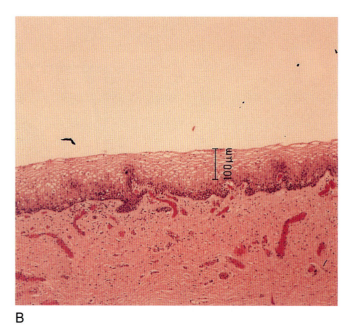

B

FIGURE 12-12 A, The vaginal epithelium consists of well-organized stratified squamous epithelium. Stromal penetration by the rete pegs is shallow. The underlying connective tissue consists of collagen and smooth muscle, with a generous vascular supply. **B,** In a postmenopausal woman, the vaginal epithelial layer is 100 to 200 μm thick.

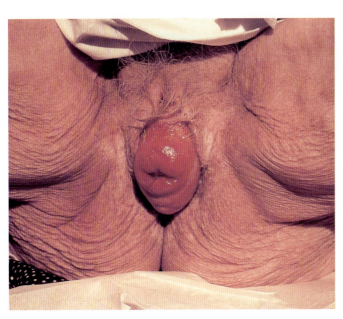

FIGURE 12-13 The normal vagina does not have a layer of keratin. However, when the vagina is exposed to the external environment, hyperkeratosis typically is present. The biopsy specimen of this vagina showed a thick later of keratin. The patient has complete vaginal prolapse.

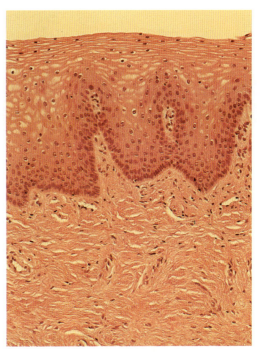

FIGURE 12-14 A normal vagina is 20 to 30 cell layers thick. A single layer of basal cells forms a dark line at the bottom of the epithelium. Approximately five layers of prickle cells lie above the basal layer. A zone of large, clear glycogen-containing cells gives way to the flattened squamous cells seen at the top of the epithelium.

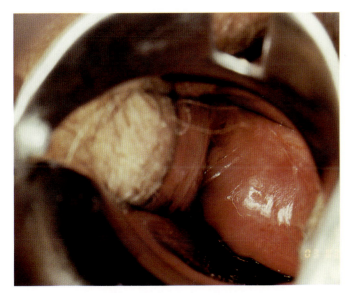

FIGURE 12-15 Atrophy of the vagina is caused by estrogen deprivation. This vagina is smooth, thin-walled, and red, with no rugal pattern. The red color is caused by decreased filtration of the underlying blood flow as a result of reduced epithelium and stroma.

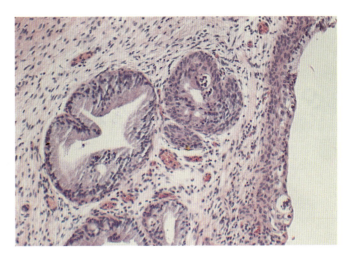

FIGURE 12-16 This vaginal wall is thin as a result of prenatal exposure to diethylstilbestrol and the subsequent formation of adenosis. Mucous glands in the underlying stroma show active squamous metaplasia. The surface glandular tissue is largely gone and has been replaced with six to eight layers of young, metaplastic squamous cells.

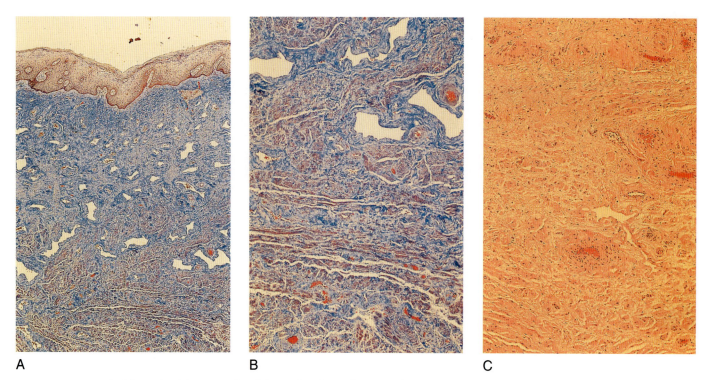

A   B   C

FIGURE 12-17 A, Masson's trichrome stain of the vagina shows the stromal composition of collagen (blue) and smooth muscle (red). **B,** A magnified view of the section seen in *A* shows at least two layers of red-staining smooth muscle, circular and longitudinal, in the outermost portion of the vaginal wall. **C,** A hematoxylin and eosin section of the vaginal muscularis shows circular and longitudinal bundles of smooth muscle.

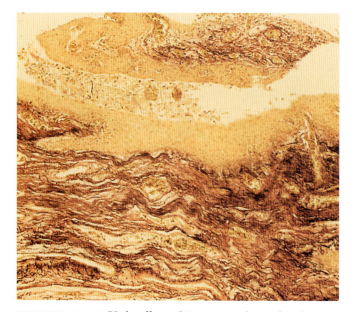

FIGURE 12-18 Verhoeff-van Gieson stain shows abundant black elastic tissue within the vaginal lamina propria.

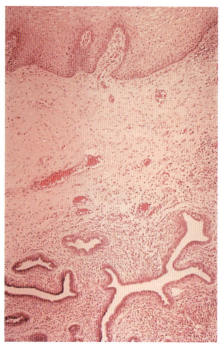

FIGURE 12-19 The glandular structures shown deep within the vaginal wall are remnants of the Wolffian, or mesonephric, duct. The epithelium is cuboidal and non-mucus-secreting.

CHAPTER 13
Pathology of the Vagina

Infection is both the major source of vaginal pathology and the cause of most gynecologic office visits (Figs. 13-1 to 13-3). Many infections are associated with coliform organisms that emanate from the large intestine and travel into the vagina by way of the perineum (see Fig. 13-2). Other infections are introduced by the fingers, mouth, or penis. Whatever the route of introduction, the vagina offers a dark, moist environment for infectious microorganisms. Infections cause vaginal discharge and are associated with inflammation (see Fig. 13-3).

Directly viewing the vagina often gives the examiner clues about the etiology of infection (Fig. 13-4A). The magnified view offered by the colposcope is especially helpful in identifying the type of infection (Fig. 13-4B). High-power magnification may be pathognomonic of a specific type of infection (Fig. 13-4C). For example, the colposcopic finding of the superficial ulcers and disk-like inflammation associated with *Trichomonas* infection confirms the results of a cytologic or saline slide preparation (Fig. 13-4D). Similarly, common fungal infections may be diagnosed cytologically as well as with potassium hydroxide slide preparations (Figs. 13-4E to G).

Vaginal intraepithelial neoplasia often is discovered after a patient has an abnormal result on vaginal cytologic screening. The cells shed from the neoplastic tissue typically are of the large keratinizing type (Figs. 13-5A and B). Because the vagina normally does not contain columnar mucous cells, adenocarcinoma cells rarely are seen. However, glandular epithelium is present in the vagina of patients who had intrauterine exposure to diethylstilbestrol (Figs. 13-6A and B). Vaginal intraepithelial neoplasia is the least common precancerous lesion of the lower genital tract and is much less common than cervical or vulvar neoplasia. These lesions rarely are visible to the naked eye and cannot be located accurately without the aid of colposcopic magnification.

Vaginal colposcopy typically is performed after a patient has abnormal cytologic findings. Commonly, intraepithelial neoplasia causes flat, warty, multicentric lesions (Figs. 13-7A and B). After the application of 3%

to 4% acetic acid, the lesions appear as white, raised, papillomatous islands. Vascular abnormalities, such as punctation, are not common (Figs. 13-8A to D). Multiple biopsies are performed to map the extent of the neoplastic process.

Microscopically, vaginal intraepithelial neoplasia is graded similarly to cervical intraepithelial neoplasia, with three grades used to indicate mild, moderate, and severe dysplasia (Figs. 13-9A to C). Grade 1 includes condylomatous atypia (Figs. 13-10A and B). Grade 3 is defined as neoplastic cells that affect more than 50% of the epithelial surface. This grade includes both severe dysplasia and carcinoma in situ (full-thickness, or through-and-through, neoplasia of the vaginal epithelium) (Figs. 13-11A and B).

Adenosis of the vagina is glandular epithelium located within the vaginal epithelium (Figs. 13-12A and B). The glandular cells are mucous, columnar types. Grossly, the adenosis appears as red, grape-like clusters or scattered red defects in the otherwise continuous pink squamous epithelium (Fig. 13-13). Adenosis usually is associated with cervical deformities. Biopsy usually shows glandular epithelium associated with varying degrees of squamous metaplasia (Fig. 13-14). Adenosis leads to multiple squamocolumnar transformation zones and therefore greater risk of squamous intraepithelial neoplasia (Figs. 13-15A and B). Additionally, diethylstilbestrol-exposed women are at increased greater risk for adenocarcinoma. Clear cell adenocarcinoma most often is associated with intrauterine exposure to diethylstilbestrol (Figs. 13-16A to C). In addition to the increased risk of neoplasia, diethylstilbestrol-exposed women have structural abnormalities, including narrowing of the vaginal vault, a T-shaped uterus, and tubo-ovarian abnormalities.

Several sexually transmitted viral diseases are seen in the vagina. Most noteworthy are herpes simplex and condylomata acuminata (Figs. 13-17A to D). Occasionally, bizarre vascular ectasia is seen when atrophic vaginal tissues are treated with massive topical administration of estrogen (Fig. 13-18).

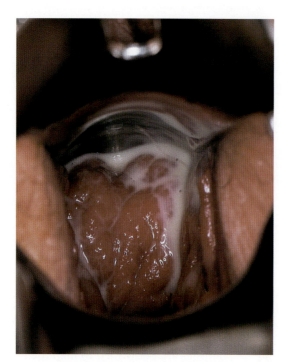

FIGURE 13-1 The copious white, milky discharge and red, beefy epithelium are characteristic of coliform infection.

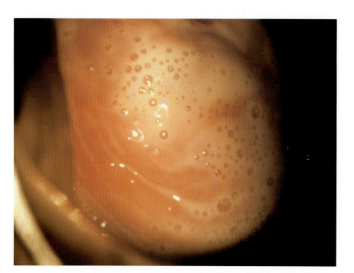

FIGURE 13-2 This foamy, yellow discharge and inflamed vagina were associated with malodor. Saline microscopic examination showed pus cells and clue cells, and subsequent culture showed infection with *Gardnerella* species.

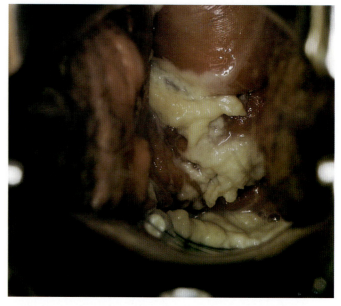

FIGURE 13-3 This patient had vaginal and vulvar pruritus accompanied by a thick, yellow-white discharge. The thick, clumped, "curdled" discharge is characteristic of fungal vaginitis.

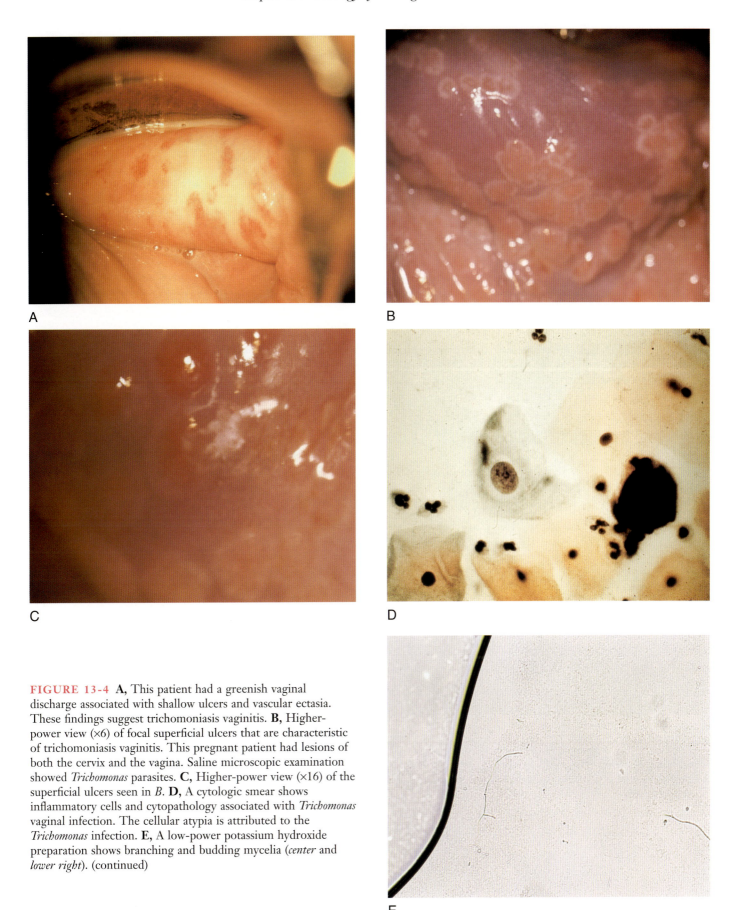

FIGURE 13-4 **A,** This patient had a greenish vaginal discharge associated with shallow ulcers and vascular ectasia. These findings suggest trichomoniasis vaginitis. **B,** Higher-power view (×6) of focal superficial ulcers that are characteristic of trichomoniasis vaginitis. This pregnant patient had lesions of both the cervix and the vagina. Saline microscopic examination showed *Trichomonas* parasites. **C,** Higher-power view (×16) of the superficial ulcers seen in *B*. **D,** A cytologic smear shows inflammatory cells and cytopathology associated with *Trichomonas* vaginal infection. The cellular atypia is attributed to the *Trichomonas* infection. **E,** A low-power potassium hydroxide preparation shows branching and budding mycelia (*center* and *lower right*). (continued)

F

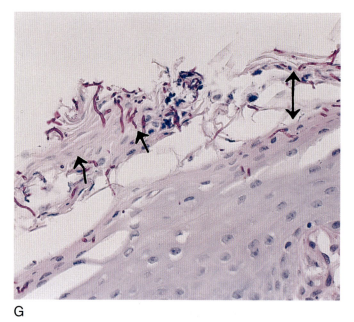

G

FIGURE 13-4 **F,** A high-power potassium hydroxide preparation shows mycelia. **G,** A vaginal biopsy specimen was stained with periodic acid-Schiff to detect fungi. Dark pink fungal mycelia are seen in the upper epithelial layers (*arrows*).

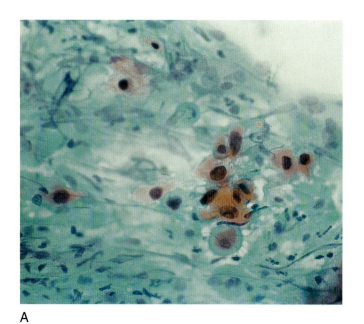

A

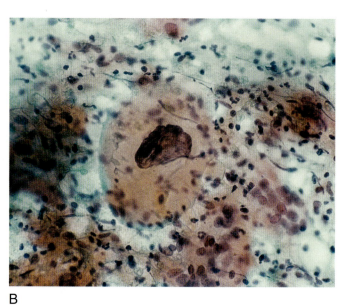

B

FIGURE 13-5 **A,** Pap smear of the vagina shows clumps of red-staining squamous cells that have large hyperchromatic nuclei. These cells are clearly dysplastic. **B,** The finding of a huge, keratinized, pleomorphic cell surrounded by smaller, atypical cells was interpreted as compatible with keratinizing squamous cell carcinoma in situ.

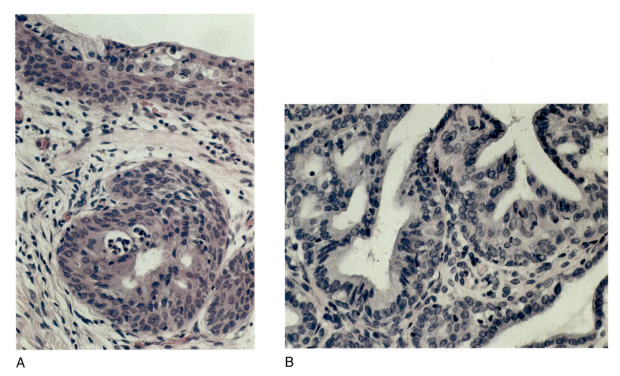

A   B

FIGURE 13-6 **A,** Vaginal biopsy from an area of gross adenosis. The surface epithelium shows remnants of glandular epithelium on the left side of the picture. The majority of the glandular cells have been replaced by squamous metaplastic cells. The underlying glandular structure is filled with young, metaplastic squamous cells. **B,** A vaginal biopsy specimen shows columnar mucus-secreting epithelium with significant areas of squamous metaplasia. This glandular tissue within the vagina is diagnostic of adenosis.

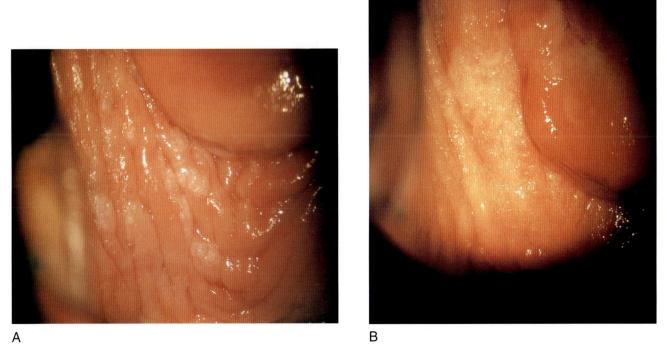

A   B

FIGURE 13-7 **A,** These flat, warty lesions show multicentric foci of dense, white epithelium, and are diagnostic of vaginal intraepithelial neoplasia. **B,** A confluent, flat, warty lesion occupies the vaginal vault. Directed biopsy showed vaginal intraepithelial neoplasia grade 3.

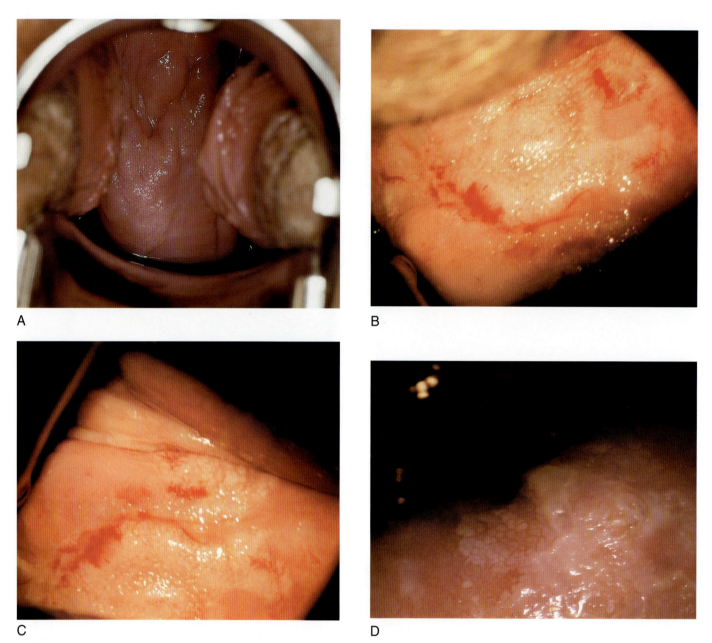

A

B

C

D

FIGURE 13-8 A, A scanning (×4) colposcopic view of the vagina obtained before the application of acetic acid shows raised, pebbly vaginal mucosa. **B,** Spicules of dense, warty epithelium create a microvillous pattern that is characteristic of a high-grade vaginal intraepithelial lesion. Biopsy showed carcinoma in situ. **C,** High-power (×16) view of *B.* **D,** Abnormal vascular patterns are not commonly seen with vaginal intraepithelial neoplasia. However, this case was associated with a well-defined mosaic pattern (×16).

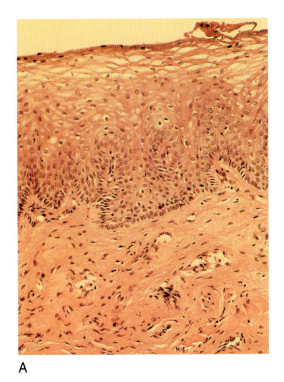

A

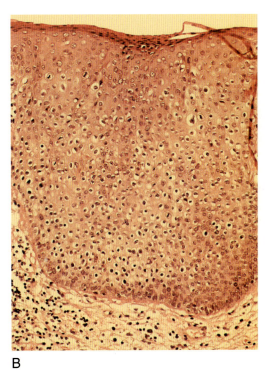

B

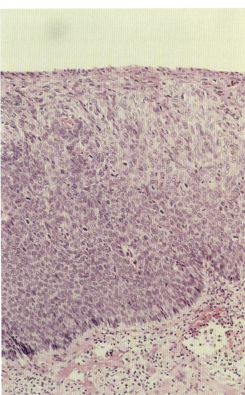

C

FIGURE 13-9 A, Vaginal intraepithelial neoplasia grade 1 is associated with atypical cellular maturation that involves the lower third of the epithelium. More than 50% of the epithelial thickness shows normal maturation and organization.
B, Extensive koilocytosis and atypical metaplastic cells are associated with acanthosis and parakeratosis. This section was diagnosed as vaginal intraepithelial neoplasia grade 2.
C, Neoplastic cells extend from the top to the bottom of the epithelium. No maturation or organization is seen. This section was interpreted as vaginal intraepithelial neoplasia grade 3.

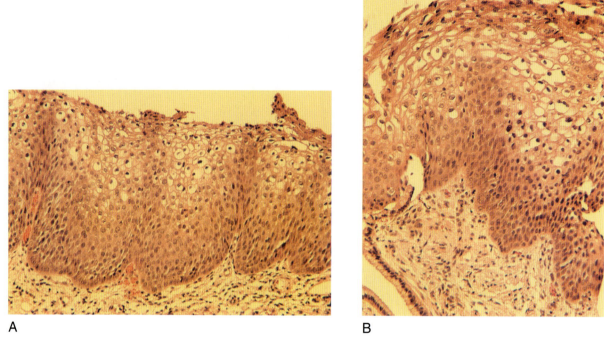

A   B

FIGURE 13-10 A, Atypical condylomatous epithelium is seen. Extensive koilocytic changes affect the upper third to half of the epithelium. The changes are characteristic of human papillomavirus infection. **B,** A high-power view of Figure 10*A* shows balloon cells with multiple hyperchromatic nuclei. These changes are associated with additional cellular abnormalities and were interpreted as vaginal intraepithelial neoplasia grade 1 to 2.

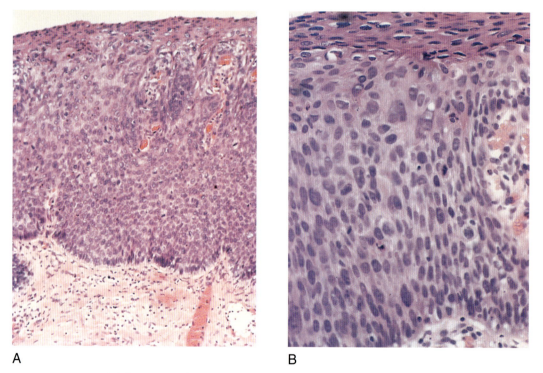

A   B

FIGURE 13-11 A, This section shows vaginal carcinoma in situ as well as atypical vascular channels within the epithelium. Colposcopic examination showed punctation. **B,** A high-power view of full-thickness neoplastic epithelial cells shows parakeratosis in the upper layers of maturation. Keratinization of individual cells in the center of the field and atypical mitotic figures are seen.

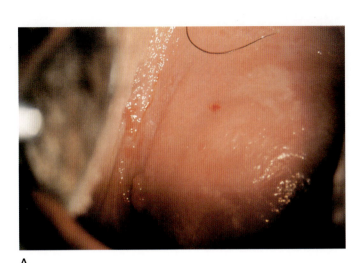

A

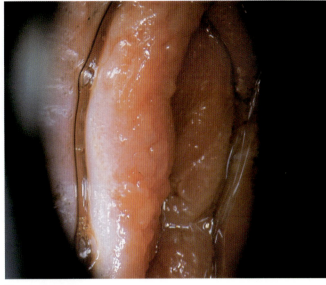

B

FIGURE 13-12 **A,** This patient was exposed to diethylstilbestrol and has vaginal abnormalities that show vaginal adenosis. The red glandular tissue contrasts with the pink squamous epithelium (*center*). **B,** A magnified view shows vaginal adenosis with a papillary pattern and crypt-like crevices produced by proliferating glandular cells. These findings are similar to the configuration seen in the endocervix.

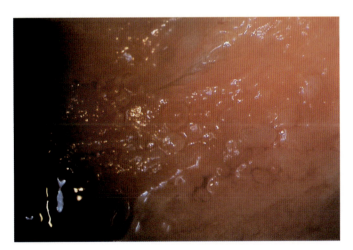

FIGURE 13-13 After acetic acid is applied to the vagina of the patient shown in Figures 12*A* and 12*B*, the glandular epithelium that covers the cervices and areas of vaginal adenosis shows a grape-like pattern.

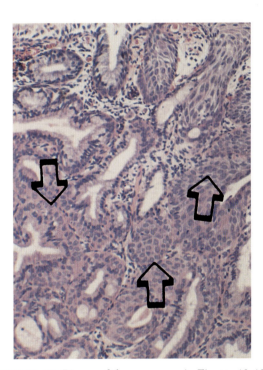

FIGURE 13-14 Biopsy of the areas seen in Figures 13-12*A*, *B*, and 13-13 shows crypts lined by columnar mucous epithelial cells and areas of immature squamous metaplasia (*arrows*).

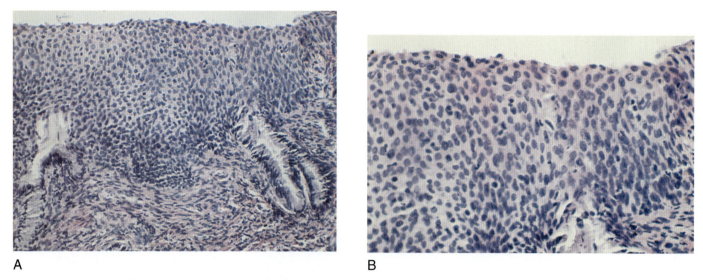

A   B

FIGURE 13-15 **A,** This section was obtained through a transformation zone between areas of vaginal adenosis and the squamous epithelium of neighboring nonadenotic vagina in the patient shown in Figures 13-12*A* and *B;* 13-13. Exposure to diethylstilbestrol and the subsequent development of adenosis creates extensive vaginal transformation zones. The metaplastic squamous cells produced a significantly dysplastic epithelium. **B,** A high-power view of *A* shows nearly full-thickness neoplastic cellular changes and lack of maturation, even at the surface. These findings are consistent with vaginal intraepithelial neoplasia grade 3 arising in adenosis.

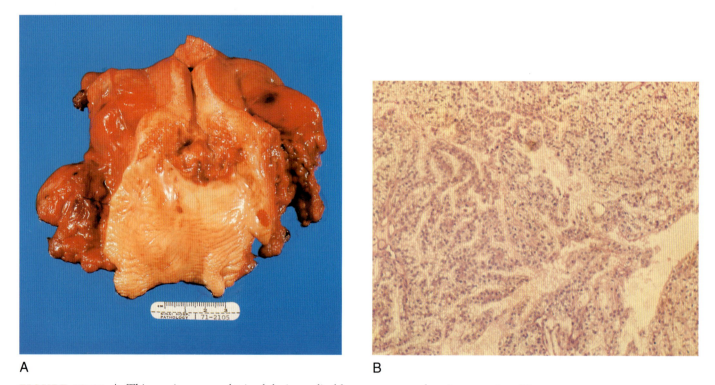

A   B

FIGURE 13-16 **A,** This specimen was obtained during radical hysterectomy and vaginectomy in a 20-year-old woman. The lesion occupies the upper vagina and cervix. Until the advent of diethylstilbestrol-induced abnormalities, adenocarcinoma of the vagina and cervix in this age group was a medical rarity. **B,** The histologic features of diethylstilbestrol-associated cervicovaginal malignancy are consistent and repetitive. Glandular proliferation includes malignant clear cells. (continued)

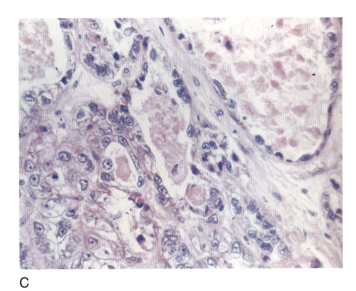

FIGURE 13-16 C, A high-power view shows the metamesonephric pattern of diethylstilbestrol-associated adenocarcinoma. The crypts are lined by hobnail cells (*top right*) and clear cells (*center right*).

C

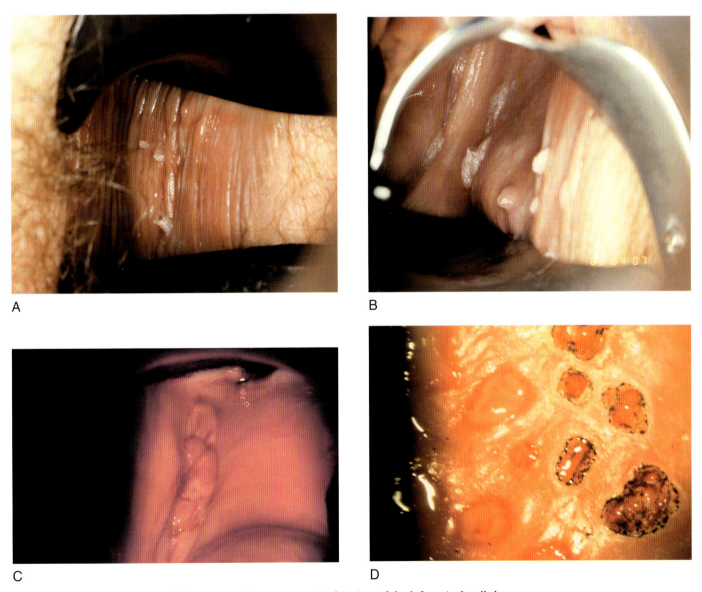

A

B

C

D

FIGURE 13-17 A, Many condylomata acuminata are seen in this view of the left vaginal wall that was obtained between the opened speculum blades. **B,** A close-up view of vaginal warts shows the difference between warts and a projection of normal vaginal mucosa. **C,** Herpes simplex of the upper vagina. Two to three ulcers are seen on a vaginal epithelial fold. Fibrin within the crater of the ulcer creates the white appearance. **D,** Close-up view of multiple herpes simplex ulcers. Several ulcers have been laser vaporized (*right*).

CHAPTER 15
Colposcopic Technique

Within the lower genital tract, the vagina is the most difficult location to examine colposcopically. The rugae of the vagina both increase its surface area and complicate its examination (Fig. 15-1A). Because the vagina is a potential space, a speculum must be inserted to allow the examiner to view it (Figs. 15-1B and C). In contrast to the cervix, which is viewed easily as the blades of the speculum are opened, the vaginal fornices are partially obscured by the cervix. Further, the anterior and posterior walls of the vagina are obscured by the speculum blades (Figs. 15-1D to F). The lateral walls can be seen only by angulating the speculum to the right or left and viewing the lateral walls through the opened blades. The anterior and posterior walls are seen only when the speculum is withdrawn (Figs. 15-2A and B). Because of these difficulties, vaginal lesions may be missed, even during colposcopic examination. A long-handled, fine hook is required to manipulate the vaginal mucosa and cervix and provide a view of the entire structure (Figs. 15-3A and B).

The patient is placed in the lithotomy position on a mechanical gynecology examination table. The table is elevated to a height that is comfortable for the examiner, and the colposcope is swung into position. The objective lens is set at a focal distance of 300 mm, and magnification is at its lowest power (scanning).

A bivalve speculum is placed into the vagina, and the cervix is located. The blades of the speculum are opened gradually to their full extent (Figs. 15-4A and B). A titanium manipulating hook is placed on the anterior lip of the cervix, and this lip is pulled down (posteriorly) sharply to expose the anterior vaginal fornix (Figs. 15-5A and B). The anterior fornix is viewed under scanning power and then at higher magnification (×6 and ×10).

Next, a large cotton swab (Proctoswab) soaked in 3% or 4% acetic acid is placed onto the mucosa of the anterior fornix (Fig. 15-6). After 30 to 40 seconds, the anterior fornix is examined again (×4, ×6, ×10, and ×16). Abnormalities are noted or are photographed with a cervicoscope or a camera mounted on a beam splitter. This examination is repeated for the posterior, left, and right vaginal fornices by shifting the hook and manipulating the speculum.

Next, the upper half of the vagina is examined by withdrawing the speculum partially and placing the anterior and posterior walls of the vagina on stretch with a skin hook (Fig. 15-7). The walls are examined (×4, ×6, and ×10) before acetic acid is applied. Acetic acid is applied with a large, cotton-tipped applicator, and the walls of the vagina are examined again (×4, ×6, ×10, and ×16). Then the speculum is angled to the right to allow the left vaginal wall to be examined (Figs. 15-8A and B). This process is repeated as the speculum is retracted until the entire vagina is examined (Fig. 15-9).

If a biopsy is required, it is performed under direct colposcopic guidance. Biopsy is best performed at low magnification (×4 or ×6) (Fig. 15-10).

If the patient has a heavy discharge or possible infection, samples of the discharge are obtained for culture or microscopic evaluation before acetic acid is applied. At the end of the examination, the examiner should create a schematic map of the vagina. This map can be used for future follow-up and comparison (Fig. 15-11).

The vagina is sensitive to stretch and pressure, and colposcopic examination is uncomfortable for most women. Discomfort can be minimized through gradual stretching and the use of a narrow-bladed speculum (Pederson) rather than a medium (Graves) speculum.

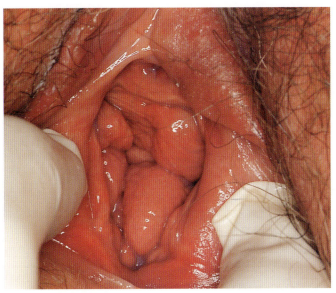

A

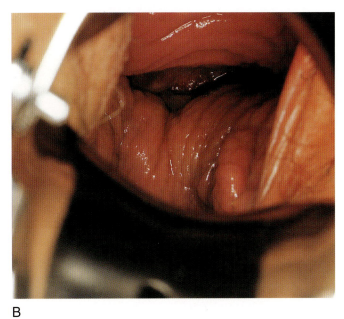

B

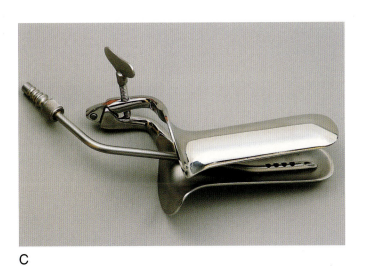

C

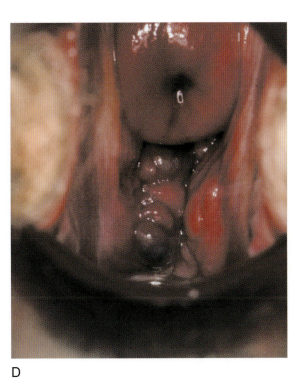

D

FIGURE 15-1 A, The vagina is a difficult area to examine because it is a potential rather than a true space, its walls have a tendency to collapse, and its surface area is large because it contains rugae. **B,** The anterior and posterior walls constrict the view of the vagina. In this case, the view is further compromised by a collapsing left lateral wall, which is characteristic of a paravaginal fascial tear. **C,** A single-hinged speculum is ideal for vaginal examination because the open side facilitates examination of the lateral vaginal walls. **D,** The cervix obstructs the view of the upper vagina. When the speculum is angled, unusual bluish cysts are seen on the anterior vaginal wall, beneath the bladder. (continued)

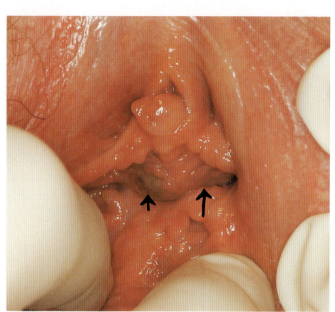

E

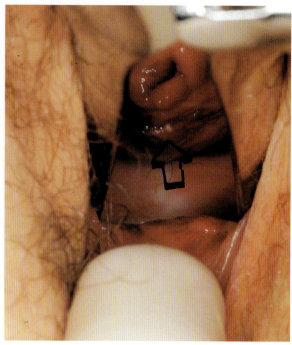

F

FIGURE 15-1 E, The cysts are seen under the urethra in the lower vagina (*arrows*). **F,** The speculum is rotated 90 degrees to flatten the anterior vaginal wall. A bluish cystic mass is seen just beneath the urethra (*open arrow*). The speculum opens the external urethral meatus widely.

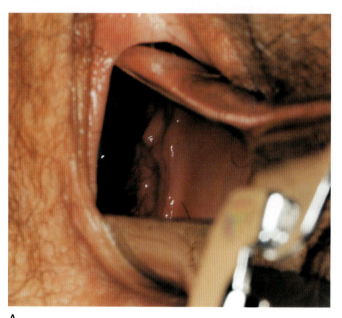

A

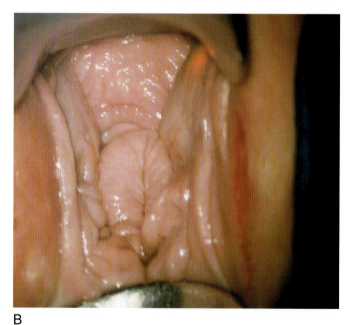

B

FIGURE 15-2 A, The lateral wall of the vagina is seen when the colposcope is angled to aim the light between the blades of the speculum. **B,** The anterior and posterior walls are viewed by withdrawing the speculum slowly while viewing the collapsing walls.

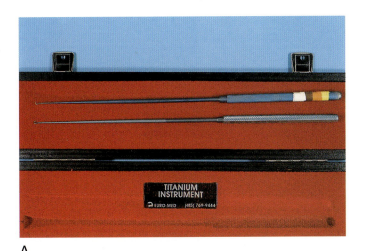

A

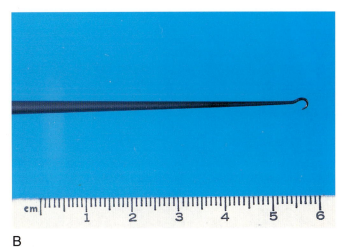

B

FIGURE 15-3 **A,** Titanium skin hooks designed for use with laser surgery on the cervix and vagina are ideal for intravaginal manipulation. The hooks are both strong and lightweight. **B,** Magnified view of the titanium skin hook shown in *A*. The entire hook is 10 inches long. The long, narrow hook does not impede colposcopic evaluation and allows atraumatic exploration.

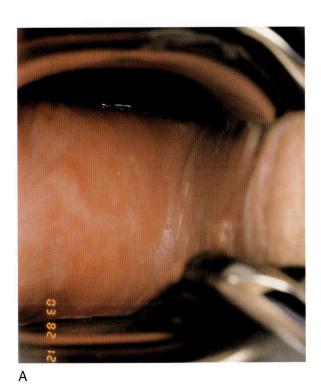

A

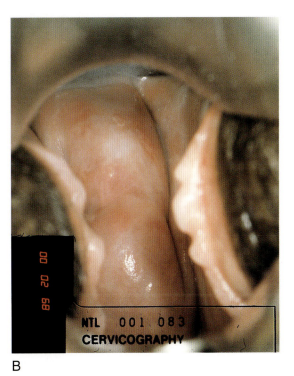

B

FIGURE 15-4 **A,** After the speculum is inserted fully, the blades are opened widely. The speculum is pressed inward, creating light pressure on the vaginal vault and flattening the mucosa. **B,** After the inward pressure on the speculum is relaxed, the vaginal vault balloons toward the examiner's colposcopic objective lens.

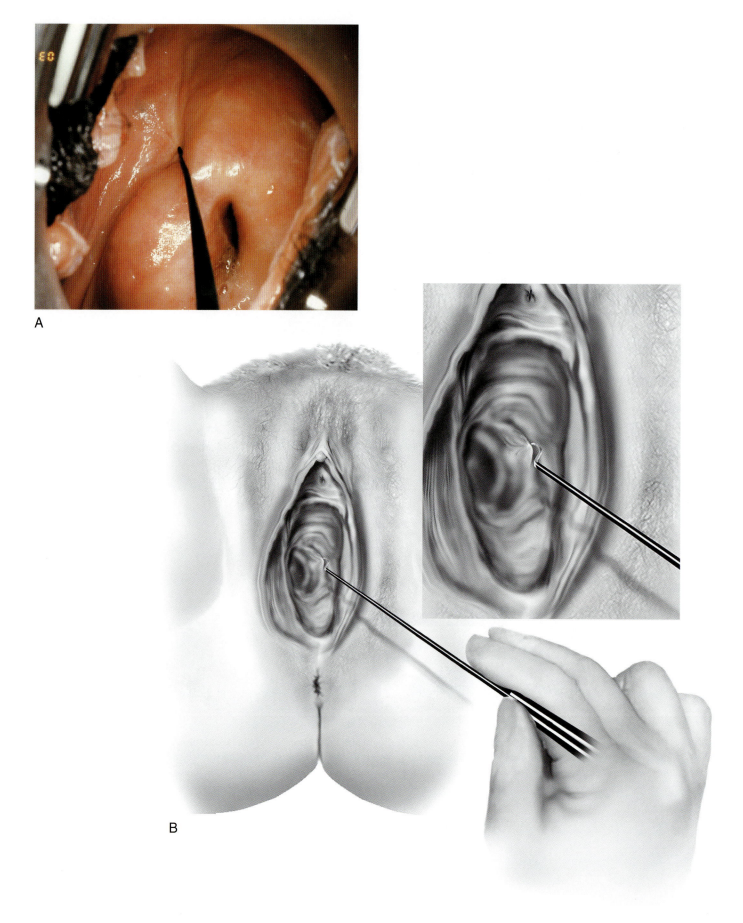

A

B

FIGURE 15-5 A, The titanium hook places traction on the cervix and exposes the anterolateral fornix on the right. This hook provides an unimpeded view of an otherwise recessed area of the vagina without causing trauma to the tissue. **B,** A titanium hook is used to place traction on the vagina.

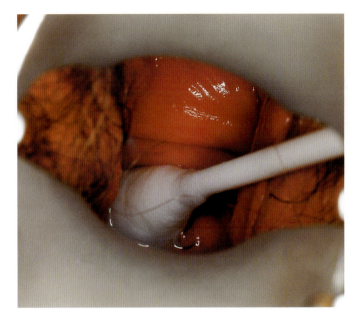

FIGURE 15-6 A large, cotton-tipped applicator (Proctoswab) is used to swab away vaginal discharge and apply acetic acid to the vagina. The swab also serves as a manipulating tool.

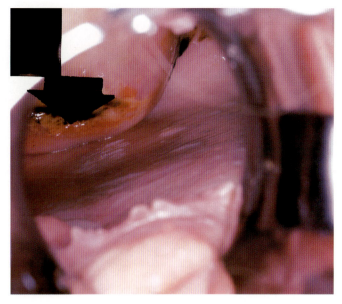

FIGURE 15-7 The posterior wall of the vagina (*arrow*) is flattened and placed on traction by rotating the speculum 90 degrees.

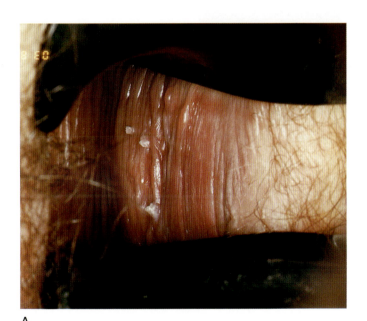

A

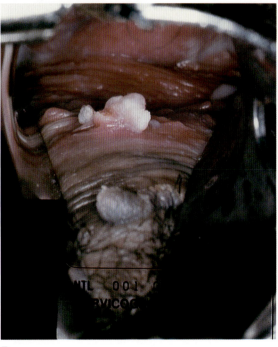

B

FIGURE 15-8 **A,** The speculum is angled, and the examiner views the area between the opened blades. Warts are seen on the introitus and lateral walls of the vagina. **B,** Deeper insertion of the speculum shows warts extending throughout the lower half of the vagina.

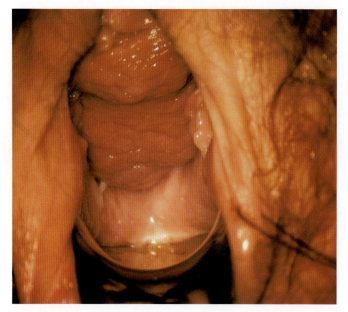

FIGURE 15-9 The speculum is withdrawn, and the lower third of the anterior and posterior vaginal walls are examined.

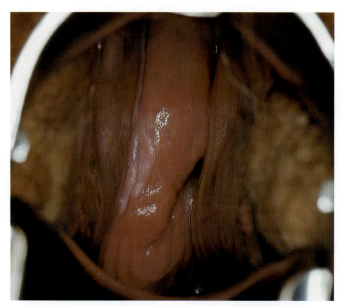

FIGURE 15-10 Suspected vaginal intraepithelial neoplasia is seen on the patient's right anterolateral wall. To perform a directed biopsy, colposcopic magnification is decreased to scanning power (×4).

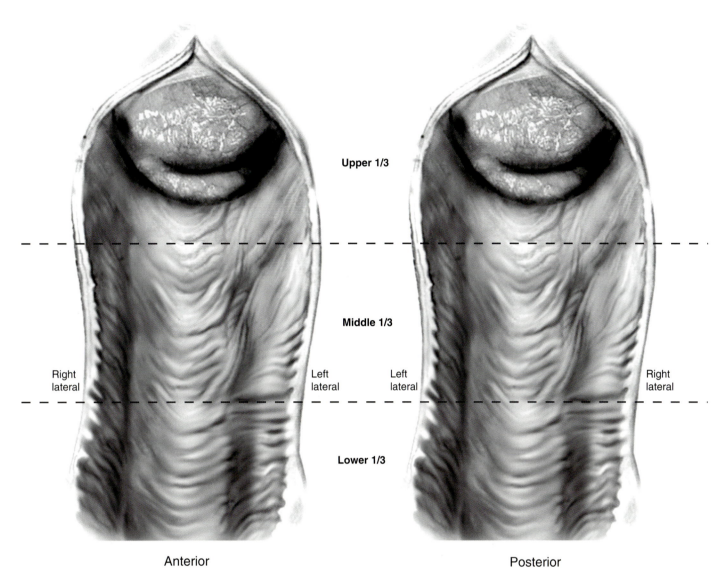

Upper 1/3

Middle 1/3

Right
lateral

Left
lateral

Left
lateral

Right
lateral

Lower 1/3

Anterior

Posterior

FIGURE 15-11 The examiner can use a schematic map of the vagina to document the colposcopic findings and record the location of colposcopically directed biopsy.

CHAPTER 16
Sampling Techniques

Biopsy of the vagina is performed with the same type of sharp long-handled punch biopsy forceps that is used for cervical biopsy (Figs. 16-1*A* and *B*). The vagina is sensitive to pressure, and a biopsy performed without anesthesia causes an uncomfortable pinching sensation. To increase patient comfort, 1 to 2 mL 1% lidocaine (Xylocaine) is injected into the vagina or a cotton-tipped swab is used to apply a small amount of lidocaine and prilocaine cream (EMLA) to the vaginal mucosa at the proposed biopsy site. All vaginal biopsies should be performed under colposcopic guidance because this technique greatly increases accuracy (Figs. 16-2*A* to *E*).

During biopsy, the examiner must exercise caution and avoid unnecessary damage to the tissue, particularly in older women who have atrophy of the vagina (Fig. 16-3). In some cases, the peritoneal cavity has been entered during vault biopsy and the bladder has been entered during anterior wall biopsy (Figs. 16-4*A* and *B*). The examiner must adjust the volume of tissue grasped by the biopsy clamp to accommodate the conditions observed.

When the biopsy is completed, a small, cotton-tipped applicator is soaked in Monsel solution and applied immediately to the biopsy crater to obtain hemostasis (Fig. 16-5*A*). If Monsel solution does not stop the bleeding, a 3–0 Vicryl suture is placed to close the wound and stop the bleeding.

When a larger biopsy specimen is needed or when an excisional biopsy is required, the patient is taken to an operating theater and anesthetized. The biopsy site is exposed with retractors, and the subepithelial connective tissue is infiltrated with a 1:100 solution of vasopressin and sharply excised with a scalpel. Hemostasis is maintained with suture ligatures, and the wound is closed with interrupted 3–0 Vicryl sutures (Figs. 16-5*B* and *C*).

The use of electrosurgery in the vagina is not recommended because the distances between the peritoneum (vault), rectum (posterior wall), and bladder (anterior wall) are small. Because the depth of potential thermal injury to adjacent tissue is difficult to predict, the risk of inadvertent conduction damage outweighs the advantages of electrosurgical hemostasis.

Vascular-appearing lesions in the vagina may be hemangiomas, metastatic choriocarcinoma, or endometrial carcinoma, and biopsy of these lesions could cause severe bleeding. Therefore, biopsy of vascular-appearing vaginal lesions must be performed in an operating room after a blood sample is sent to the blood bank for type and hold (Fig. 16-6). After the surgery is completed, 2–0 to 3–0 Vicryl sutures are placed around the periphery of the lesion for immediate hemostasis.

If cystic lesions are seen within the vagina, sonographic or radiographic examination is performed to determine their origin and contents before biopsy is performed. These lesions may be Gartner's duct cysts, inclusion cysts, enteroceles, or angiomas (Fig. 16-7).

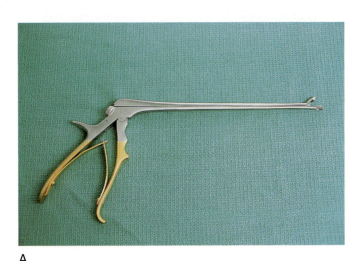

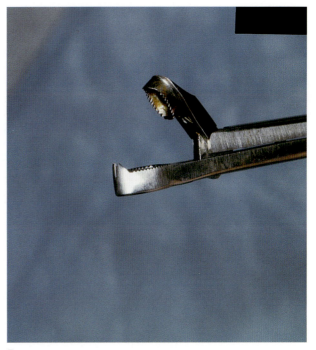

A

B

FIGURE 16-1 **A,** This contemporary biopsy clamp is identical to the instrument used for cervical biopsy. The long, narrow shank is ideal for colposcopically directed vaginal biopsy. **B,** The jaws of the biopsy forceps are sharp and serrated to permit rapid cutting and minimize patient discomfort.

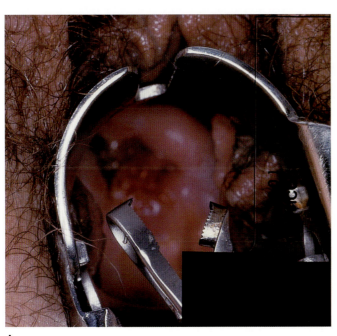

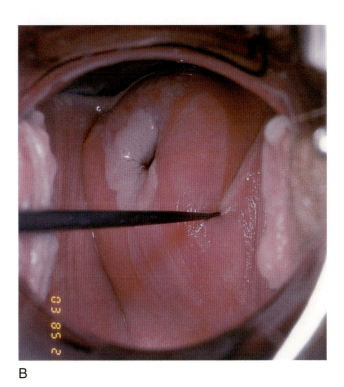

A

B

FIGURE 16-2 **A,** Biopsy is performed under direct colposcopic guidance to improve the accuracy of the procedure. **B,** A hook is used to retract the tissue and expose the biopsy site. (continued)

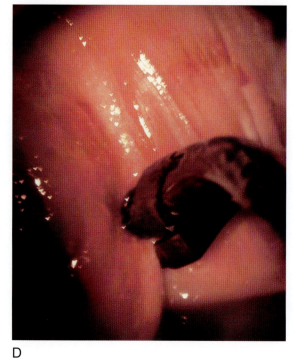

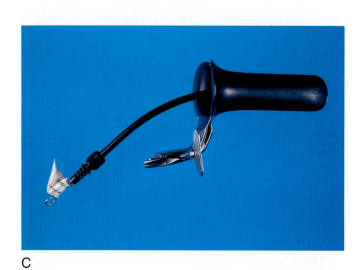

C

D

E

FIGURE 16-2 C, A laser-coated, single-hinged speculum is ideal for biopsy or for any surgical procedure within the vagina. If suturing is required, the open side of the speculum permits the stitch to be cinched down. **D,** The biopsy is performed at low power (×4 to ×6). The operative field is clear as the jaws of the biopsy clamp are closed. **E,** Before the biopsy is performed, a high-power view (×10) may be obtained to ensure that the most severe abnormality is sampled.

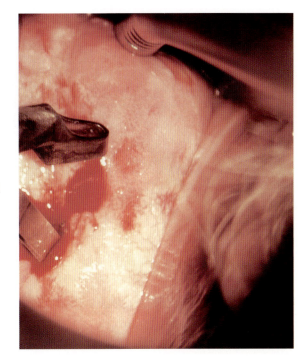

FIGURE 16-3 In an atrophic vagina, the epithelium and stromal wall are thin. Therefore, a superficial biopsy specimen is obtained to avoid injury to adjacent structures.

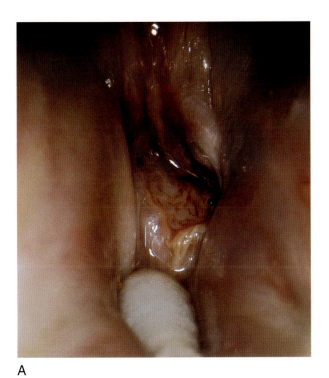

A

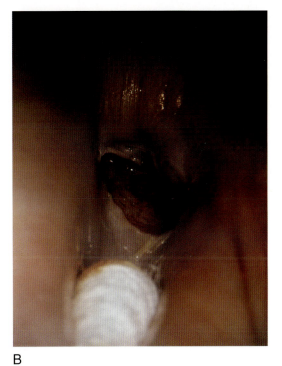

B

FIGURE 16-4 **A,** In this 80-year-old woman with vaginal atrophy, the peritoneum was entered, just above the cotton-tipped applicator, during full-thickness vaginal biopsy. **B,** A magnified view of *A* shows the hazards of overzealous biopsy in a patient who has vaginal atrophy.

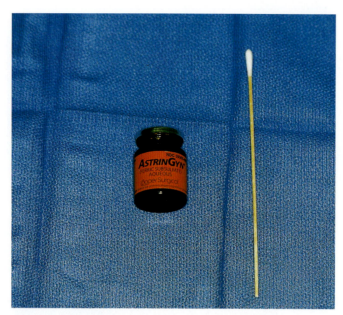

A

FIGURE 16-5 A, After vaginal biopsy is performed, a small amount of Monsel solution is applied to the crater for hemostasis. **B,** Prior to biopsy, 1% Xylocaine with epinephrine or 1:100 vasopressin solution diluted with 1% Xylocaine is injected just beneath the vaginal mucosa. The punch biopsy is then painlessly performed. (continued)

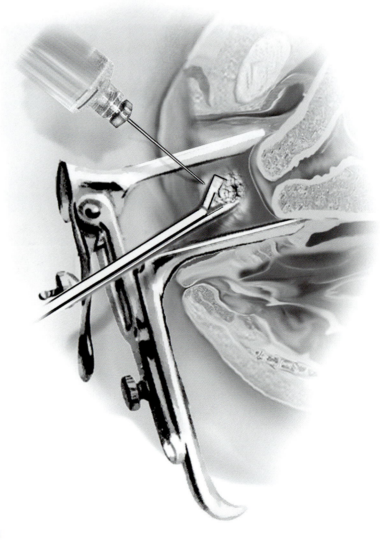

B

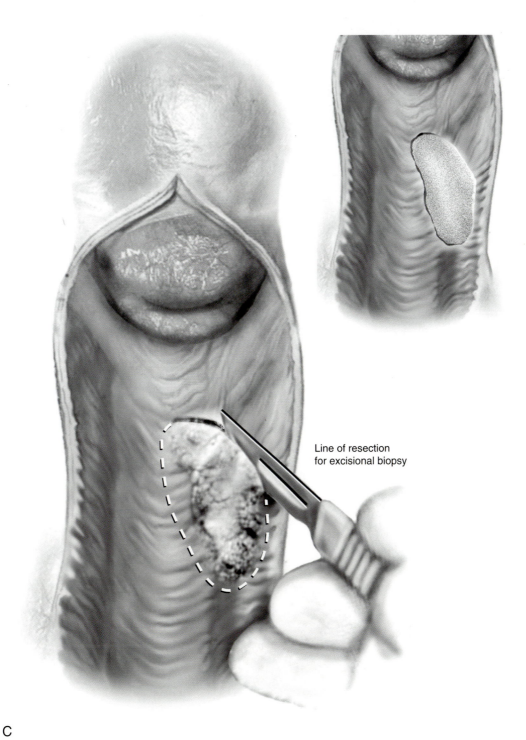

Line of resection
for excisional biopsy

C

FIGURE 16-5 C, When a layer biopsy is required, the vagina is infiltrated with a 1:100 diluted vasopressin solution, which is injected subepithelially in order to balloon the mucosa at the biopsy location. A scalpel is used to excise a portion of the vagina containing the suspicious lesion. The defect is closed with 3-0 vicryl sutures.

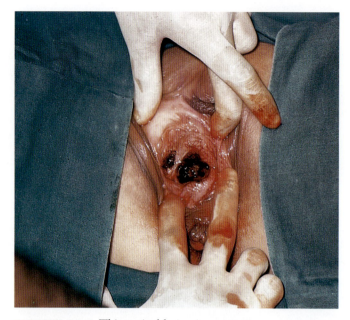

FIGURE 16-6 This vaginal lesion is metastatic choriocarcinoma. When biopsy was performed in an operating room, severe bleeding occurred. Vascular-appearing lesions within the vagina typically are deep red, purple, or blue. Because of the risk of bleeding, biopsy of these lesions should not be performed in the office setting.

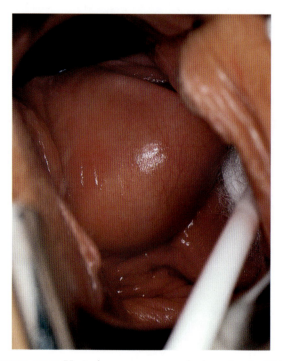

FIGURE 16-7 Vaginal cysts are approached cautiously. This Gartner's duct cyst occupies the anterolateral fornix and is in close proximity to the urinary bladder and right ureter.

CHAPTER 17
Case Examples

Vaginal Intraepithelial Neoplasia

Case 1

A 40-year-old woman who had two pregnancies and two children underwent renal transplant because of polycystic kidney disease. She received standard maintenance immunosuppressive medications. She was treated three times for cervical intraepithelial neoplasia (CIN), but had a recurrence each time (Fig. 17-1).

Case 2

A 48-year-old woman underwent vaginal hysterectomy to treat prolapse and CIN grade 3. An annual Pap smear 6 years after the hysterectomy showed dysplastic squamous cells that suggested VAIN grade 2 (Figs. 17-2*A* and *B*).

Case 3

A 27-year-old nulligravid woman had a Pap smear that showed cells consistent with VAIN grade 1. Examination showed islands of flat, white epithelium on the ectocervix as well as denser, white epithelium in the posterior fornix of the vagina (Fig. 17-3).

Case 4

A 33-year-old woman with five pregnancies, one abortion, and four children underwent a hysterectomy at 30 years of age because of CIN grade 3. A subsequent annual Pap smear showed atypical squamous cells (Fig. 17-4).

Case 5

A 42-year-old woman had five Pap smears that showed atypical squamous cells of undetermined significance over a 2.5-year period. Repeated colposcopic examinations of the cervix showed no colposcopic or histologic

abnormalities. She underwent colposcopy of the cervix and vagina (Fig. 17-5).

Case 6

A 50-year-old woman had a history of vaginal hysterectomy that was performed for unknown reasons. Pap smear showed severe dysplasia and additional changes compatible with human papillomavirus infection (Fig. 17-6).

Case 7

A 35-year-old woman underwent CO_2 laser treatment by a gynecologic oncologist for VAIN grade 2. Within 1 year, Pap smears showed mild to moderate dysplasia. She was treated with sharp excision, laser vaporization, and grafting. For 6 months after surgery, the patient was injected with interferon 1,000,000 units three times per week (Figs. 17-7*A* and *B*).

Case 8

A 36-year-old woman underwent CO_2 laser vaporization for VAIN grade 1 to 2. The lesions persisted (Fig. 17-8).

Case 9

A 43-year-old woman had a Pap smear that showed severely atypical, large, keratinizing squamous cells. Colposcopy and directed biopsy showed carcinoma in situ (Figs. 17-9*A* and *B*).

Case 10

A 25-year-old woman had six pregnancies, the first at 16 years of age. Her first sexual experience occurred at 13 years of age. After she underwent hysterectomy for carcinoma in situ of the cervix, she had vaginal bleeding.

Colposcopic examination and cytologic smears of the vagina were performed (Fig. 17-10).

Case 11

A 24-year-old woman who had prenatal exposure to diethylstilbestrol was diagnosed with adenosis at 20 years of age. She undergoes annual colposcopic examination and cytologic smears of the cervix and vagina. The last smear showed dysplastic squamous cells in the vagina (Figs. 17-11*A* and *B*).

Case 12

A 60-year-old woman who had undergone an abdominal hysterectomy for myomata uteri 12 years earlier had a Pap smear that showed atypical squamous cells of undetermined significance. A Pap smear 3 months later showed the same results. The patient was referred for vaginal colposcopy. In the interim, she was treated with vaginal estrogen cream (estrace or premarin, one full applicator inserted into the vagina daily) (Fig. 17-12).

Case 13

A 62-year-old woman had a history of cervical carcinoma in situ and had undergone vaginal hysterectomy at 48 years of age. She underwent vaginal colposcopy because a recent Pap smear showed dysplasia. The results of previous annual Pap smears had been normal. The vaginal epithelium is smooth, devoid of rugae, and light pink. These findings are characteristic of atrophy. No focal lesions are seen; however, geographic areas in the vault show lightly colored, flat, white epithelium. Superficial biopsy showed VAIN grade 1. The patient was treated with estrogen cream for 1 month. The results of a repeat Pap smear were normal. Results of repeat colposcopy and biopsy 8 weeks later also were normal (Fig. 17-13).

Case 14

A 48-year-old woman underwent loop electrical excision of the cervix for CIN grade 1. Two years later, Pap smear showed atypical squamous cells of undetermined significance. After the patient was treated for bacterial vaginitis, another Pap smear showed dysplasia, and she was referred for colposcopy (Fig. 17-14).

Diethylstilbestrol-Related Abnormalities

Case 15

A 17-year-old patient and her twin sister had prenatal exposure to high doses of diethylstilbestrol during the first and second trimesters. The sisters underwent routine colposcopic examination from the time they were

16 years of age to assess the cervicovaginal abnormalities (Figs. 17-15*A* and *B*).

Case 16

A 19-year-old woman underwent colposcopic examination because her cervix appeared abnormal. The patient's mother received diethylstilbestrol during her first trimester of pregnancy because of threatened abortion. The medication was increased incrementally according to the Smith regimen (Figs. 17-16*A* and *B*).

Case 17

A 21-year-old woman whose mother received an unknown quantity of diethylstilbestrol during pregnancy sought medical advice after reading a newspaper account of cancer associated with diethylstilbestrol administration in pregnancy (Fig. 17-17).

Case 18

A 25-year-old woman was referred for colposcopy because her mother received diethylstilbestrol more than 100 mg daily during the first and early second trimesters of pregnancy (Fig. 17-18).

Case 19

A 30-year-old woman underwent colposcopic examination because of atypical Pap smear findings. The patient's mother had sustained pregnancy losses before successfully carrying the patient to term. Her mother received medication during the pregnancy, but could not recall the type, duration, or dose (Figs. 17-19*A* and *B*).

Case 20

A 17-year-old girl was referred for colposcopy because of prenatal exposure to diethylstilbestrol (Figs. 17-20*A* and *B*).

Case 21

A 21-year-old woman had prenatal exposure to diethylstilbestrol. Results of annual Pap smears were normal. One pregnancy ended in second-trimester loss after a short, painless labor (Figs. 17-21*A* and *B*).

Case 22

A 26-year-old woman who had prenatal exposure to diethylstilbestrol underwent colposcopic screening for adenosis for 6 years. She had a poor obstetric history that included three consecutive abortions. As a result of the history and physical findings, a hysterosalpingogram was performed (Figs. 17-22*A* and *B*).

Case 23

A 23-year-old woman who had prenatal exposure to diethylstilbestrol underwent colposcopic examination because of dyspareunia (Fig. 17-23).

Case 24

A 20-year-old woman was referred for colposcopic examination because a Pap smear showed mildly atypical squamous cells (Fig. 17-24).

Case 25

A 19-year-old woman was referred for evaluation because of prenatal exposure to diethylstilbestrol. Pap smear showed mild to moderately atypical squamous cells (Fig. 17-25).

Vaginal Warts and Papillomas

Case 26

A 27-year-old woman was referred for colposcopy because of "refractory condylomata acuminata." The patient was treated with trichloroacetic acid twice and with podophyllum once. The "warts" that filled the vagina did not regress (Figs. 17-26A and B).

Case 27

A 40-year-old woman underwent colposcopy because of genital warts. Colposcopic examination showed widespread human papillomavirus infection. Warts were seen on the vulva, in the vagina, and within the anus and perianal skin. In addition, cultures showed chlamydia and *Ureaplasma* species (Fig. 17-27).

Case 28

A 31-year-old woman with four pregnancies had persistent vaginal warts. She had a history of smoking cigarettes. She underwent CO_2 laser treatment, but the warts recurred or persisted (Figs. 17-28A and B).

Case 29

A 45-year-old woman with two pregnancies and two children was referred for colposcopic examination because of suspected genital warts. The patient was a nonsmoker and monogamous. Her husband of 20 years admitted visiting a house of prostitution while on a trip to Las Vegas (Fig. 17-29).

Case 30

A 30-year-old woman sought prenatal care in an obstetrics–gynecology clinic after she had a positive result on a pregnancy test. She had a foul-smelling vaginal discharge, and microscopic examination showed bacteria, white blood cells, and clue cells. She also had extensive condylomata acuminata in the vagina (Fig. 17-30).

Case 31

A 51-year-old woman had a 7-month history of irritative vaginal discharge and a question of genital warts (Figs. 17-31A and B).

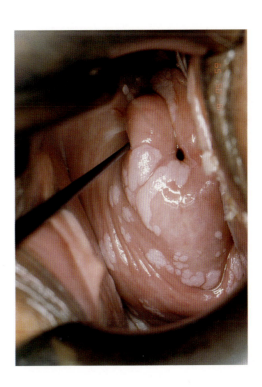

FIGURE 17-1 Colposcopic examination shows multicentric papillomatous foci of dense, white epithelium involving the upper vagina and cervix. Biopsy showed vaginal intraepithelial neoplasia (VAIN) grade 3. The cervix is retracted with a long hook to expose the lateral fornix.

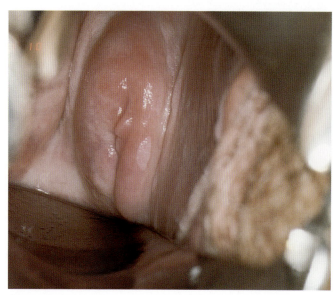

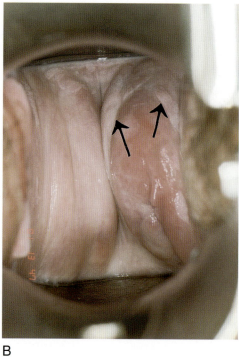

A

B

FIGURE 17-2 **A,** A colposcopic view shows relaxation of the vault and a small enterocele. The white epithelium is moderately dense and has foci with a flat, warty pattern. **B,** A higher-power colposcopic view shows the vault and the upper right wall of the vagina. Flat, white epithelium extends around the base of the prolapsed vault (*arrows*). White epithelium is seen on the upper right wall, and islands of flat, warty epithelium are seen on the right side of the anterolateral wall.

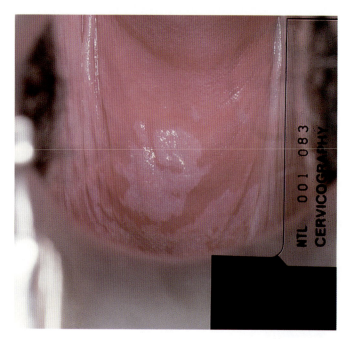

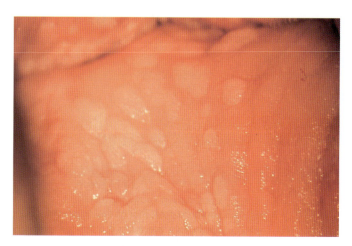

FIGURE 17-3 Many separate, confluent areas of flat, warty, white epithelium fill the posterior vaginal fornix. Multiple punch biopsies showed VAIN grade 2 with extensive koilocytosis.

FIGURE 17-4 A colposcopic view (×10) within the midvagina shows the posterior vaginal wall. The anterior wall (*background, upper left*) is slightly out of focus. Multifocal flat, warty lesions extensively occupy the anterior and posterior vaginal walls. Biopsy confirmed the diagnosis of vaginal carcinoma in situ, or VAIN grade 3.

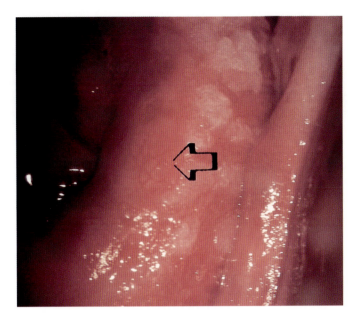

FIGURE 17-5 The left lateral fornix (×10) shows white, warty plaques. The unusual finding of a mosaic vascular pattern is seen (*arrow*). The lesion is compatible with VAIN grade 2 or 3.

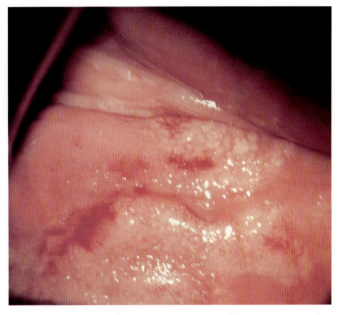

FIGURE 17-6 A colposcopic view (×16) of the upper vaginal wall shows a microvillous pattern of VAIN grade 3. The lower portion of the lesion shows a less conspicuous microvillous pattern compared to the upper part.

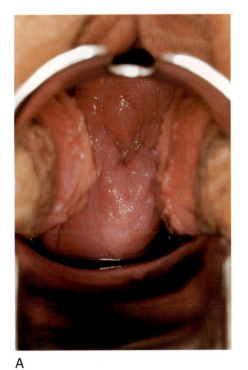

A

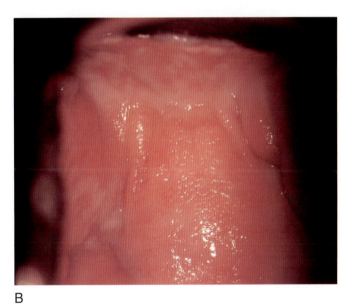

B

FIGURE 17-7 A, The uterus and cervix were removed during previous abdominal hysterectomy. The pebbly epithelium seen in the vaginal vault continues onto the upper posterior wall of the vagina. Slight white shading is seen on the upper posterior wall. **B,** A colposcopic view (×6) shows the pebble-like epithelial pattern. Vaginal biopsy showed VAIN grade 2.

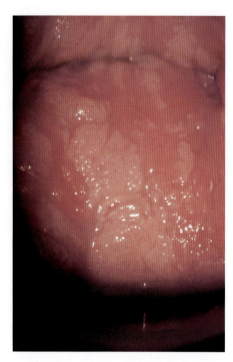

FIGURE 17-8 A colposcopic view (×10) shows extensive multifocal VAIN involving the upper two-thirds of the vagina, including the anterior and posterior walls.

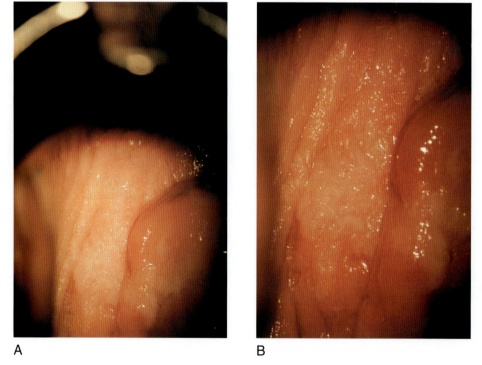

A   B

FIGURE 17-9 **A,** A colposcopic view (×6) shows that most of the vault is occupied by a dense, white lesion that shows considerable relief. The flat, condylomatous pattern is compatible with VAIN. **B,** A magnified colposcopic view (×16) shows the papillomatous relief of a large vault lesion.

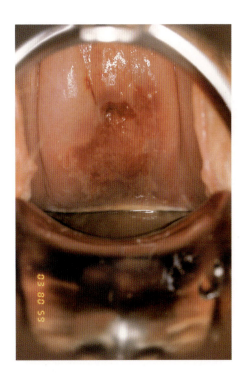

FIGURE 17-10 A scanning colposcopic view (×4) shows a large, red area involving the posterior vault. This ulcerated lesion bled on contact. The periphery of the red zone shows foci of condylomatous, or papillomatous, white epithelium. Biopsy showed a denuded vagina with acute inflammation, but no neoplasia. Multiple biopsies of the white peripheral epithelium showed VAIN grade 1. The patient admitted to masturbation with a sex toy that likely traumatized the vaginal vault.

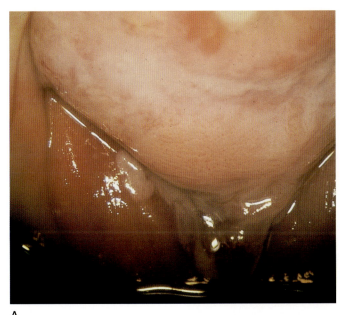

A

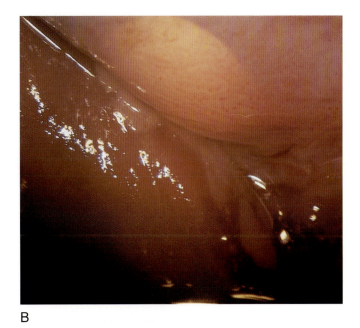

B

FIGURE 17-11 **A,** Red areas of adenosis are seen in the posterior fornix of the vagina. With the application of acetic acid, these areas show the typical grape-like clustering that is seen with endocervical mucosa. White epithelium is seen in the transformation zone between the glandular adenosis and the squamous epithelium of the vagina. Biopsy showed VAIN grade 1. **B,** A high-power view of *A* shows punctation in the ground leukoplakia of the cervicovaginal junction as well as the dense white epithelium at the periphery of the area of red adenosis.

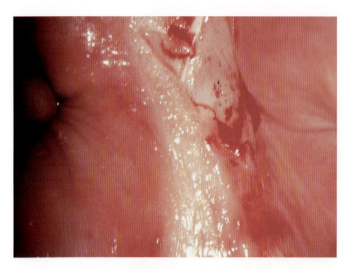

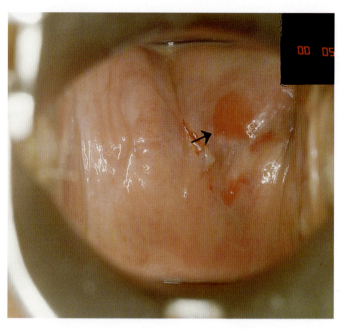

FIGURE 17-12 After the application of 3% acetic acid, colposcopic examination showed dense, white epithelium at the apex of the vagina. This area is in stark contrast to the pink, atrophic surrounding vaginal epithelium. The bleeding is caused by fissures that are created when the brittle tissue is stretched by the speculum. Biopsy of the vault showed VAIN grade 3.

FIGURE 17-13 The vagina is atrophic. Diffuse, lightly colored white epithelium is seen in the vault after the application of 3% acetic acid. The biopsy site is seen (*arrow*). Pathologic examination showed mildly dysplastic squamous epithelium and atrophy.

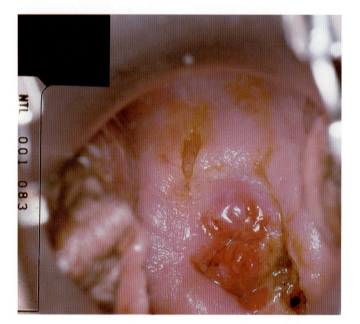

FIGURE 17-14 A colposcopic view (×4) shows a shortened cervix with ectopy. On the anterior ectocervix, extensive flat, warty, densely white epithelium is seen extending into the anterior vaginal fornix. A superficial biopsy specimen was obtained from the anterior vaginal fornix. Bleeding was controlled with Monsel solution. Pathologic examination showed VAIN grade 1.

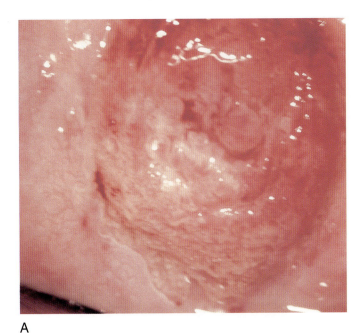
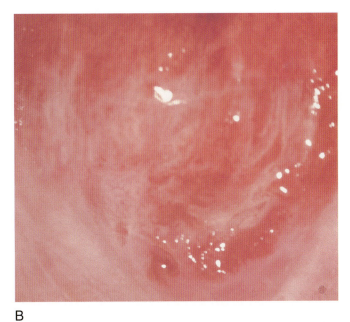

A

B

FIGURE 17-15 **A,** The central area of the cervix is devoid of native squamous epithelium and is covered with mucus-secreting glandular epithelium. The cervicovaginal junction has a thick rim that shows red areas of adenosis and cloudy, white areas of squamous metaplasia. **B,** A high-power colposcopic view of the cervicovaginal transformation zone shows cloudy, white wisps of metaplasia interspersed with glandular epithelium, or adenosis.

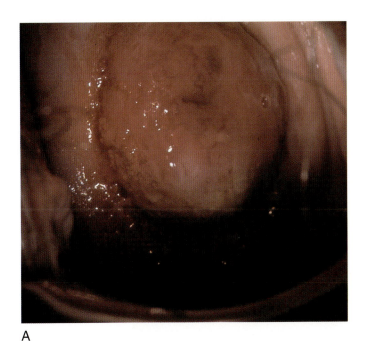
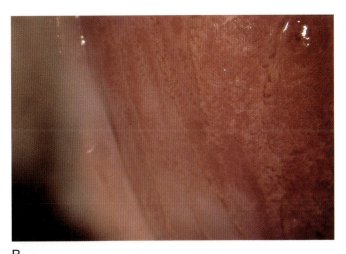

A

B

FIGURE 17-16 **A,** A colposcopic view shows a typical diethylstilbestrol-induced congenital abnormality of the cervix. The cervix is devoid of squamous epithelium, and a hood forms a boundary between the vagina and the cervix. **B,** A magnified view (×16) of the cervicovaginal junction shows extensive adenosis (red areas) and metaplasia (ground leukoplakia, or white background epithelium with punctation).

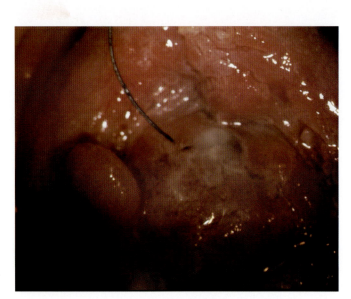

FIGURE 17-17 This nulliparous woman has a severely distorted cervix. The cervicovaginal rim is seen in the background. This patient has an intrauterine contraceptive device. When it was inserted, she was not told about the abnormalities of her cervix and vagina.

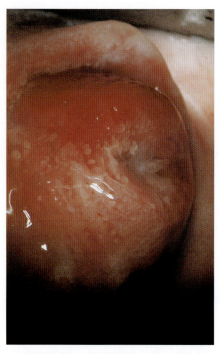

FIGURE 17-18 A classic cock's comb cervical abnormality associated with intrauterine exposure to diethylstilbestrol is seen. Grape-like endocervical mucosa covers the ectocervix.

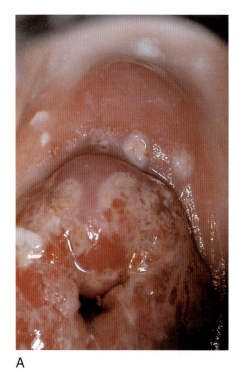

A

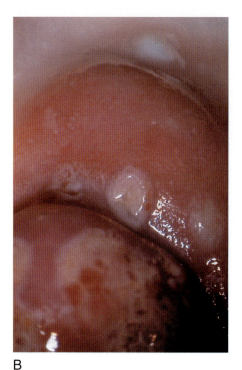

B

FIGURE 17-19 **A,** A colposcopic view shows a typical diethylstilbestrol-associated cervical deformity, with a hood and a cock's comb pattern. White epithelial areas of squamous metaplasia are seen on the cervix and cervicovaginal rim. **B,** A magnified view (×16) of the cervicovaginal hood shows a faint mosaic pattern in the background, above the foci of white epithelium. This pattern is associated with squamous metaplasia. Biopsy at the 12 o'clock position through to the hood showed no dysplasia.

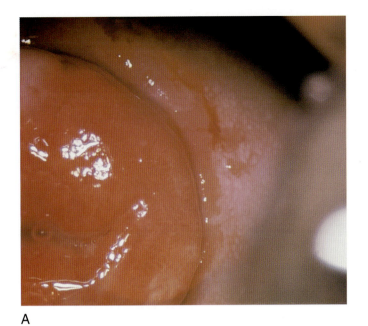
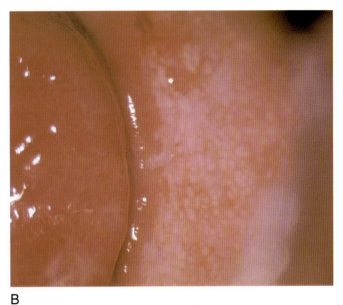

A

B

FIGURE 17-20 **A,** A scanning view (×4) shows a glandular cervix and a basally located rim. With the application of 3% acetic acid, an extensive area of white epithelium is seen from the 3 o'clock position to the 5 o'clock position. **B,** A magnified view (×10) shows a mosaic pattern within the white epithelium. Biopsy showed glandular epithelium and extensive squamous metaplasia.

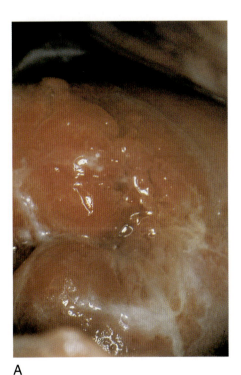
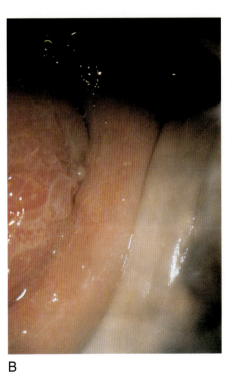

A

B

FIGURE 17-21 **A,** The cervix shows the characteristic composition of glandular epithelium. The cervicovaginal rim is seen in the background. A 27-French Pratt dilator was passed through the cervix into the uterine cavity without resistance, confirming the suspicion of an incompetent cervix. **B,** The vaginal rim shows extensive adenosis (red). A colposcopic view (×6) shows normal vaginal tissue (*far right*).

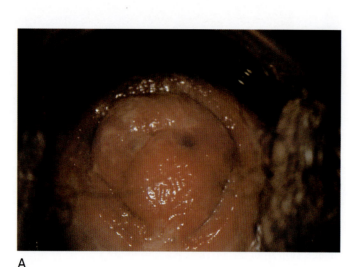

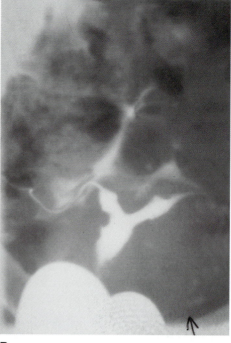

A

B

FIGURE 17-22 A, This cervix has an unusual pattern. The typical basal rim is absent, and the vagina extends upward. Adenosis is seen at the junction of the cervix and the vagina. **B,** A hysterogram of *A* shows the T-shape configuration of the uterus and ballooning at the uterotubal junction.

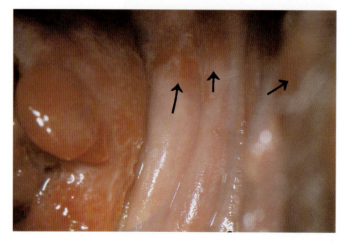

FIGURE 17-23 A colposcopic view shows extensive vaginal adenosis (*arrow*). Reddish adenotic mucosa is seen from the upper to the lower third of the vagina.

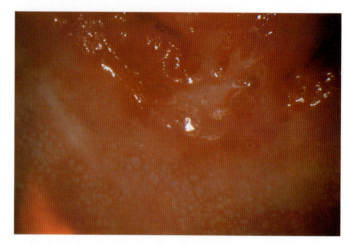

FIGURE 17-24 The cervicovaginal junction shows an extensive mosaic pattern. Biopsy showed mildly atypical metaplastic epithelium.

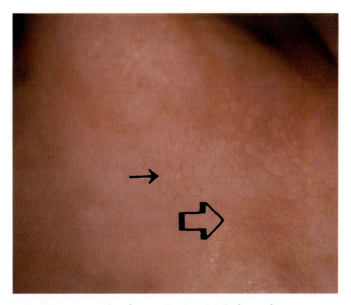

FIGURE 17-25 A colposcopic view (×16) shows the cervicovaginal junction. Extensive white epithelium, consistent with squamous metaplasia, is seen. A mosaic pattern (*arrow*) and a focus of punctation (*open arrow*) are seen. Directed biopsy showed VAIN grade 2.

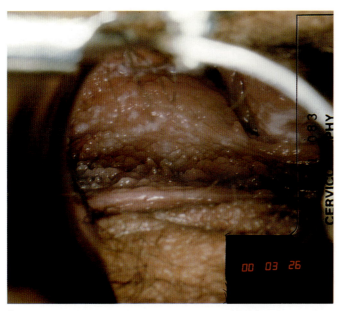

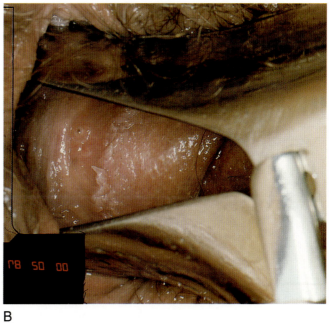

A   B

FIGURE 17-26 A, The speculum is rotated to expose the lower vagina and introitus. Many spicules are seen within the posterior vaginal mucosa and in the vestibule. These are not warts, but a normal variant known as papillosis. **B,** A colposcopic view obtained between the blades of a speculum shows papillosis at the junction of the lower lateral vaginal wall and the vestibule, approximately at the level of the hymenal ring.

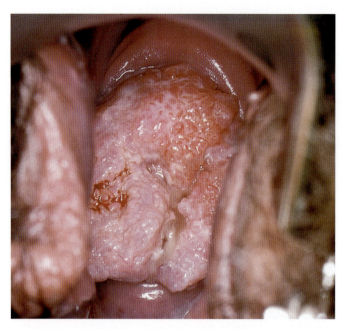

FIGURE 17-27 A colposcopic view shows that the vagina is filled with large clusters of fleshy condylomata acuminata. The lesions are well vascularized and bleed on contact.

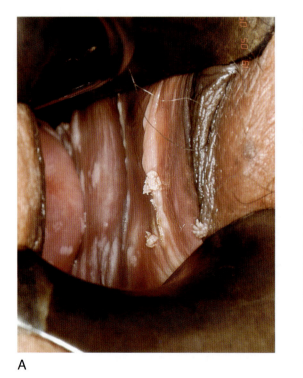

A

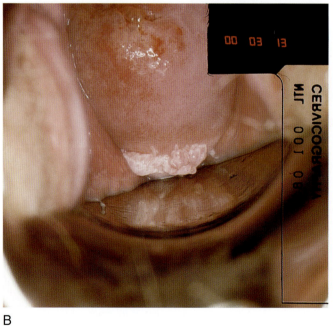

B

FIGURE 17-28 A, A colposcopic view obtained through the blades of a speculum shows scattered warts on the vestibule, vagina, and cervix. **B,** The cervix is elevated to permit an unobstructed view of the posterior vaginal fornix. A cluster of warts is seen.

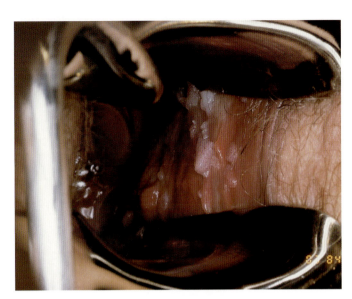

FIGURE 17-29 Colposcopic examination with a single-hinged speculum shows many warts in the lower vagina. The left lateral wall is seen.

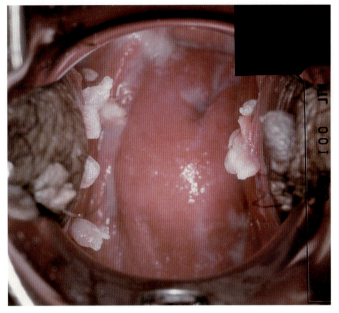

FIGURE 17-30 Colposcopic examination shows extensive vegetative warts on both lateral vaginal walls.

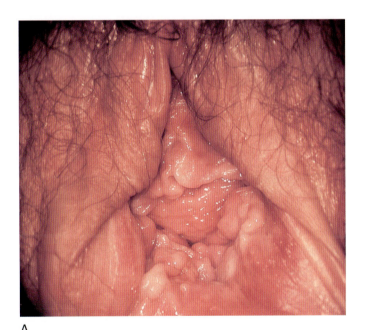

A

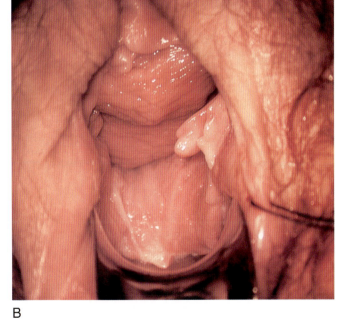

B

FIGURE 17-31 A, The posterior and lateral walls show exaggerated rugal folds that suggest condylomata acuminata. These folds are not warts. **B,** The left lower anterolateral wall shows a protrusion of vaginal mucosa that is not a wart. Biopsy showed a skin tag, or squamous papilloma.

C
Colposcopy of the Vulva

CHAPTER 18
Anatomy and Microanatomy of the Vulva

Gross Anatomy

The vulva consists of the mons veneris (pubic mound); the clitoris, together with its hood and frenulum; the labia majora and surrounding skin; the labia minora; the perineum; and the vestibule. For practical purposes, the perianal skin often is included as well (Figs. 18-1A to C).

The vulvar vestibule consists of the hymenal ring or its remnants; the vaginal opening; the ducts of the Bartholin, Skene, and paraurethral mucous glands; the external urethral meatus; and the surrounding skin (Figs. 18-2A and B).

The vulvar skin is divided into hair-bearing and non–hair-bearing areas. The major hair-bearing areas are the mons veneris, labia majora, perineum, and peripheral perianal skin (Fig. 18-3A). The non–hair-bearing areas include the interlabial sulci, labia minora, vestibule, and clitoris (Fig. 18-3B).

The vulva is the gateway to the vagina. Normally, the labia minora are in contact with each other and partly close off the vaginal opening to the outside environment (Fig. 18-4A). The rounded contour of the labia majora, in concert with the buttocks and mons veneris, lends symmetry to the lower trunk that clearly has teleologic purposes. Occasionally, accessory nipples are seen distal to the posterior and lateral aspects of the labia majora. These are remnants of the embryonic milk line (Figs. 18-4B and C).

The principal mucous glands of the vestibule are the Bartholin and paraurethral mucous glands (see Fig. 18-2B). These glands secrete mucus and provide lubrication during coital entry into the vagina. The glans clitoris, clitoral body, corpora cavernosum clitoris, and vestibular bulb consist of cavernous tissue. During sexual stimulation, these structures fill with blood and become erect (see Figs. 18-1B, 18-2B, and 18-3B).

The portion of the vestibule that is located below the hymenal ring and between the point of posterior labial fusion (posterior fourchette) is the fossa navicularis (see Fig. 18-1B). Because this area is a natural reservoir for vaginal and vulvar secretions, it is a common site of pathology. The boundary between the vestibule and the medial aspect of the labia minora is marked by an irregular line called Hart's line (Fig. 18-4D).

If the vulvar skin is stripped away, fat is exposed (Figs. 18-5A to C). Other than the tissue of the clitoris and labia minora, fat is the principal component of the vulva. The labia majora are 98% fat. Below the fat is the white, condensed layer of Colles' fascia. This layer overlies the thin muscles of the urogenital diaphragm that are located medial to the pubic and ischial rami (Fig. 18-5D). If the vestibular skin is incised peripheral to the hymenal ring, slightly lateral to the orifice of the Bartholin duct, and through Colles' fascia, a space is created along the adventitial border of the inner aspect of the vagina (Fig. 18-6A). This area is easily dissected to a depth of 2 to 3 cm (Figs. 18-6B and C). Next, Colles' fascia is incised linearly, 1.5 to 2.0 cm lateral to the previously created fossa. The fascia is stripped from the isolated block of tissue to expose the bulbocavernosus muscle (Fig. 18-6D). At the level of the Bartholin duct, the multilobed Bartholin gland clings to the undersurface of the bulbocavernosus muscle (Figs. 18-7A and B). The bulb of the vestibule is located above and deep to these structures (Fig. 18-8). The lowest portion of the bulbocavernosus leads the dissector to the medial portion of the transverse perineal muscle.

Closely applied to the pubic ramus is the thin ischiocavernosus muscle (Fig. 18-9A). Beneath the muscle is the large, bluish crus, or corpora cavernosum, of the clitoris (Fig. 18-9B). Between the cavernous structures is a well-developed fascial membrane known as the inferior fascia of the pelvic diaphragm (Fig. 18-9C). Incision through this perineal membrane shows a thin layer of fat and the levator ani muscle (Figs. 18-9D and E).

The anal sphincter occupies the area beneath the fat and fascia of the perineum (Fig. 18-9F). The anal sphincter is easily seen by inserting a gloved fifth finger into the anus and asking the patient to squeeze and release the muscles. The sphincter extends upward to the distal rectovaginal septum (Figs. 18-10*A* and *B*).

Microanatomy

The vulvar skin is similar to skin found elsewhere on the body. The skin has the following layers: epidermis, papillary dermis, reticular dermis, and fat (Figs. 18-11*A* to *C*).

The epidermis consists of multilayered squamous epithelium arranged in organized strata (Fig. 18-12*A*). As in the cervix and vagina, the deepest layer is the basal cell layer, which abuts the underlying dermal connective tissue. The basal cell layer consists of cuboidal cells that have large, regular nuclei. The basal cells lie on a basement membrane that easily is seen with periodic acid-Schiff stain. The basement membrane stains a characteristic magenta color. The next level has five or more layers of cells and is called variously the stratum spinosum, stratum germinativum, or prickle cell layer. These cells are larger than the basal cells and are connected by intercellular bridges, or spines. The third layer has one or two layers of clear cells that have smaller nuclei. Unlike the corresponding area in the cervix and vagina, the fourth layer contains pre-eleidin. As the mature squamous cells flatten, coarse granules (eleidin) are seen within the cytoplasm. This layer is appropriately called the granular cell layer. At the top of the epithelial layers is a pinkish layer of anucleate keratin, or stratum corneum. The epidermis also contains melanocytes and Langerhans' cells (Fig. 18-12*B*).

Epidermal fingers of cells that project into the dermis are known as rete pegs. Between the rete pegs are dermal papillae that project into the epidermis and carry blood vessels and lymphatics (Fig. 18-13*A*). The thin layer of dermis, or connective tissue, beneath the epidermis is known as the papillary dermis. Within this layer are found the reserve cells. The rest of the deeper, more plentiful dermis is known as reticular dermis (Fig. 18-13*B*). Within the dermis are several skin appendages that include sebaceous glands, sweat glands (eccrine), and specialized sweat glands (apocrine) (Figs. 18-14*A* to *G*). Hair shafts and follicles are seen in hair-bearing areas (Figs. 18-14*H* and *I*). Sections obtained through the labia minora show primarily sebaceous glands and no hair follicles or shafts (Figs. 18-15*A* to *C*). The appendages may reach as deep as 3.5 to 4.0 mm below the surface and may continue into the subcutaneous fat. The mean thickness of normal epidermis is 0.31 mm. The mean depth of papillary dermis is 0.15 mm. The mean depth of reticular dermis is 2.0 mm. The mean depth of skin appendages is 1.63 mm. The full thickness of normal skin is 3.0 to 5.0 mm. The skin of hair-bearing areas is thicker than that of non–hair-bearing regions. For example, the skin of the labium minus is barely 1 mm thick (see Fig. 18-15*D*).

Gland ducts are seen within the vulvar vestibule. The largest of these are the Bartholin gland ducts, which are lined by transitional epithelium (Fig. 18-16*A*). As the duct nears the actual gland, columnar mucous cells are seen with the duct epithelium (Fig. 18-16*B*). The gland is a true racemose mucous gland that has lobules of columnar cells that are organized into a tight glandular structure (Figs. 18-16*C* and *D*). Minor vestibular glands are characterized by gland acini that are lined with mucus-secreting columnar epithelium and scattered throughout the vestibule.

The clitoris has a thin covering of stratified squamous epithelium. Beneath this covering are large, cavernous spaces that contain red blood cells and are lined by elastic tissue, collagen, and smooth muscle.

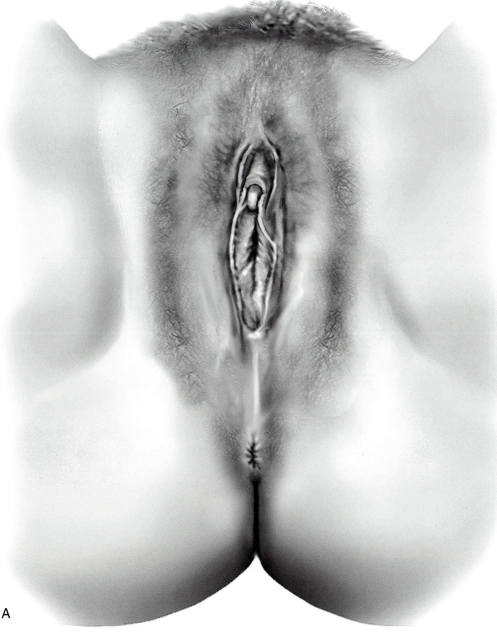

A

FIGURE 18-1 **A,** A normal vulva. The junction between the abdomen and the vulva is marked by a collection of subcutaneous fat that produces a mound of hair-bearing tissue, the mons veneris. The rounded contour of the hair-bearing labia majora is another landmark, as are the perineum and anal orifice. (continued)

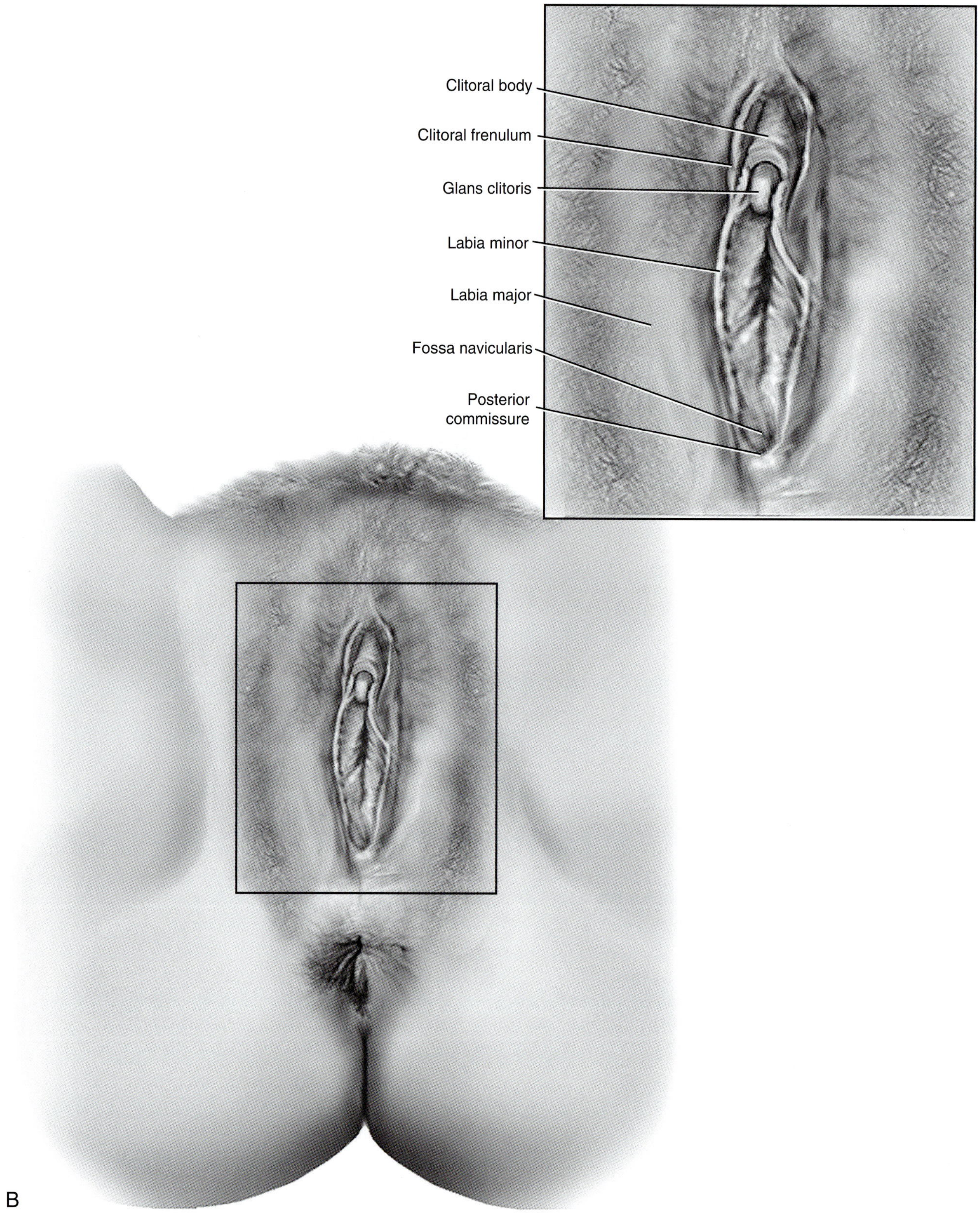

Clitoral body

Clitoral frenulum

Glans clitoris

Labia minor

Labia major

Fossa navicularis

Posterior
commissure

B

FIGURE 18-1 B, The labia majora, labia minora, and clitoral apparatus are seen (*inset*). Lesions in the vagina usually cause secondary abnormalities on the medial aspects of the labia minora, the vestibule, and particularly, the fossa navicularis. Because lesions also occur in natural recesses, such as the interlabial sulci and clitoral hood, all of these areas must be viewed during colposcopic examination. (continued)

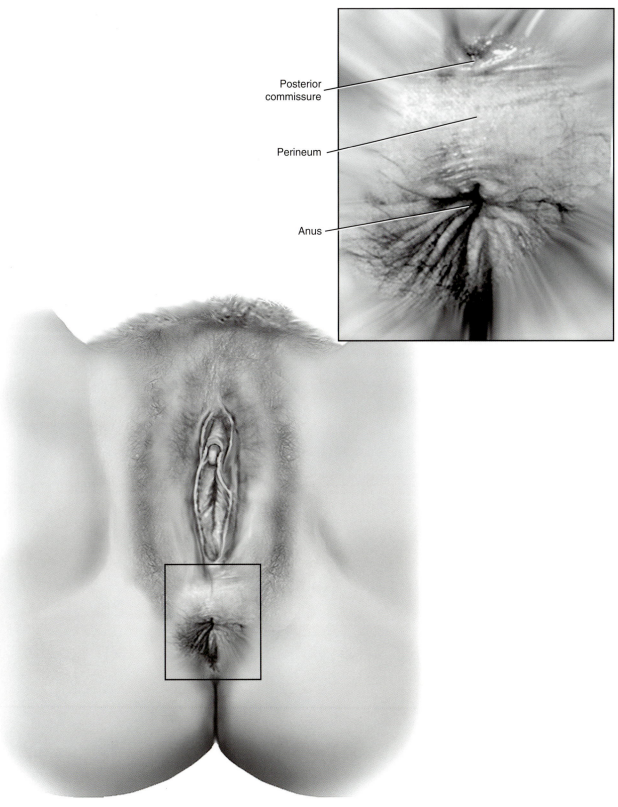

C

FIGURE 18-1 C, As seen in *C*, vaginal and cervical fluid, mucus, and cellular debris flow into the vestibule and spill onto the perineum and perianal skin. Further, fecal material travels upward from the anus, from the perianal skin to the perineum, and from the vestibule into the vagina.

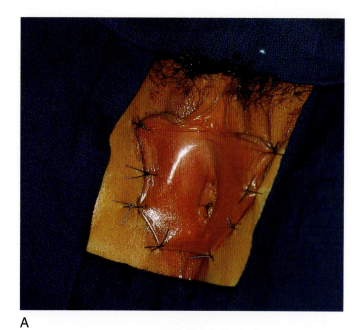

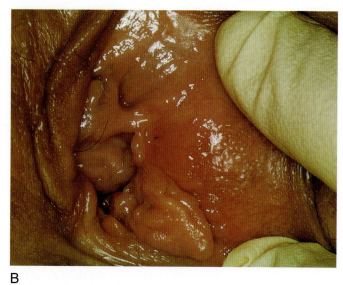

A

B

FIGURE 18-2 A, The labia are sutured to the skin of the medial thigh, widely exposing the vulvar vestibule. The boundaries of the vestibule are: anteriorly, the clitoris; laterally, the inner, or medial, aspects of the labia minora; and posteriorly, the fossa navicularis and posterior commissure. **B,** The urethra, vagina, Skene ducts, paraurethral ducts, and Bartholin gland duct (small hole lateral to hymenal ring) open into the vestibule.

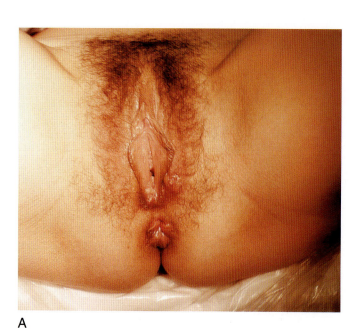

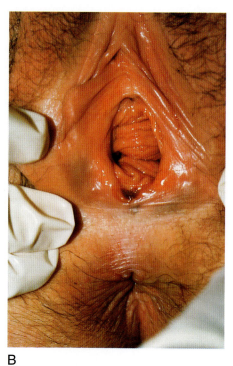

A

B

FIGURE 18-3 A, Hair-bearing areas of the vulva include the mons veneris, labia majora, perineum, and perianal skin. **B,** Non–hair-bearing areas include the labia minora, interlabial sulci, and vestibule.

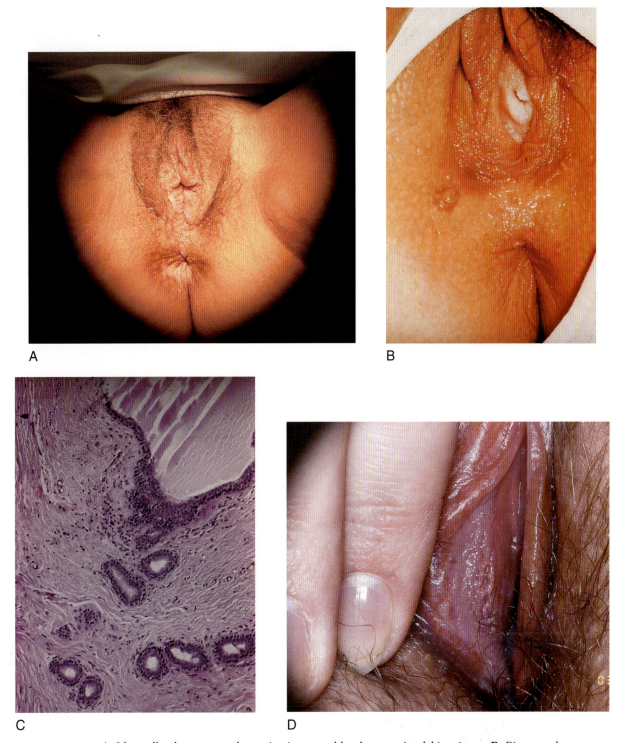

FIGURE 18-4 A, Normally, the entry to the vagina is covered by the opposing labia minora. **B,** Pigmented papillary tissue may be seen on the skin between the thigh and the vulva. This tissue is a remnant of the embryonic milk line. **C,** Biopsy of the structure seen in *B* shows that it is an accessory nipple. This tissue contains the typical apocrine glands and duct that are seen in the mammary gland tissue that normally is located on the ventral wall of the chest. **D,** A sharp, irregular line is seen on the medial aspect of the labium minus. The dentate line, or Hart's line, forms the boundary between the labium minus and the vestibule.

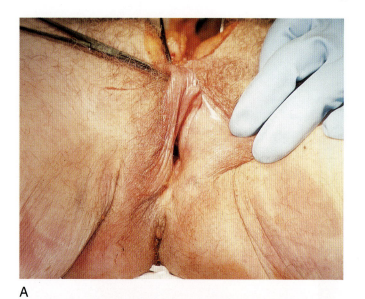

A

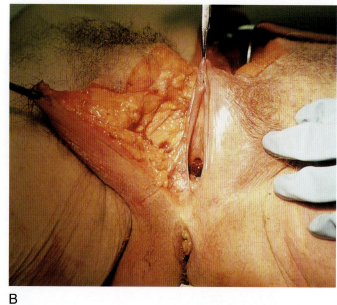

B

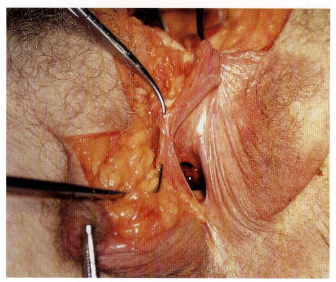

C

FIGURE 18-5 A, The vulva of a fresh cadaver is exposed. The clamp points to the area where a flap will be created on the right labium majus. **B,** The vulvar flap is cut beneath the skin of the labium majus. Fat comprises 98% of the underlying structural support. **C,** At the medial aspect of the labium minus and immediately lateral to the hymenal ring, dissection is performed to identify deeper structures. (continued)

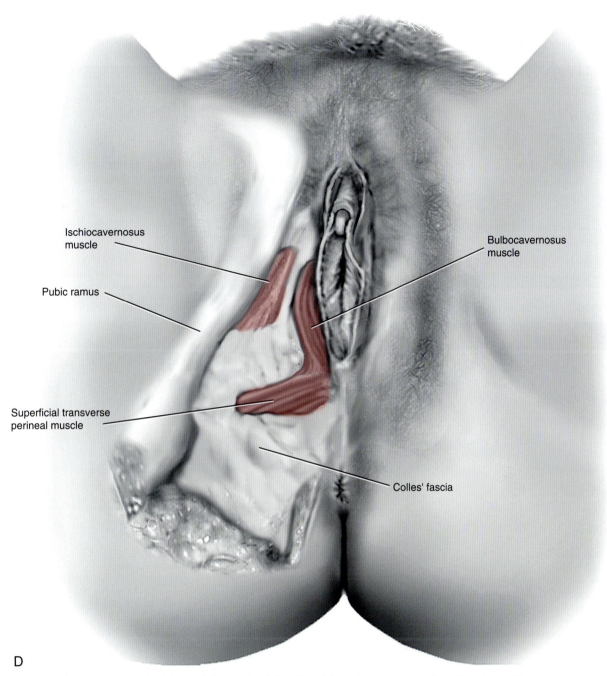

Ischiocavernosus
muscle

Pubic ramus

Bulbocavernosus
muscle

Superficial transverse
perineal muscle

Colles' fascia

D

FIGURE 18-5 D, After the labia and fat on the right side of the vulva are removed, a glistening, white membrane is seen (Colles' fascia). Beneath Colles' fascia, three superficial muscles are seen: the bulbocavernosus muscle, transverse perineal muscle, and ischiocavernosus muscle.

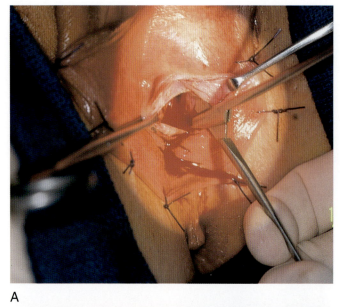

A

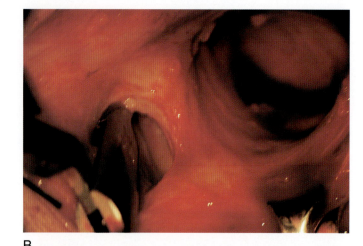

B

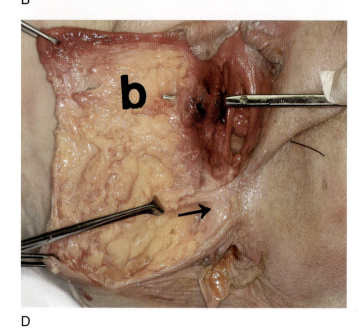

C

D

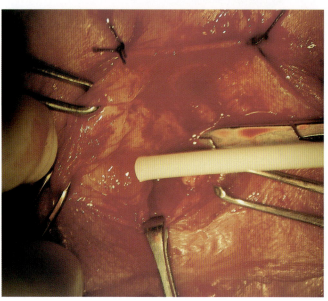

E

FIGURE 18-6 A, A fossa is created parallel to the adventitial, or lateral, wall of the vagina by incising Colles' fascia and dissecting the tissue medial to the bulbocavernosus muscle. Blood flows from the cavernous vessels of the bulb and vagina. **B,** Two fossae are dissected on each side of the bulbocavernosus muscle. **C,** A mosquito clamp is placed in the medial fossa and shows the depth of the space relative to the lateral wall of the vagina as well as the bulge produced by the tip of the clamp. **D,** In a fresh cadaver dissection, the reddish bulbocavernosus muscle (b) is seen stretched by the underlying scissors. Note its position relative to the vagina. **E,** Operative dissection showing the bulbocavernosus muscle partially exposed by opening colles fascia. The tip of the cardboard swab points to the red muscle. The mosquito clamp beneath the swab has opened into the fossa just lateral to the hymenal ring. The arrow points to the vaginal interiors.

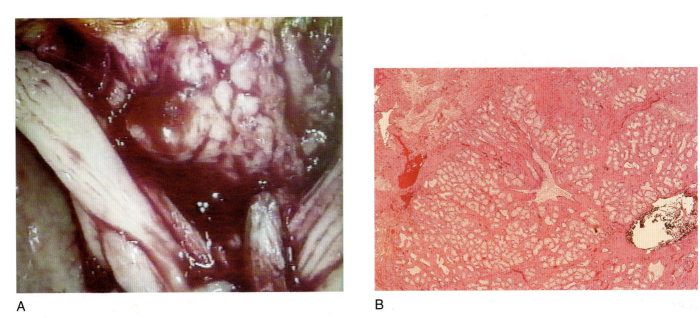

A   B

FIGURE 18-7 **A,** In a living patient, the undersurface of the bulbocavernosus muscle is exposed to show the lobular detail of the Bartholin gland. **B,** Histologic examination of the tissue shown in *A* shows the racemose lobes that contain the mucous acini that comprise the greater vestibular gland, or Bartholin gland.

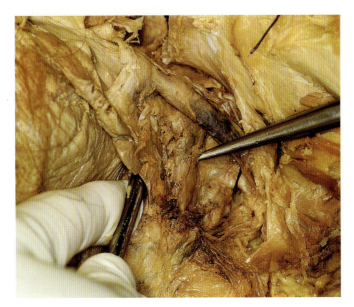

FIGURE 18-8 In a fixed cadaver dissection, the superficial perineal muscles and Colles' fascia are removed. The bulb of the vestibule is identified by the tip of the scissors.

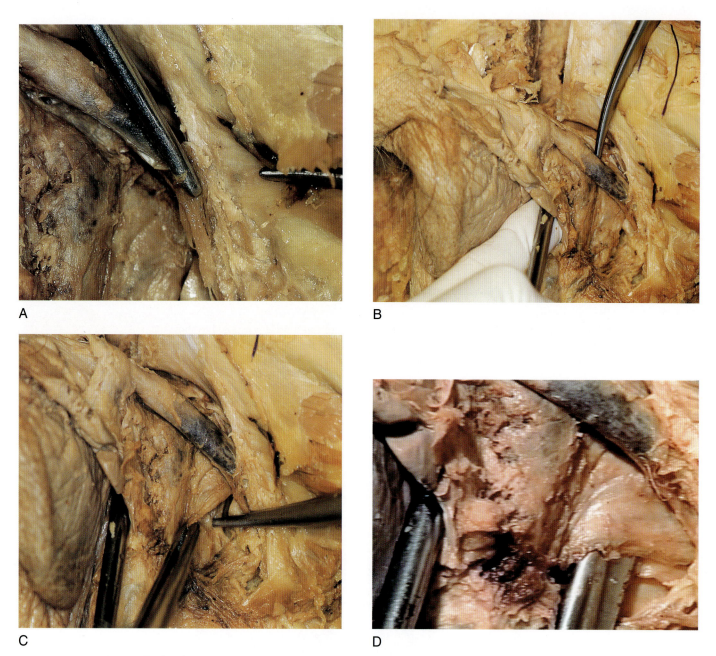

A

B

C

D

FIGURE 18-9 **A,** In a fixed cadaver dissection, a Kocher clamp is used to grasp the remnant of the ischiocavernosus muscle that clings to the ischial ramus. **B,** In a fixed cadaver dissection, the scissors point to a prominent slate blue structure, the corpus cavernosum clitoris. **C,** In a fixed cadaver dissection, the scissors cut the deep fascia between the corpus cavernosum clitoris and the bulb of the vestibule and rest on the levator ani muscle. The body of the clitoris and its juncture with the left clitoral crus are seen. A metal cannula has been placed in the vagina. **D,** In a fixed cadaver dissection, a magnified view shows the fascia overlying the levator ani muscle. (continued)

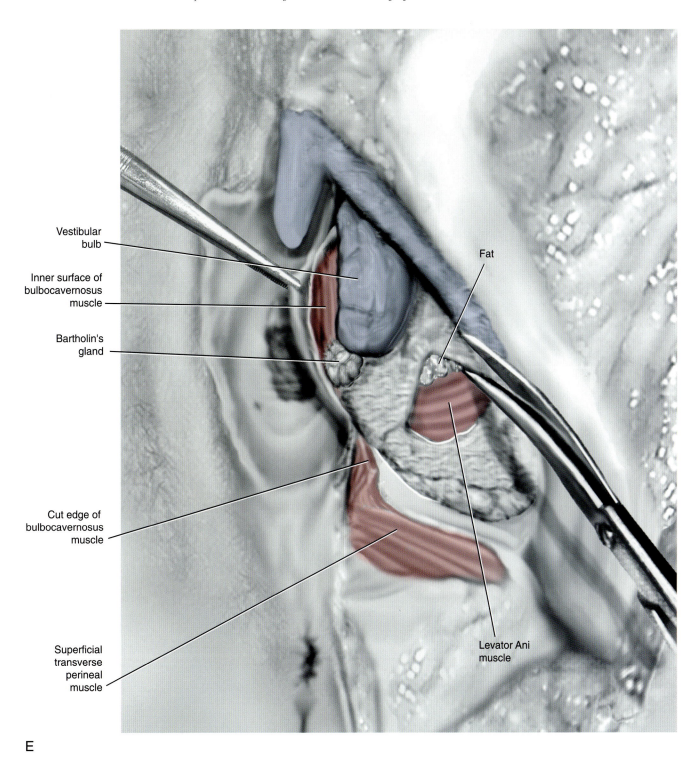

Vestibular bulb

Inner surface of bulbocavernosus muscle

Bartholin's gland

Fat

Cut edge of bulbocavernosus muscle

Levator Ani muscle

Superficial transverse perineal muscle

E

FIGURE 18-9 **E,** The scissors point to the levator ani muscle that is emerging from beneath the pubic ramus. (continued)

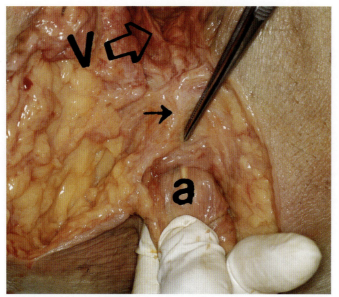

F

FIGURE 18-9 F, Fresh cadaver dissection shows detail of the external sphincter ani. The author's finger is inserted into the anal canal and the external (outer) wall of the anus (a) is exposed. The arrow and the forceps point to the sphincter ani muscle. The open arrow points to the vagina (v).

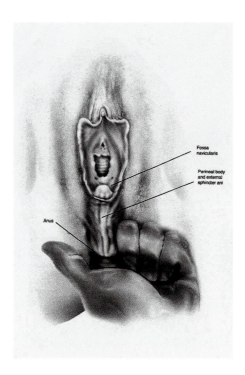

A

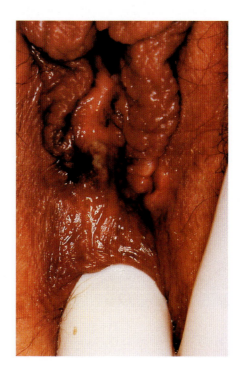

B

FIGURE 18-10 A, The course of the rectum relative to the perineum and the posterior wall of the vagina. **B,** In a live patient, a gloved finger is inserted into the rectum. Beneath the perineal skin, fat, and fascia lies the wide anterior portion of the anal sphincter. The sphincter is located directly in the course of a potential midline episiotomy.

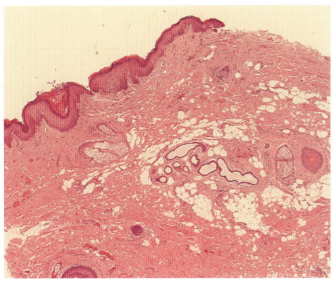

A

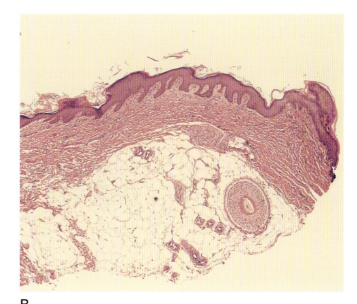

B

FIGURE 18-11 A, A scanning photomicrograph (×2) of a section of normal vulvar skin shows the thin, stratified squamous epithelium that overlies the dermal connective tissue. Skin appendages are seen within the reticular dermis. **B,** A scanning photomicrograph (×2) of a full-thickness section of vulvar skin shows the epidermis, papillary dermis, reticular dermis, and fat. A cross-section of a hair shaft is seen within the fat layer. **C,** A photomicrograph (×4) of the upper portion of vulvar skin shows the epidermis. A rete peg extends into the papillary dermis. On each side are the papillae that reach into the epidermis (*far right*). The papillae are derived from papillary dermis.

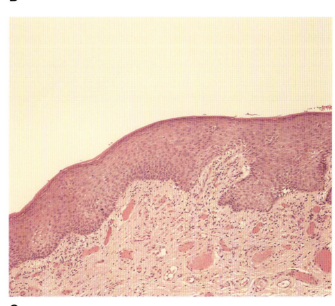

C

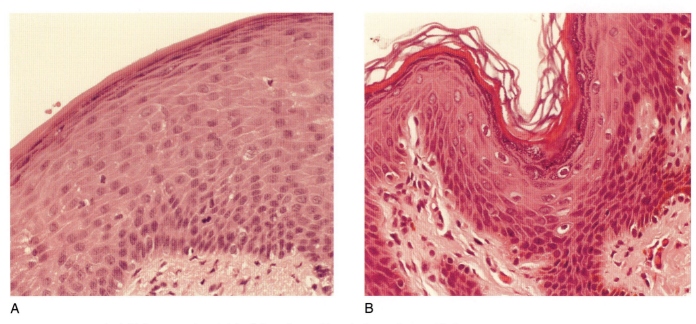

A

B

FIGURE 18-12 **A,** A high-power view (×16) of the vulvar epidermis shows the stratified squamous epithelium, which consists of more than 20 layers of cells. Just above the dermis is a single layer of basal cells. The prickle cells, or intercellular bridges, extend upward for several layers. As these cells mature toward the surface, they gain cytoplasm. The three uppermost layers of cells contain dark, keratohyaline granules, or stratum granulosum. These granules contribute to the uppermost keratinized, or hyalinized, acellular layer. **B,** The basal cell layer (×10) shows a brownish pigmented layer of melanocytes. The rete pegs of the epidermis and the dermal papillae are seen as well.

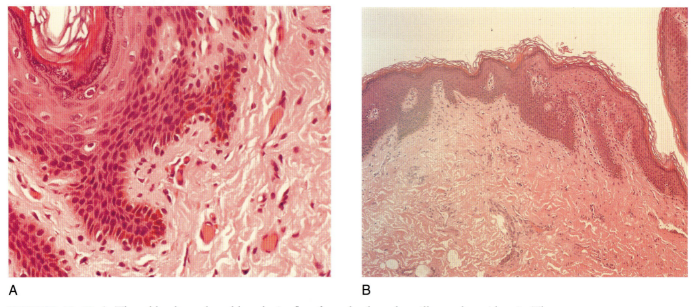

A

B

FIGURE 18-13 **A,** These blood vessels and lymphatics flow from the dermal papillae to the epidermis. The granular and keratin layers also are seen (×10). **B,** This section (×4) shows the papillary dermis immediately underlying the epidermis and the reticular dermis beneath the papillary dermis.

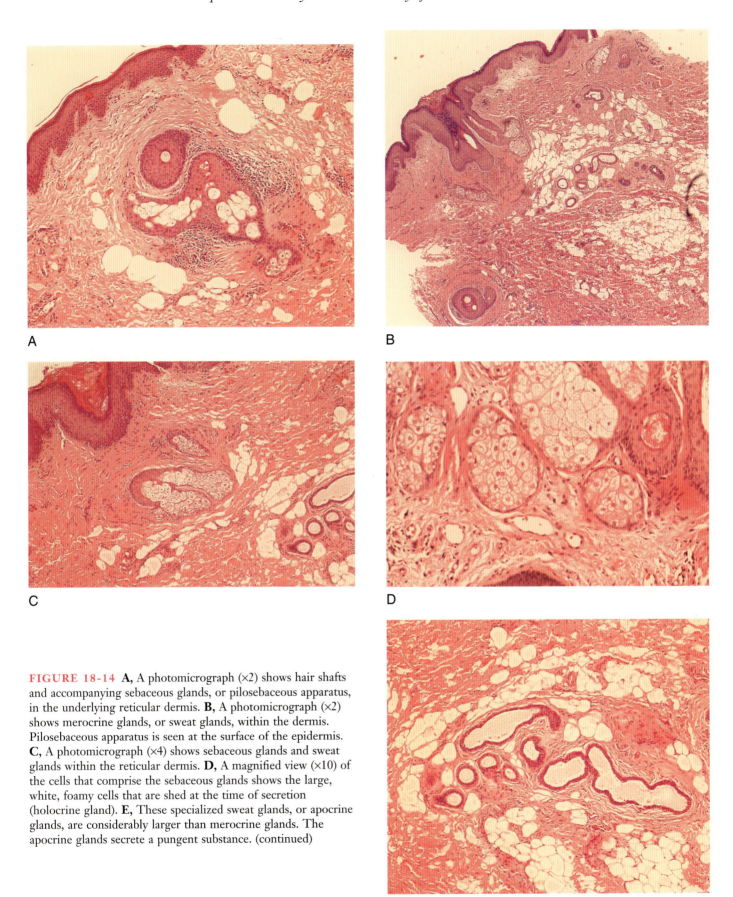

A

B

C

D

E

FIGURE 18-14 **A,** A photomicrograph (×2) shows hair shafts and accompanying sebaceous glands, or pilosebaceous apparatus, in the underlying reticular dermis. **B,** A photomicrograph (×2) shows merocrine glands, or sweat glands, within the dermis. Pilosebaceous apparatus is seen at the surface of the epidermis. **C,** A photomicrograph (×4) shows sebaceous glands and sweat glands within the reticular dermis. **D,** A magnified view (×10) of the cells that comprise the sebaceous glands shows the large, white, foamy cells that are shed at the time of secretion (holocrine gland). **E,** These specialized sweat glands, or apocrine glands, are considerably larger than merocrine glands. The apocrine glands secrete a pungent substance. (continued)

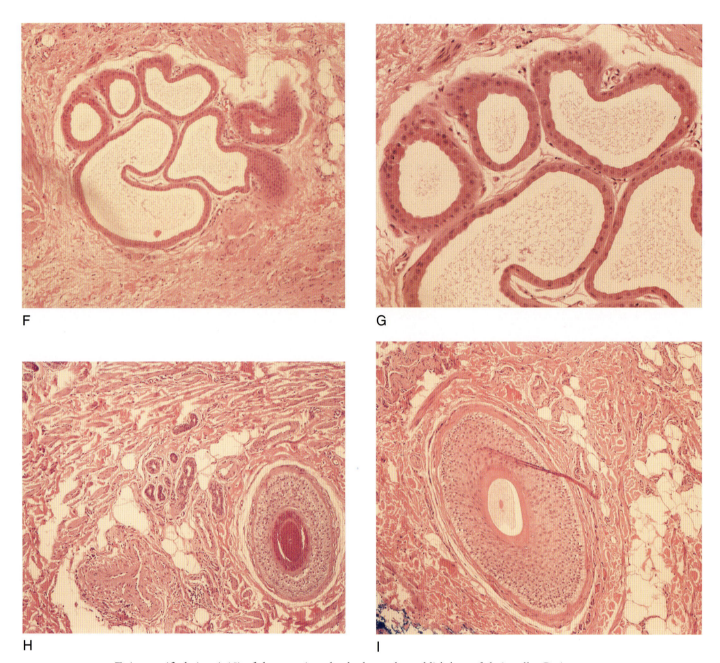

F

G

H

I

FIGURE 18-14 **F,** A magnified view (×10) of the apocrine glands shows the reddish hue of their cells. **G,** A photomicrograph (×16) of apocrine sweat glands. The largest apocrine glands in the human body are the paired mammary glands. **H,** A hair shaft is seen deep in the reticular dermis. **I,** A high-power view of a vulvar hair follicle shows concentric stratification of the cells. The stratified squamous epithelium is analogous to that of the epidermis.

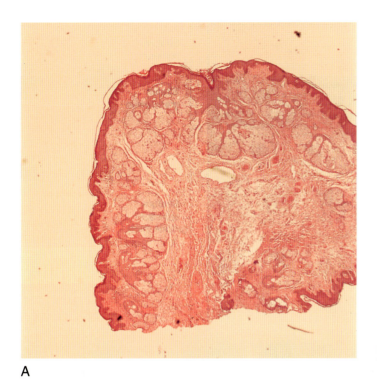

A

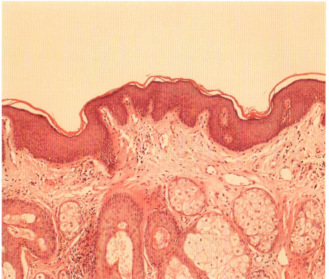

B

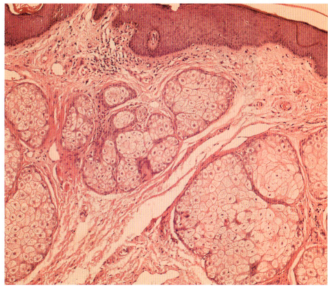

C

FIGURE 18-15 A, A section of the labium minus shows the epidermis and the underlying appendages of glandular configuration. **B,** A magnified view (×4) shows no hair follicles in the labium minus. **C,** Plentiful sebaceous glands occupy the underlying dermis of the labium minus. The epidermis is less than 1 mm thick. (continued)

Contact dermatitis is associated with chemical, drug, or cosmetic exposure and causes itching, irritation, and erythema. Nonspecific erythema responds to withdrawal of the noxious agent (Figs. 19-9F and 19-9G).

Lichenification Disorders

The most common lichen disorder of the vulva is lichen sclerosus, formerly known as lichen sclerosus et atrophicus. Although its cause is unknown, patients have intense pruritus that usually is most severe at night. The disease causes stromal inflammation as shown by the inevitable agglutination of the vulvar components (Fig. 19-10A). The labia minora may be virtually glued to the labia majora (Fig. 19-10B). The clitoral frenulum usually is obliterated, and the clitoral hood adheres to the glans of the clitoris (Fig. 19-10C). Scanning colposcopy shows unusual pallor of the vulva, particularly around the clitoris and at the interlabial sulci (Figs. 19-10D and E). The perineum, posterior fourchette, and perianal skin also may be involved. The affected skin is thickened and lacks elasticity (Fig. 19-10F). When skin stretch is critical to function, the affected skin splits, creating painful fissures. The natural course of disease leads to severe shrinkage of the vulva and sealing up of the vaginal introitus (Fig. 19-10G). The perineum is white and wrinkled as a result of dermal scarring (Fig. 19-10H). This change, known as cigarette paper skin, is seen under colposcopic examination (×10) (see Fig. 19-10B). Clitoral scar formation causes clitoral phymosis (see Fig. 19-10C).

Microscopically, the changes caused by lichen sclerosus are conclusive. The papillary dermis is completely collagenized, or scarred. The epidermis is thin, with five or six layers of cells. The basal layer is fractured: the line of basal cells is broken up and distorted. Hyperkeratosis is seen in some areas, whereas in others, little or no keratin is observed (Fig. 19-10I).

Erosive lichen planus causes significant pain and disability (Fig. 19-11A). The vestibule and entire vagina may be denuded of the epidermal layer, and as a result, the underlying dermis, with its nerves and blood vessels, may be exposed (Fig. 19-11B). Colposcopic examination may show attempts by a thin layer of metaplastic squamous epithelium to form the exposed stromal bed (Fig. 19-11C). The stroma is acutely inflamed. The reticular support structures are damaged, and the framework for repair is lost. Because this condition is so painful, nothing can be placed into the vagina without eliciting a digital pain score of 10/10. The cause of this disorder is not known, but like lichen sclerosus, it has characteristics of an autoimmune disorder. Similar spotty lesions may be seen in the mouth, particularly on the buccal mucosa.

Microscopically, ulceration, or erosion, and acute stromal infiltration of inflammatory cells are seen (Figs. 19-11D and E). Reticulum stain shows defective reticulum formation.

Lichen simplex chronicus is the antithesis of lichen sclerosus. Rather than atrophy, chronic inflammation and extensive thick, white areas of hyperkeratosis are seen (Figs. 19-12A and B). The vulvar skin is thickened, but not as a result of dermal scar formation.

Lichen simplex chronicus is characterized by intense pruritus. Scratching causes secondary bacterial infection. Microscopically, thick layers of keratin dominate the section and degrees of acanthosis are seen. Areas of thickened, hyperkeratic skin are interspersed with normal-appearing skin.

Hyperplastic Vulvitis

Hyperplasia may be typical or atypical. Typical hyperplasia has many of the same features as chronic lichen simplex, and atypical hyperplasia is similar to vulvar intraepithelial neoplasia (Figs. 19-13A and B). The major differences are in the organization and differentiation of cells within the rete pegs (Figs. 19-13C to E).

Cystic Lesions

The most common cyst seen in the vulva is the inclusion, or sebaceous, cyst, which is caused by obstruction of one or more sebaceous gland ducts. These cysts usually create painful nodules on the labia majora or minora. Infection causes a small abscess (Fig. 19-14A).

Within the vestibule, the most common cyst is the Bartholin duct cyst. An obstructed duct may become infected and produce a Bartholin gland abscess (Figs. 19-14B and C).

Fox-Fordyce disease causes intense itching and small cysts in the area of the mons veneris and on the labia majora. The pruritus may lead to secondary ulceration. Fox-Fordyce disease is caused by obstruction of apocrine sweat gland ducts (Fig. 19-14D).

Lymphangioma is an unusual cystic disorder that typically affects the labia majora and causes clusters of microcysts (Figs. 19-14E to G). Microscopically, distension of the subepidermal lymphatics confirms the diagnosis.

Bullous-Ulcerative Lesions, Including Tubercular Lesions

Behçet's disease is a recurrent disorder that begins as a painful bleb and may be misdiagnosed as herpes (Fig. 19-15A). The bleb usually is much larger than a herpetic vesicle. Necrosis soon occurs and leads to a painful ulcer (Figs. 19-15B to D). Similar, smaller aphthous ulcers may be seen in the mouth, typically on the buccal mucosa (Fig. 19-15E).

Although tuberculosis of the vulva is rare in the United States, it is a public health problem in developing countries throughout the world. Large ulcers and caseous necrosis are characteristics of this disease (Fig. 19-16*A*). More common in the United States is sarcoidosis, which causes plaques and shallow ulcers (Fig. 19-16*B*). Histopathologic examination shows granuloma formation as well as Langhans' giant cells (Fig. 19-16*C*).

Intraepithelial and Invasive Neoplasia

Gross findings

As with cervical and vaginal intraepithelial disease, vulvar intraepithelial neoplasia (VIN) is classified as mild, moderate, or severe, corresponding to VIN grades 1 to 3. VIN grade 3, carcinoma in situ, and Bowen's disease are different names for the same disease. The most common intraepithelial neoplastic lesion in the vulva is VIN grade 3, or carcinoma in situ. Vulvar intraepithelial neoplasia is easily mistaken for a variety of benign disorders, most often condylomata acuminata (Fig. 19-17*A*). Colposcopic examination may show distinguishing features that suggest neoplasia (Figs. 19-17*B* and *C*).

VIN may cause no symptoms or may be associated with chronic pruritus. Because vulvar itching often is mistakenly assumed to indicate a yeast infection, most women with pruritus are treated without examination or culture, and an accurate diagnosis may be delayed as a result.

VIN often appears as flat, warty lesions (Fig. 19-17*D*). Dark pigmentation suggests a neoplastic process (Figs. 19-17*E* and *F*). Colposcopic examination shows a raised, pebbled appearance that is typical of warty disease (Fig. 19-17*G*). Abnormal vascular patterns usually are not seen. Application of 3% acetic acid may increase the white appearance of these lesions. As in the vagina, VIN is a multifocal disorder and areas of normal-appearing skin may be seen between raised areas of neoplasia (Figs. 19-17*H* and *I*). When parakeratosis rather than hyperkeratosis is present, a plateau of red lesions may be seen (Fig. 19-17*J*). Discrete differences in the pigmentary pattern compared with the surrounding skin suggests neoplasia, and the gynecologist should describe the location, pattern, color, size, and focus of the lesions (Fig. 19-17*K*).

Paget's disease of the vulva is a variant of carcinoma in situ. It is not a disorder of the squamous epithelium, but is a neoplastic disorder of the apocrine glands. Paget's disease causes a characteristic red lesion (Figs. 19-17*L* and *M*). The affected vulvar skin appears ragged, irregular, and raw (Figs. 19-17*N* and *O*).

Microscopic findings

In vulvar intraepithelial neoplasia disease, the organization of epithelial maturation is disturbed. The number of cell layers in the prickle cell layer is increased, creating deep, thickened rete pegs (Fig. 19-17*P*). Mitotic activity is increased, particularly within the pegs. The quantity of nuclear material is increased, and this material appears darker as a result of increased chromation content and ploidy (Figs. 19-17*Q* and *R*). Keratinization of individual cells deep within the epithelium is a common form of malignant dyskeratosis (Fig. 19-17*S*). In the mature form of VIN grade 3, corps ronds may be seen. These cells are characterized by clear cytoplasm that contains round, black nuclei (Fig. 19-17*T*). These cells resemble miniature targets. The epithelium is thickened compared with normal, or non-neoplastic, epidermis. Dark lines of pigmentation are seen in the basal layers (Fig. 19-17*U*). The upper epidermal strata contain either thickened keratin or parakeratosis (Fig. 19-17*V*).

Paget's disease is identified by the presence of large, clear cells that infiltrate the various epidermal layers (Figs. 19-17*W* and *X*). Parakeratosis is seen in the uppermost layers of the epidermis. Mucicarmine staining is helpful in identifying pagetoid cells. Paget's disease may with time become invasive (Fig. 19-17*Y*).

The dermis, particularly the skin appendages, must be examined carefully because they show infiltration by neoplastic epithelium in 38% of cases (Fig. 19-17*Y*). For women older than 50 years of age, the involvement of skin appendages approaches 50% (Fig. 19-17*Z*). Because the appendages may extend deeply into the reticular dermis or even into the underlying fat, the neoplastic extension must be considered when designing a treatment plan. The regeneration of destroyed epidermis is initiated from the undamaged skin appendages. Generation of neoplastic cells from these appendages causes persisting disease. Therefore, the appendages may be considered in the same category as the endocervical glands.

Invasive cancer of the vulva

Invasive carcinoma of the vulva usually is squamous in origin. Glandular cancer is rare, but may originate from either sweat glands or Bartholin glands. Paraurethral gland cancer is rare.

Invasive cancer may be indicated by the presence of a large, fungating or ulcerating lesion (Figs. 19-18*A* and *B*). Some lesions are more subtle (Fig. 19-18*C*). If neoplasia is suspected, biopsy should be performed promptly. The diagnosis must be established by directed biopsy (Figs. 19-18*D* and *E*).

The vulva is an area of increased risk for malignant melanoma (Fig. 19-18*F*). Nevi are excised and sent for histopathologic evaluation (Figs. 19-18*G* and *H*). Biopsy should be performed on suspicious lesions because amelanotic melanoma may occur in this area (Figs. 19-18*I* and *J*). Microscopically, invasive cancer is characterized by nests or columns of cells that invade the vulvar stroma (Figs. 19-18*K* and *L*). Occasionally, adenocarcinoma metastasizes onto the vulvar skin from neighboring (e.g., Bartholin gland) or distant primary sites (Figs. 19-18*M* and *N*).

Blood Vascular Lesions

Vulvar varicosities vary in significance (Fig. 19-19*A*). They cause distended bluish subepidermal or surface vessels. Hemangiomas also affect the vulva and cause cyanotic discoloration and surface vessels (Figs. 19-19*B* to *D*). Because of the risk of excessive bleeding, biopsy of these lesions should not be performed in a clinic. Small, scattered papules seen on the vulva may consist of small, dilated surface vessels encased in surrounding squamous mucosa. These lesions are angiokeratomas (Fig. 19-19*E*).

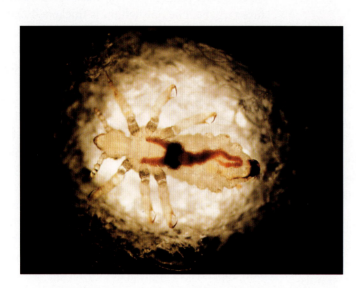

FIGURE 19-1 A small, moving white speck was seen in the pubic hair. A magnified view showed a crab louse.

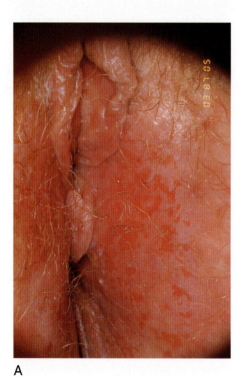

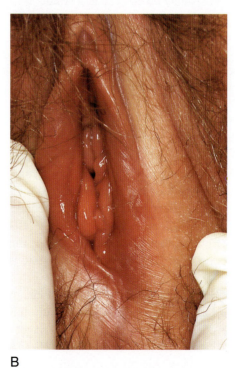

A

B

FIGURE 19-2 **A,** These striking red inflammatory skin changes diffusely affect the entire vulva, typifying acute vulvitis. **B,** These deep wine-red skin changes involve the labia minora, labia majora, and vestibule, and are associated with contact vulvitis. These lesions caused itching that progressed to burning. (continued)

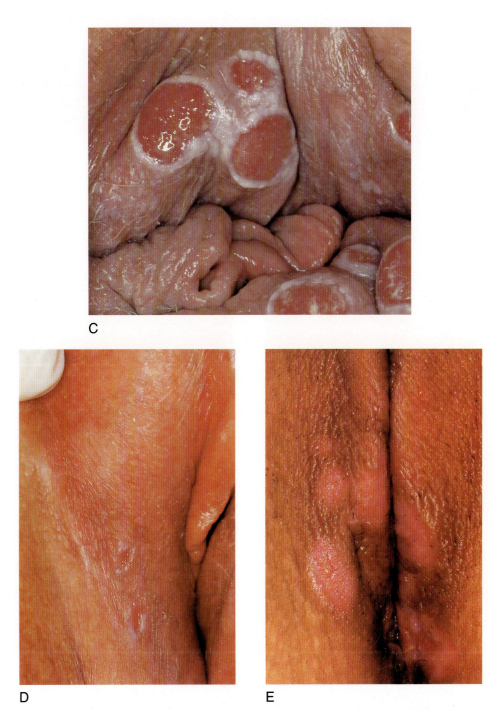

C

D

E

FIGURE 19-2 C, These large, sharp, bright red ulcers cause intense vulvar itching. Culture showed a predominantly staphylococcal infection. The differential diagnosis included pemphigus. **D,** The patient seen in *C,* 1 week after the initiation of treatment. **E,** The patient seen in *C* and *D,* 2 weeks after the initiation of treatment. Healing is apparent; the redness is diminished and the ulcers have filled in.

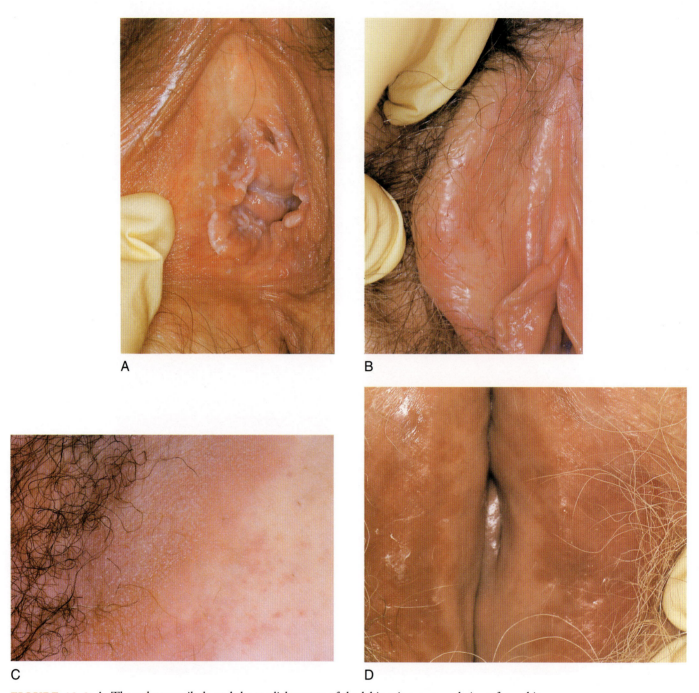

FIGURE 19-3 A, The vulvar vestibule and the medial aspects of the labia minora are red. A profuse white discharge covers the introitus, hymenal ring, and urethral meatus. **B,** The labium majus is inflamed. Redness is seen around the hair follicles. Folliculitis may be seen with fungal or bacterial vulvitis. **C,** Folliculitis and scaling associated with erythema are characteristic of chronic fungal infection. **D,** Acute fungal vulvitis causes pruritus followed by burning discomfort. (continued)

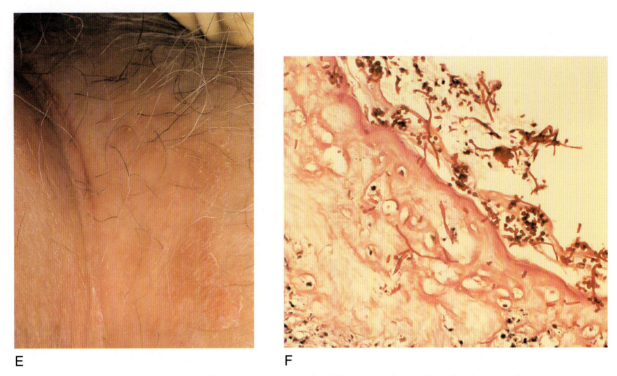

E   F

FIGURE 19-3 **E,** Lesions that show fissures and scaling should be scraped onto fungal culture medium to establish the diagnosis. **F,** Vulvar biopsy can be used to diagnose fungal vulvitis. Periodic acid-Schiff stain shows mycelia in the stratum corneum.

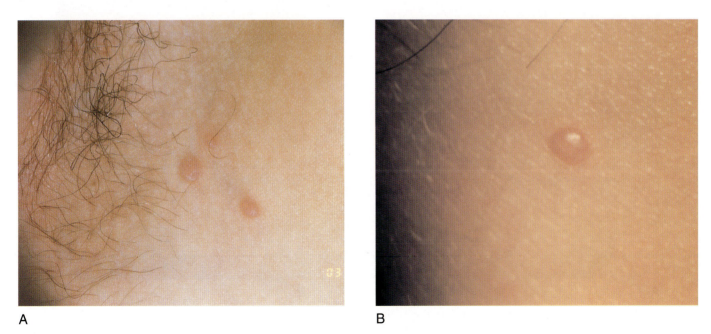

A   B

FIGURE 19-4 **A,** Multiple pink papules involve the vulva, including the mons veneris, the neighboring medial aspect of the crural region, and the thigh. **B,** A magnified colposcopic view of the lesions seen in *A* shows a waxy, umbilicated appearance consistent with molluscum contagiosum. (continued)

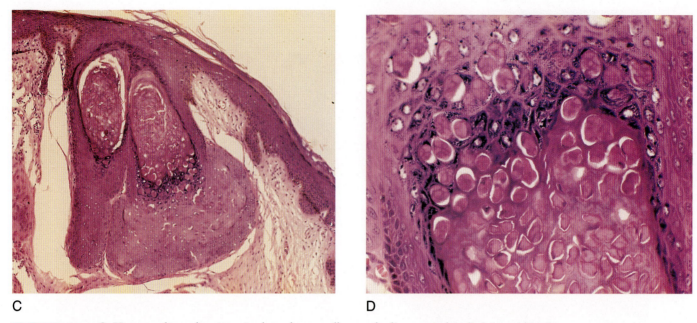

C

D

FIGURE 19-4 **C,** Hematoxylin and eosin stain shows large molluscum bodies, or viral inclusions, within the epidermis. **D,** A high-power view of *C* shows the eosinophilic viral inclusions that are diagnostic of molluscum contagiosum.

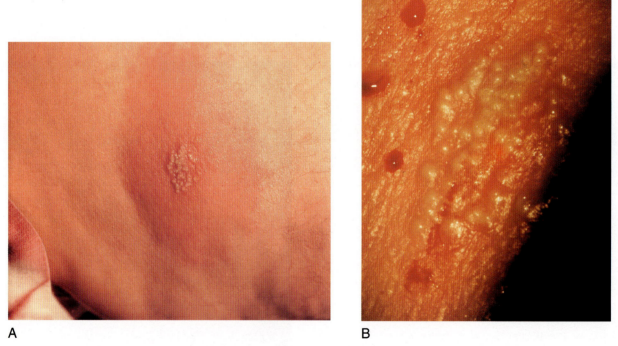

A

B

FIGURE 19-5 **A,** Early herpes simplex infection of the vulva begins with vesicle formation. Extensive inflammatory erythema surrounds the vesicles. **B,** A high-power colposcopic view shows the viral vesicles. **C,** Multiple generations of vulvar ulcers associated with herpes simplex infection. **D,** Cytopathic changes in the vulvar skin associated with herpes simplex infection show cellular destruction (*right*) and the acute inflammatory response (*bottom*). **E,** A magnified view of *D* shows the multinucleated cell with viral inclusions (*arrow*). **F,** Acute herpes simplex of the labia, vestibule, and perineum. A typical herpes ulcer has a peripheral red border and a yellow (fibrin) center. **G,** A high-power colposcopic view of the herpes simplex ulcers shown in *C* shows their sharp, red outline. **H,** A cytologic preparation obtained from a herpes ulcer shows a bizarre, enlarged cell that has four nuclei. The viral inclusion is seen within the nucleus.

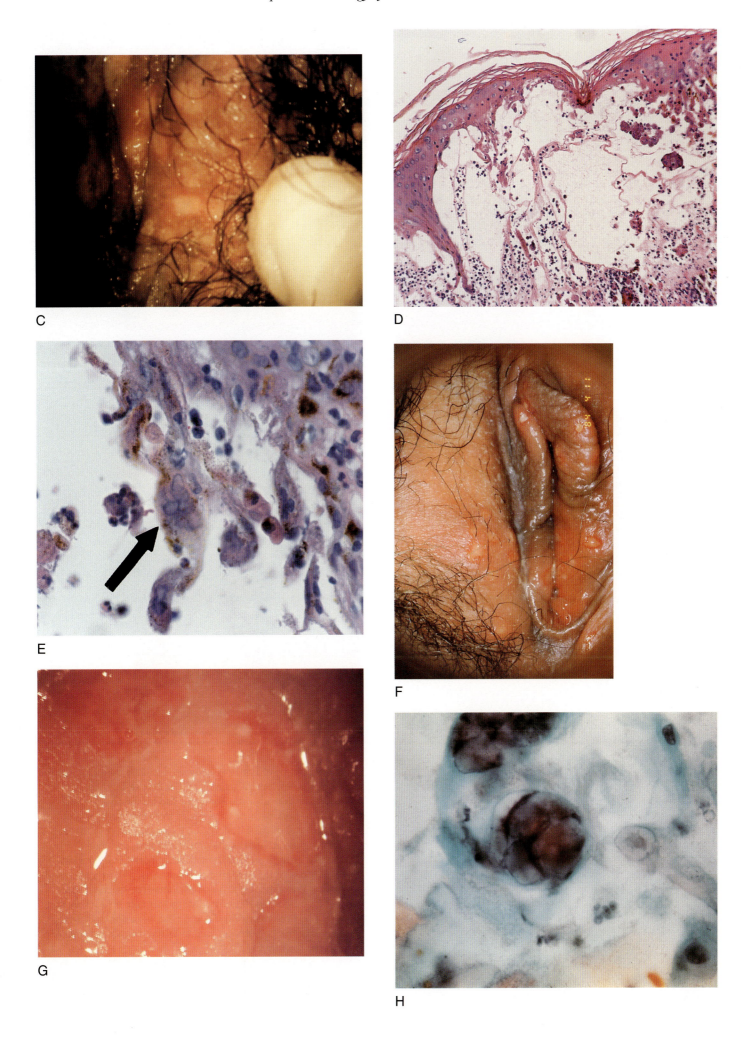

C

D

E

F

G

H

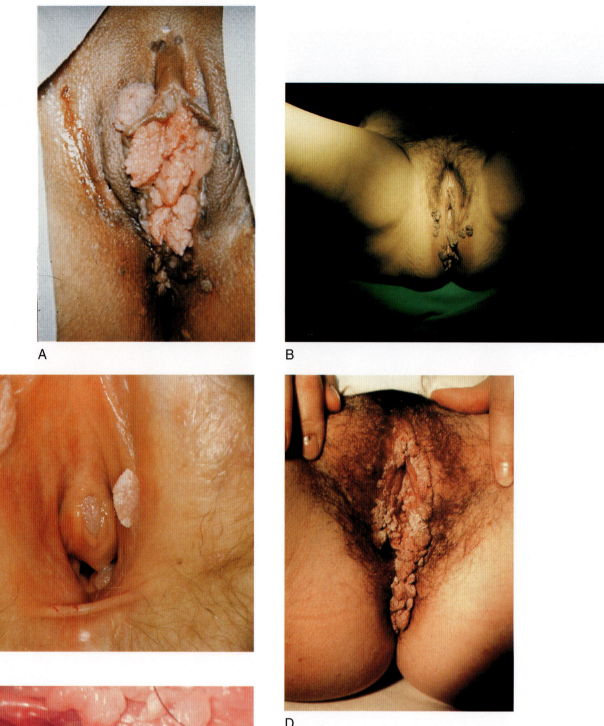

FIGURE 19-6 A, The area between the labia minora is filled with fleshy condylomata acuminata. Satellite lesions are seen elsewhere on the vulva. **B,** A woman had vulvar and perianal warts for 9 years. Because of pressure from her husband, she sought removal of these lesions. **C,** Condylomata may involve neighboring areas, such as the urethra, vagina, and anus. **D,** Massive growth of condylomata acuminata occurs during pregnancy as a result of immune compromise. At 24 weeks of pregnancy, this patient had no condyloma-free space on the vulva. **E,** The finding of perianal warts virtually guarantees that warts will be present within the anus. An anoscopic speculum, coupled with the colposcope, facilitates the diagnosis of rectal, or anal, warts. (continued)

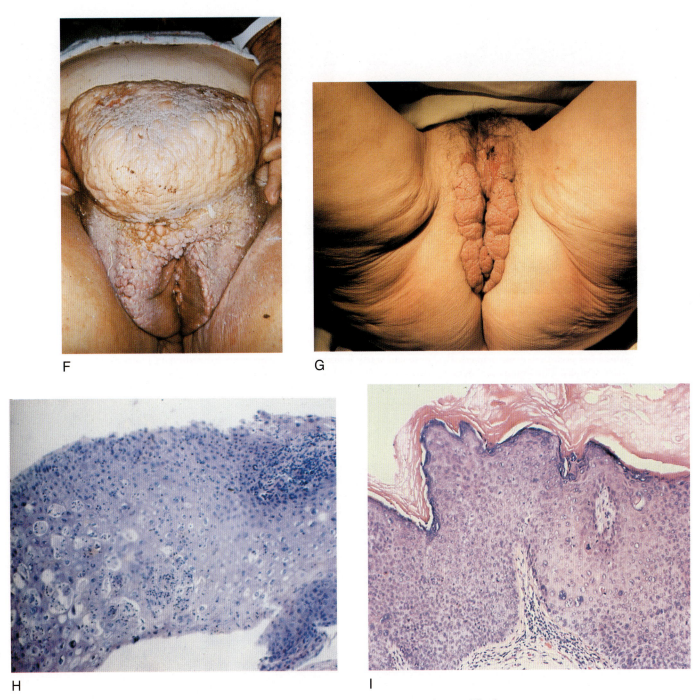

F

G

H

I

FIGURE 19-6 **F,** This atypical giant condylomatous lesion suggests verrucous carcinoma. The large mass should be sharply excised and multiply sampled. **G,** The beefy, red condylomatous lesions on the labia majora show carcinoma in situ and atypical condylomatous changes, with koilocytosis. **H,** This strip of epithelium shows acanthosis, parakeratosis, and extensive koilocytosis. Acute inflammatory cell infiltration is seen within the epidermis. **I,** This section shows carcinoma in situ arising within a condylomatous pattern. The section was obtained from a biopsy specimen of the vulva of the patient seen in *G.* It shows the classic findings of condylomata acuminata, including papillomatosis, acanthosis, and hyperkeratosis or parakeratosis, as well as neoplastic cellular changes (*left*).

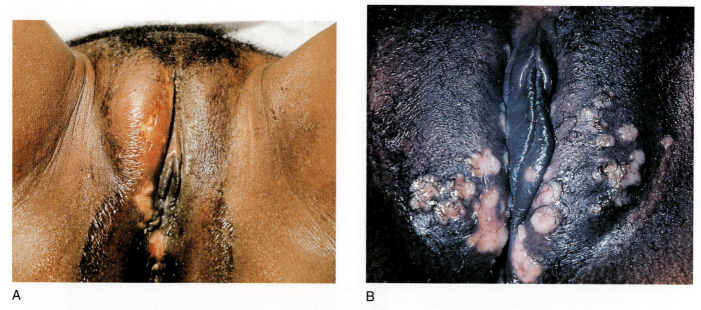

A   B

FIGURE 19-7 A, This patient has a ragged ulcer, a swollen vulva, and unilateral enlargement of the groin lymph nodes. Primary syphilis was considered in the differential diagnosis. Darkfield examination of the chancre confirmed the presence of spirochetes. **B,** These flat, warty lesions are consistent with condylomata lata, or secondary syphilis. The lesions are teeming with spirochetes. Results of serologic tests for syphilis were positive.

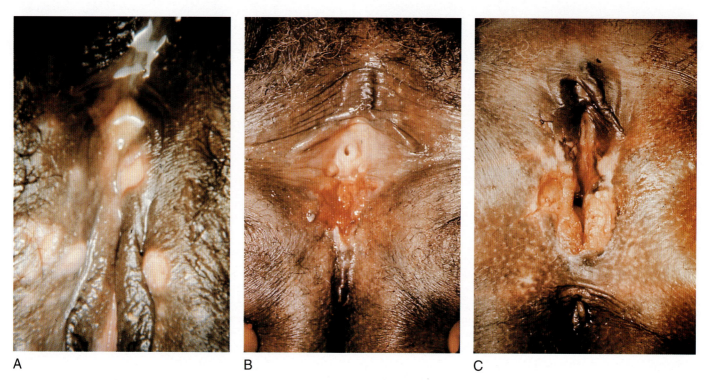

A   B   C

FIGURE 19-8 A, Multiple, nonindurated chancroid ulcers must be differentiated from ulcers caused by herpes simplex and syphilis. Chancroid ulcers cause discomfort and may be associated with inguinal lymphadenopathy. The diagnosis is made by culturing *Haemophilus ducreyi* from the ulcer.
B, Granuloma inguinale causes a festering, fungating lesion. Multiple biopsies may be needed to distinguish this condition from invasive carcinoma. Invasive squamous cell carcinoma may coexist with or follow granuloma inguinale. **C,** Chronic granuloma inguinale. (continued)

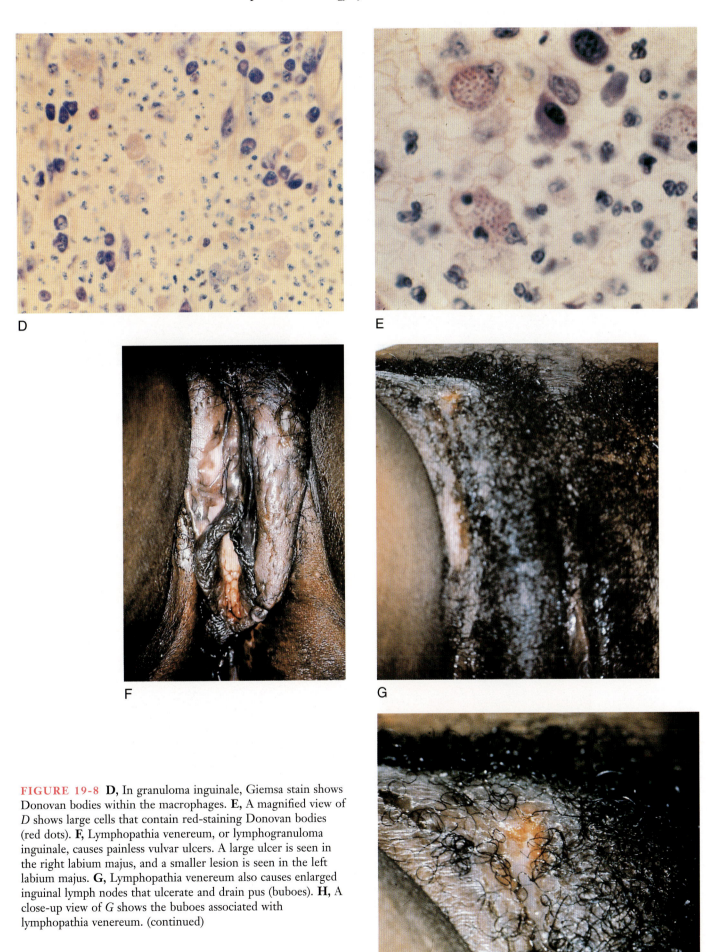

FIGURE 19-8 D, In granuloma inguinale, Giemsa stain shows Donovan bodies within the macrophages. **E,** A magnified view of *D* shows large cells that contain red-staining Donovan bodies (red dots). **F,** Lymphopathia venereum, or lymphogranuloma inguinale, causes painless vulvar ulcers. A large ulcer is seen in the right labium majus, and a smaller lesion is seen in the left labium majus. **G,** Lymphopathia venereum also causes enlarged inguinal lymph nodes that ulcerate and drain pus (buboes). **H,** A close-up view of *G* shows the buboes associated with lymphopathia venereum. (continued)

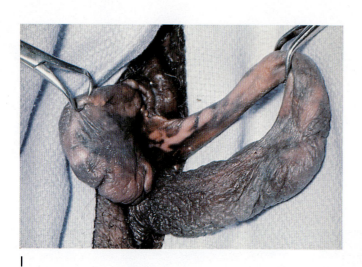

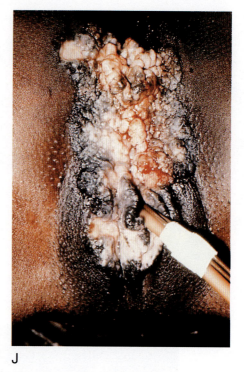

I

J

FIGURE 19-8 I, The chronic phase is characterized by vulvar deformities that include fenestrations, elephantiasis, and systemic sequelae, such as rectal strictures. **J,** Invasive squamous cell carcinoma of the vulva may coexist with lymphopathia venereum.

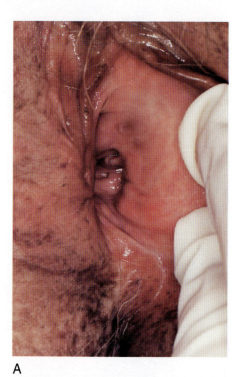

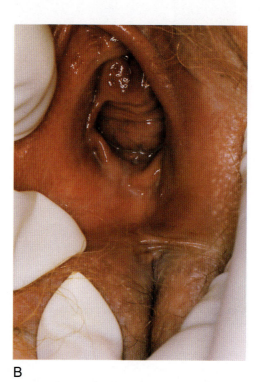

A

B

FIGURE 19-9 A, This patient had progressive burning pain and a thin, red vestibule. Fissures occurred with stretch at stress points. This abnormality was the result of vaginal deodorant allergy, or contact vestibulitis. **B,** Vulvar vestibulitis syndrome causes erythema and burning discomfort. The most intense erythema is seen around the openings of the Bartholin glands. (continued)

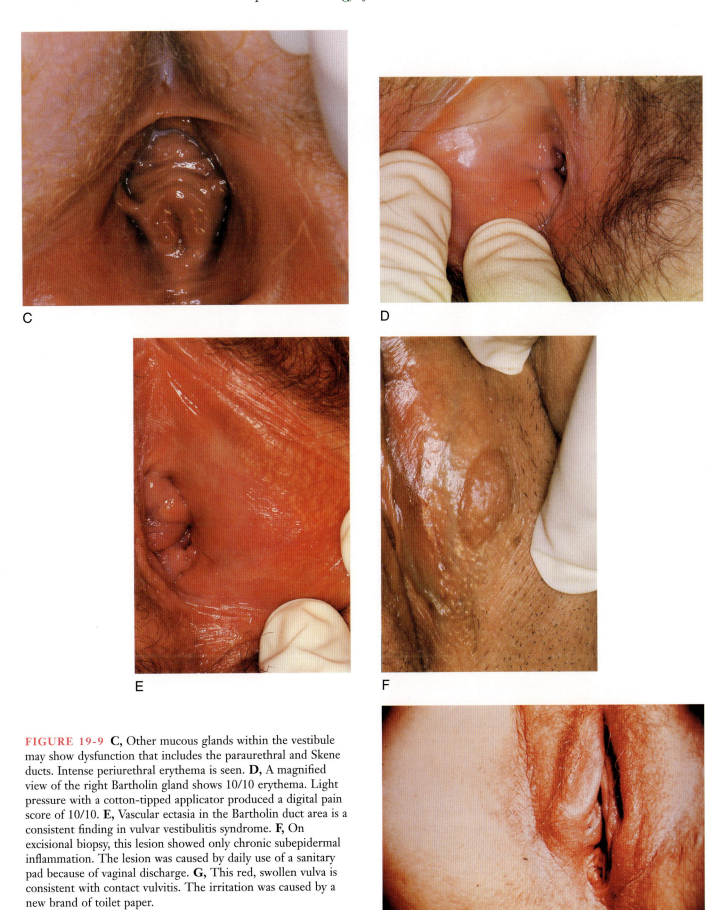

FIGURE 19-9 C, Other mucous glands within the vestibule may show dysfunction that includes the paraurethral and Skene ducts. Intense periurethral erythema is seen. **D,** A magnified view of the right Bartholin gland shows 10/10 erythema. Light pressure with a cotton-tipped applicator produced a digital pain score of 10/10. **E,** Vascular ectasia in the Bartholin duct area is a consistent finding in vulvar vestibulitis syndrome. **F,** On excisional biopsy, this lesion showed only chronic subepidermal inflammation. The lesion was caused by daily use of a sanitary pad because of vaginal discharge. **G,** This red, swollen vulva is consistent with contact vulvitis. The irritation was caused by a new brand of toilet paper.

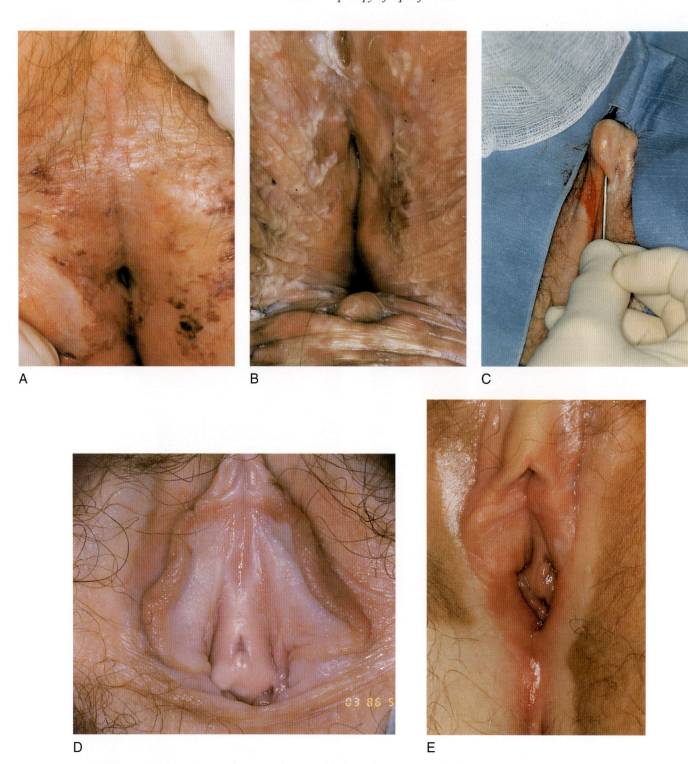

FIGURE 19-10 A, Long-standing, poorly treated lichen sclerosus caused adhesions of all of the vulvar components. The vestibule was reduced to a pencil-sized opening. The patient experienced leakage of urine as a result of urine pooling in the vagina. **B,** Several features of lichen sclerosus are seen: the white plaques (lichenification); the thin, atrophic skin; and the cigarette paper skin changes (wrinkling). **C,** Inflammatory scars in and around the clitoral hood may seal off the clitoris. Clitoral phymosis creates swelling and sometimes infection within the hood. A fine probe is placed under the hood of the phymotic clitoris. **D,** Lichen sclerosus affects all age groups. This 24-year-old woman has vulvar pallor that is diagnostic of lichen sclerosus. **E,** This patient has biopsy-proven lichen sclerosus and vitiligo. Fissures are seen at the posterior commissure. (continued)

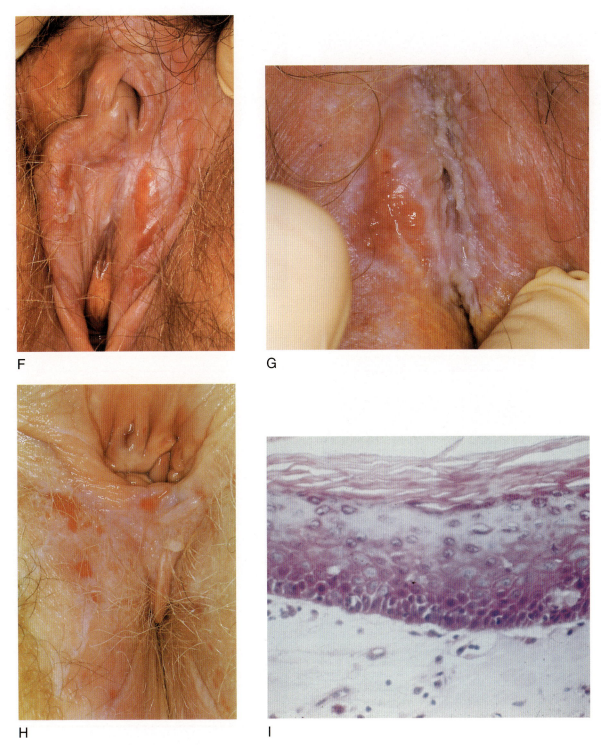

F

G

H

I

FIGURE 19-10 **F,** This patient has severe lichen sclerosus and associated intense pruritus. As a result, she has scratched at her vulva, especially at night, and the scratching has caused ulceration and a superficial bacterial infection. **G,** A magnified view of *F* shows ulceration, fissure formation, and tearing of the inflamed, scarred tissue. Lack of elasticity is the primary cause of skin split, or fissure. **H,** Lichen sclerosus may involve the perineum and perianal skin as well as the vestibule, labia, and clitoral and periclitoral tissues. **I,** The diagnosis of lichen sclerosus is made by directed biopsy. The microscopic criteria include thinning and atrophy of the vulvar epidermis; fracture, or dishevelment of the basal cell layer; collagenation of the underlying dermis; and hyperkeratosis.

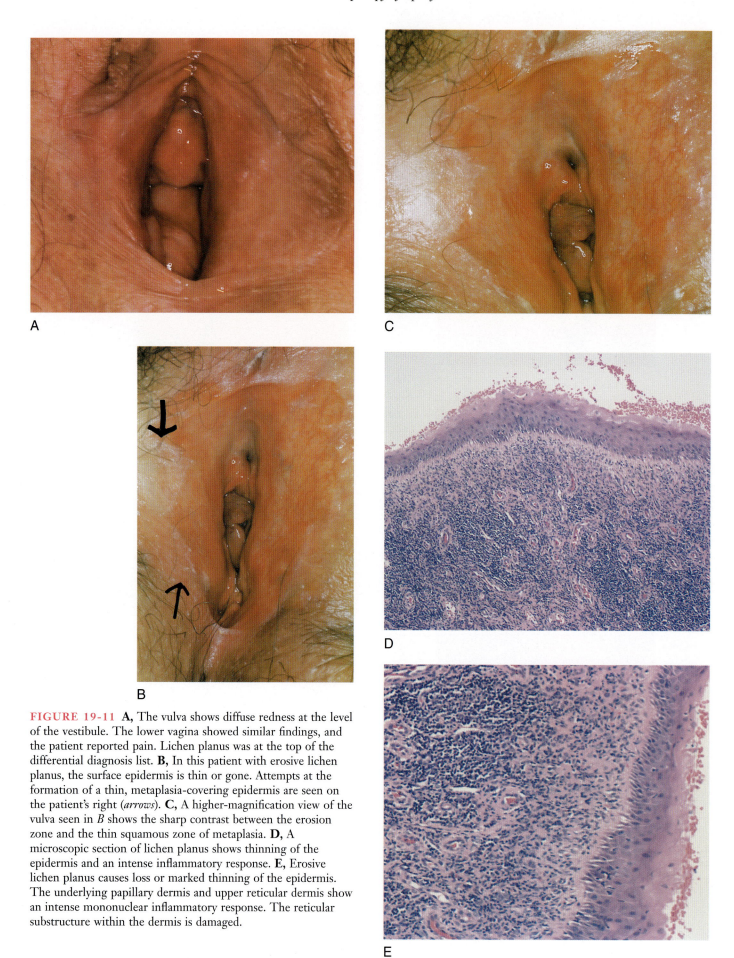

FIGURE 19-11 **A,** The vulva shows diffuse redness at the level of the vestibule. The lower vagina showed similar findings, and the patient reported pain. Lichen planus was at the top of the differential diagnosis list. **B,** In this patient with erosive lichen planus, the surface epidermis is thin or gone. Attempts at the formation of a thin, metaplasia-covering epidermis are seen on the patient's right (*arrows*). **C,** A higher-magnification view of the vulva seen in *B* shows the sharp contrast between the erosion zone and the thin squamous zone of metaplasia. **D,** A microscopic section of lichen planus shows thinning of the epidermis and an intense inflammatory response. **E,** Erosive lichen planus causes loss or marked thinning of the epidermis. The underlying papillary dermis and upper reticular dermis show an intense mononuclear inflammatory response. The reticular substructure within the dermis is damaged.

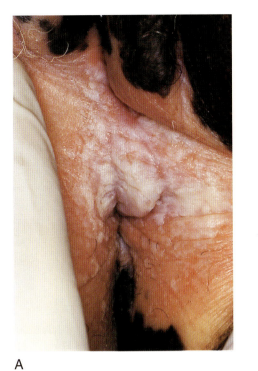
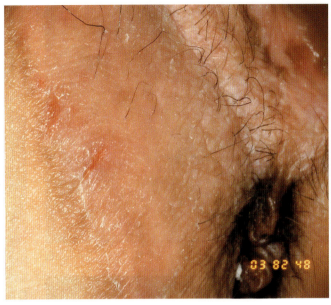

A   B

FIGURE 19-12 **A,** Extensive hyperkeratosis associated with itching is characteristic of lichen simplex chronicus. The perianal and perineal skin also shows vitiligo. **B,** The skin changes seen at the periphery of the perineum are associated with fissures. The differential diagnosis included lichen sclerosus and lichen simplex. The biopsy findings were consistent with lichen simplex.

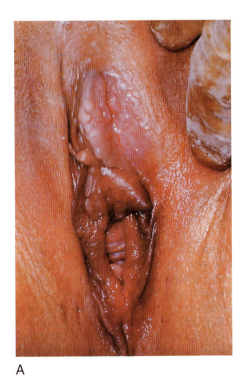
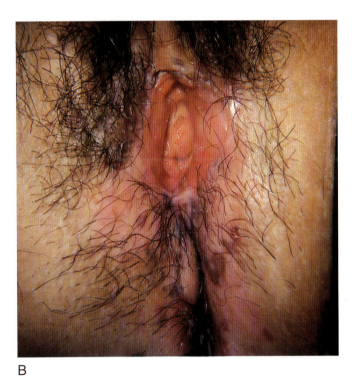

A   B

FIGURE 19-13 **A,** Abnormal thickening and whitening, or hyperkeratosis, is seen on the clitoral hood, the frenulum, and the neighboring upper left labium minus. **B,** Whitening of the lower labia minora, perineum, and perianal skin is seen. Dark pigmentary changes are scattered in the perineum and perianal skin; these changes suggest vulvar intraepithelial neoplasia. Biopsy showed only typical hyperplastic vulvitis. (continued)

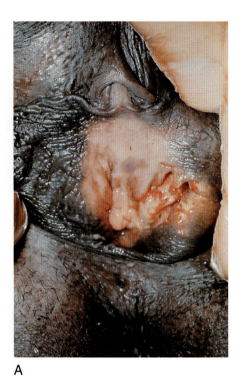

A

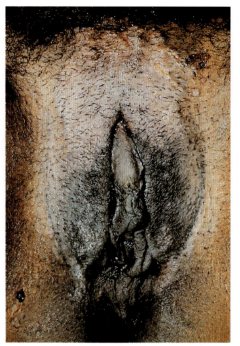

B

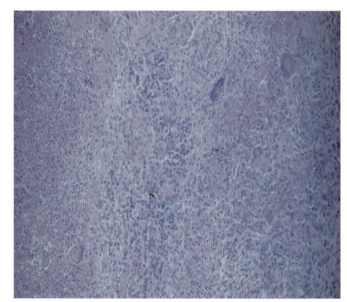

C

FIGURE 19-16 A, Culture and biopsy of this draining sinus and ulcerating lesion showed vulvar tuberculosis. **B,** Biopsy of the lesion showed granulomatous disease; however, culture findings were negative for *Mycobacterium* species. The lesion was later diagnosed as vulvar sarcoidosis. **C,** Biopsy of the lesion seen in *A* shows caseous necrosis and Langhans' giant cells. The microscopic diagnosis was granulomatous vulvitis, and vulvar tuberculosis.

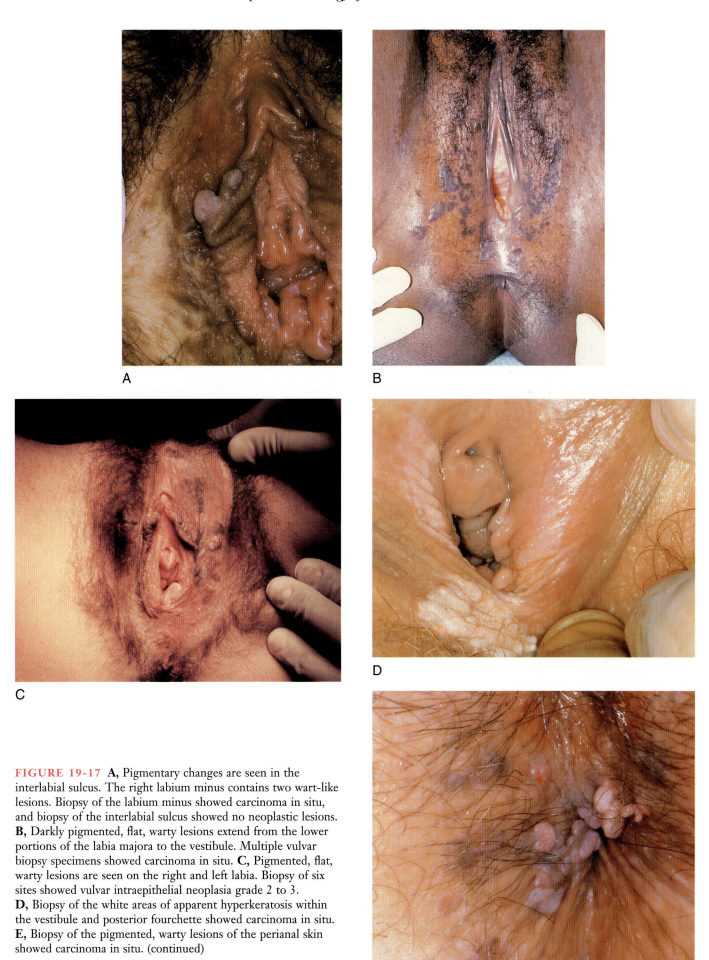

FIGURE 19-17 A, Pigmentary changes are seen in the interlabial sulcus. The right labium minus contains two wart-like lesions. Biopsy of the labium minus showed carcinoma in situ, and biopsy of the interlabial sulcus showed no neoplastic lesions. **B,** Darkly pigmented, flat, warty lesions extend from the lower portions of the labia majora to the vestibule. Multiple vulvar biopsy specimens showed carcinoma in situ. **C,** Pigmented, flat, warty lesions are seen on the right and left labia. Biopsy of six sites showed vulvar intraepithelial neoplasia grade 2 to 3. **D,** Biopsy of the white areas of apparent hyperkeratosis within the vestibule and posterior fourchette showed carcinoma in situ. **E,** Biopsy of the pigmented, warty lesions of the perianal skin showed carcinoma in situ. (continued)

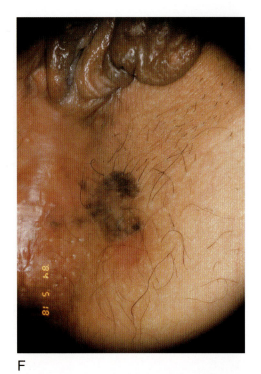

F

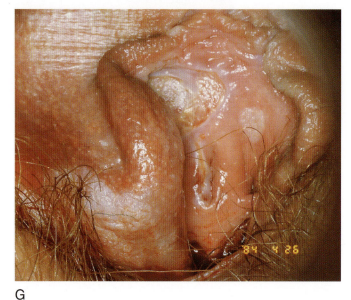

G

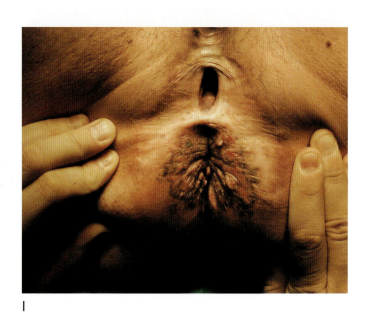

H

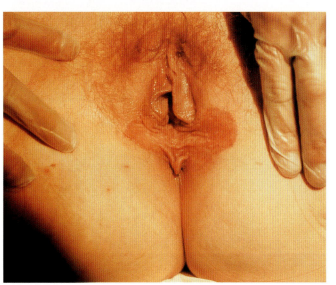

I

FIGURE 19-17 **F,** The pigmented perineal lesion is carcinoma in situ. **G,** The flat, white, warty lesions on the right labium minus and the vestibule are carcinoma in situ. **H,** In a postmenopausal patient with severe pruritus, the lower labia, perineum, and perianal skin showed raised, pigmented, multicentric lesions. Biopsy showed vulvar intraepithelial neoplasia grade 2 to 3. **I,** Raised red, brown, and black lesions are seen in a patient with perianal itching. These lesions suggest neoplasia. Multiple biopsies of the perianal lesions showed carcinoma in situ. The patient underwent vulvectomy for vulvar intraepithelial neoplasia grade 3. **J,** A red lesion involving the perineum, posterior fourchette, and perianal skin is seen in a patient with pruritus and vulvar discomfort. These lesions suggest parakeratosis or Paget's disease. Biopsy showed squamous carcinoma in situ, and the upper strata of the epidermis showed parakeratosis. (continued)

J

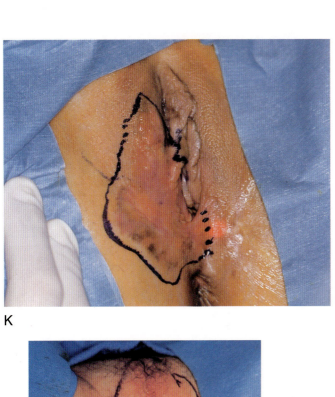

K

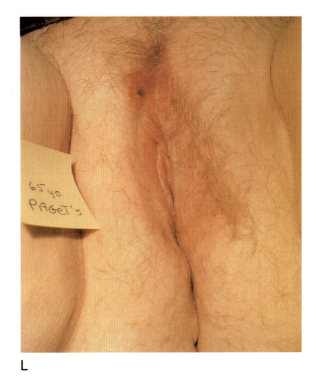

L

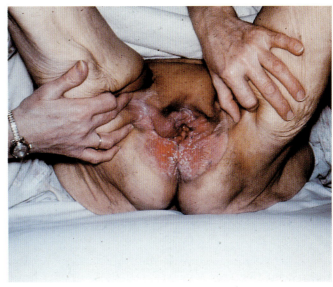

M   N

FIGURE 19-17 K, As shown by the marking pen, this lesion involved the lower right labium majus and the perineum, and extended across the midline to the left perineum. The lesion was characterized by dark brown peripheral pigmentation and reddish, raw-looking, parakeratotic skin changes. Biopsy showed carcinoma in situ. **L,** Biopsy of this persistent red lesion of the upper labium majus, labium minus, and periclitoral tissues showed Paget's disease of the vulva. **M,** Recurrent Paget's disease of the vulva. The patient will undergo vulvectomy and skin grafting. **N,** Extensive Paget's disease extends from the lower labia and perineum onto the buttocks. (continued)

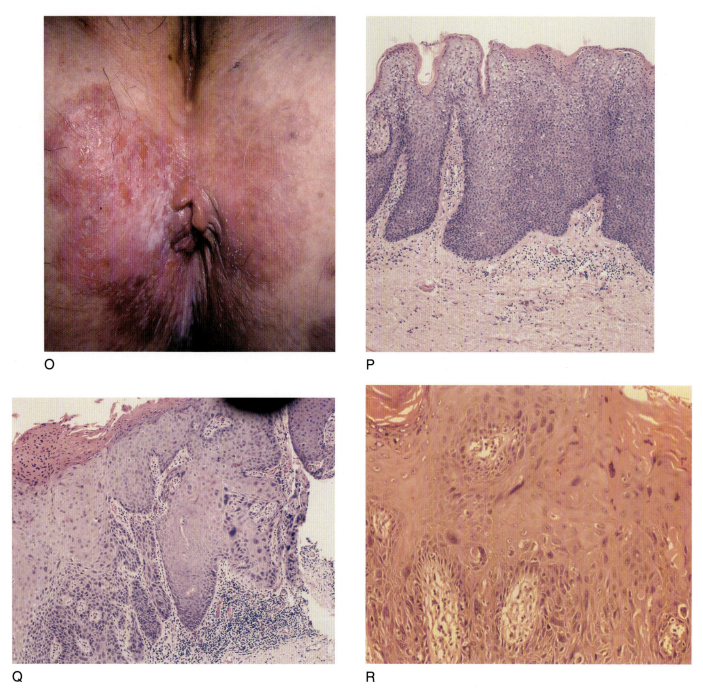

O

P

Q

R

FIGURE 19-17 O, Because extensive perianal Paget's disease may involve the anal mucosa, an adequate anal mucosal margin must be obtained during resection. **P,** A low-power view (×2) shows vulvar intraepithelial neoplasia grade 3. Bottom-to-top loss of organization and maturation is seen. The increased cell population contains many dark cells as well as bizarre parakeratotic cells. **Q,** A microscopic section (×4) taken through the area of vulvar intraepithelial neoplasia grade 3 shows enlarged, pleomorphic neoplastic cells. The nuclei are hyperchromatic and similarly enlarged. Parakeratosis shows the areas of atypical maturation. **R,** A microscopic section obtained from another site in the patient seen in *Q* shows similar cellular changes that suggest vulvar intraepithelial neoplasia grade 3. (continued)

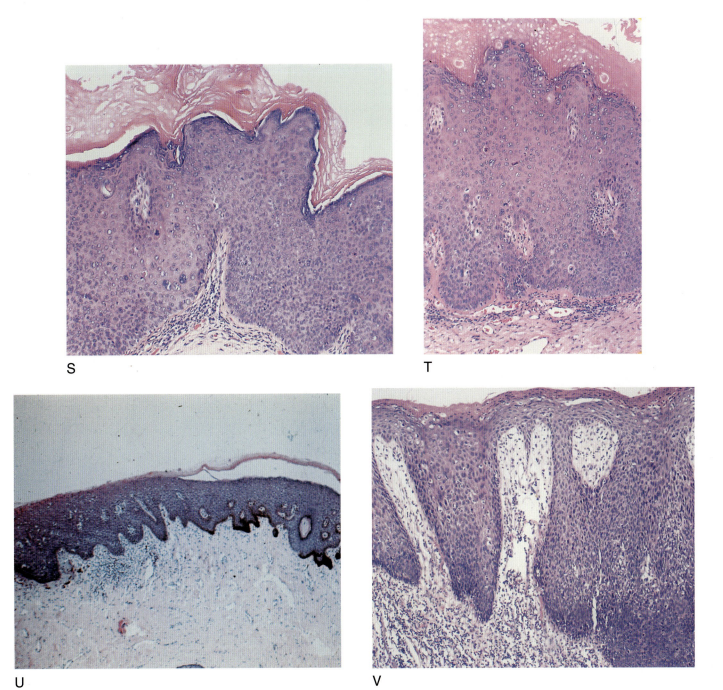

FIGURE 19-17 S, A scanning view (×4) shows the condylomatous nature of this neoplastic lesion. Histologic examination showed mature carcinoma in situ, or Bowen's disease. Several individually keratinized cells are seen within the epidermal strata, and the keratin layer is thickened, or hyperkeratotic. **T,** A scanning view (×4) of another condylomatous lesion shows unequivocal carcinoma in situ. The small cells that have dark, or hyperchromatic, nuclei surrounded by clear cytoplasm are corps ronds. These cells often are seen in Bowen's disease. **U,** This section shows the sharp boundary of pigmented epithelium between neoplastic epidermis and non-neoplastic epithelium. **V,** Increased thickness is an early change from normal to neoplastic skin that typifies intraepithelial neoplasia. The involved epidermis typically is three or more times thicker than normal vulvar skin. (continued)

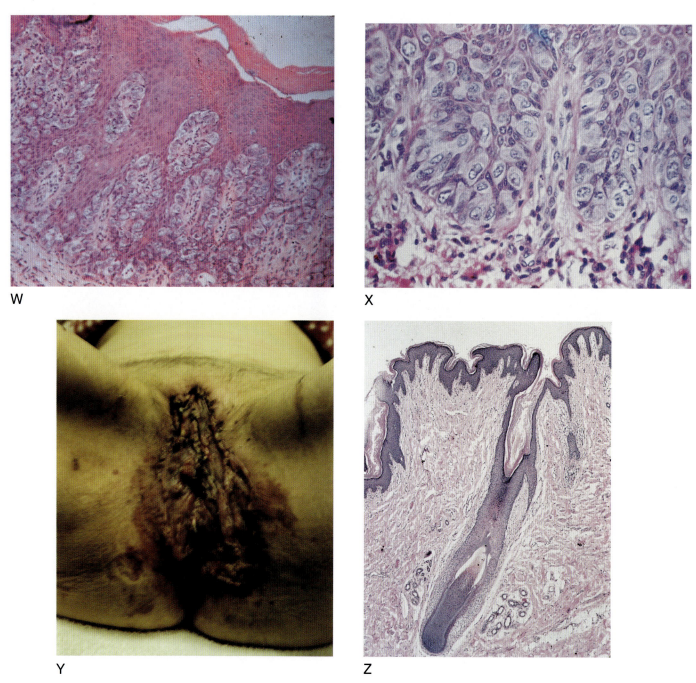

FIGURE 19-17 W, Paget's disease is diagnosed microscopically by intraepithelial proliferation of large, clear cells that arise in the basal region and move up into the prickle cell layer. **X,** A high-power view (×16) shows the clear Paget's cells within the vulvar epidermis. This tumor arises from apocrine gland cells and usually is carcinoma in situ. **Y,** This colpophotograph shows an extensive reddish colored lesion replacing the vulva. Biopsy showed invasive Paget's disease of the vulva. **Z,** At least 38% of cases of vulvar intraepithelial neoplasia involve skin appendages by direct extension. In this case, the lesion is tracking into a hair follicle. Involvement of appendages is a significant factor in the persistence or recurrence of disease after treatment.

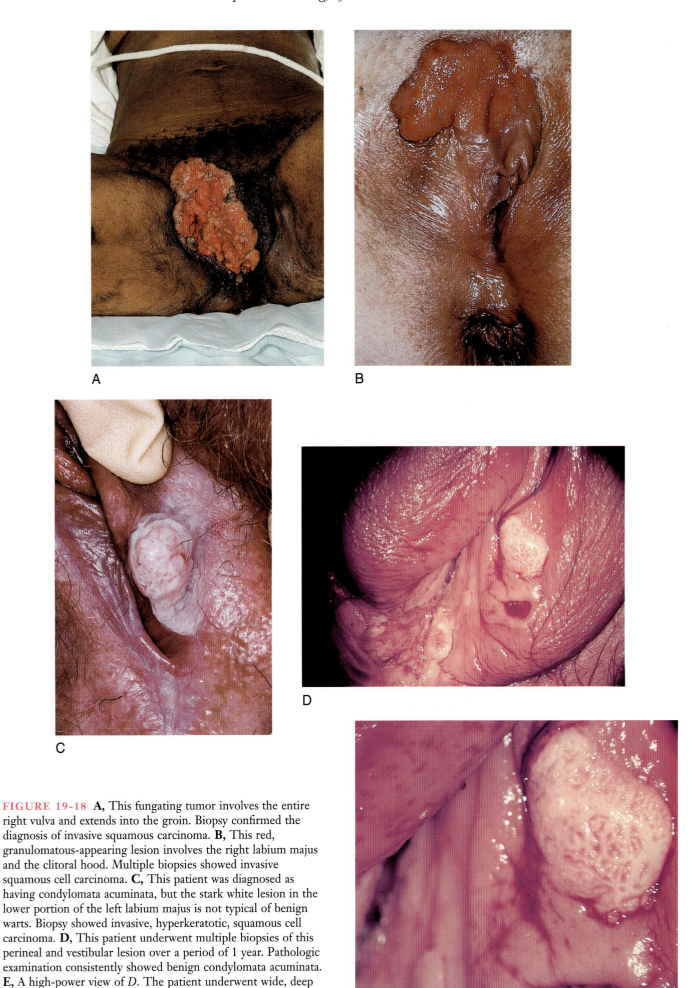

FIGURE 19-18 **A,** This fungating tumor involves the entire right vulva and extends into the groin. Biopsy confirmed the diagnosis of invasive squamous carcinoma. **B,** This red, granulomatous-appearing lesion involves the right labium majus and the clitoral hood. Multiple biopsies showed invasive squamous cell carcinoma. **C,** This patient was diagnosed as having condylomata acuminata, but the stark white lesion in the lower portion of the left labium majus is not typical of benign warts. Biopsy showed invasive, hyperkeratotic, squamous cell carcinoma. **D,** This patient underwent multiple biopsies of this perineal and vestibular lesion over a period of 1 year. Pathologic examination consistently showed benign condylomata acuminata. **E,** A high-power view of *D.* The patient underwent wide, deep excisional biopsy. Pathologic examination of the biopsy specimen showed invasive squamous cell carcinoma. (continued)

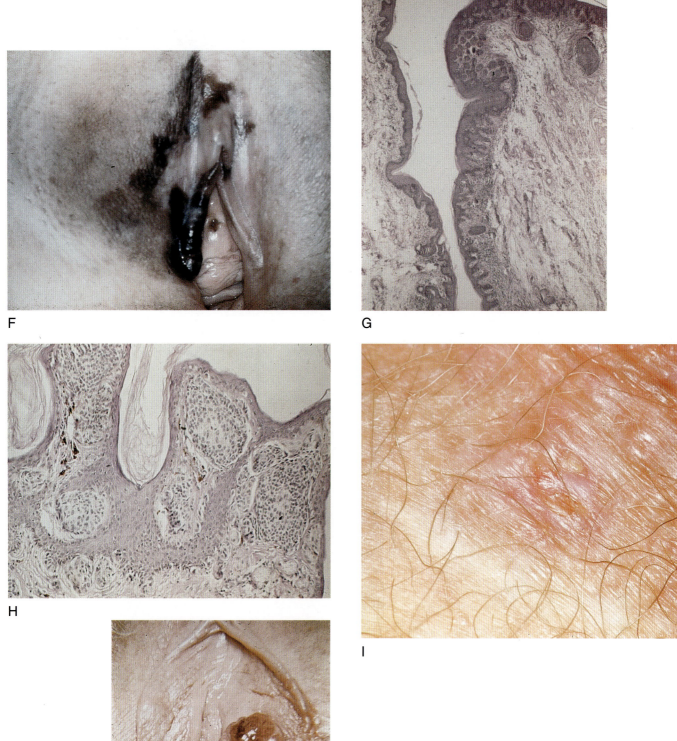

F

G

H

I

J

FIGURE 19-18 **F,** This black lesion suggests vulvar malignant melanoma. Excisional biopsy confirmed the diagnosis. **G,** A microscopic section shows nevus cells and invasive melanoma. **H,** Before the development of melanoma (*F*), the patient had a "mole" removed from the vulva. This section shows evidence of junctional nevus cells. **I,** This bland vulvar lesion was excised and showed nonpigmented melanoma cells, or malignant amelanotic melanoma. **J,** Biopsy of this ulcerative lesion of the vestibule showed amelanotic malignant melanoma. (continued)

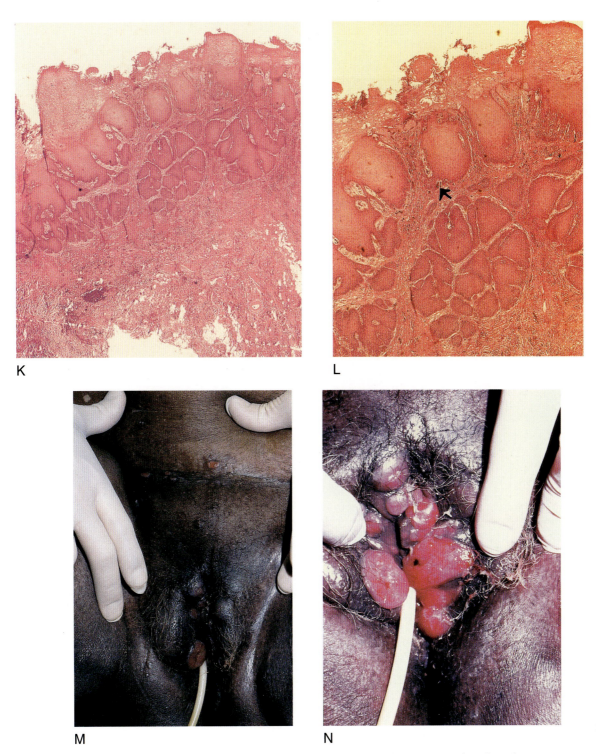

FIGURE 19-18 K, Several clumps of neoplastic squamous cells are seen within the vulvar stroma. These findings are consistent with invasive squamous cell carcinoma. **L,** A high-power view of *K* shows surface ulceration overlying the invasive carcinoma. The earliest sign of invasion is the budding of malignant epithelium from the bottom of the rete peg (*arrow*). **M,** These bright red, disk-like lesions suggest malignancy. Biopsy showed adenocarcinoma, with a gastrointestinal primary lesion. **N,** A magnified view of *M* shows a metastatic tumor infiltrating most of the vestibule.

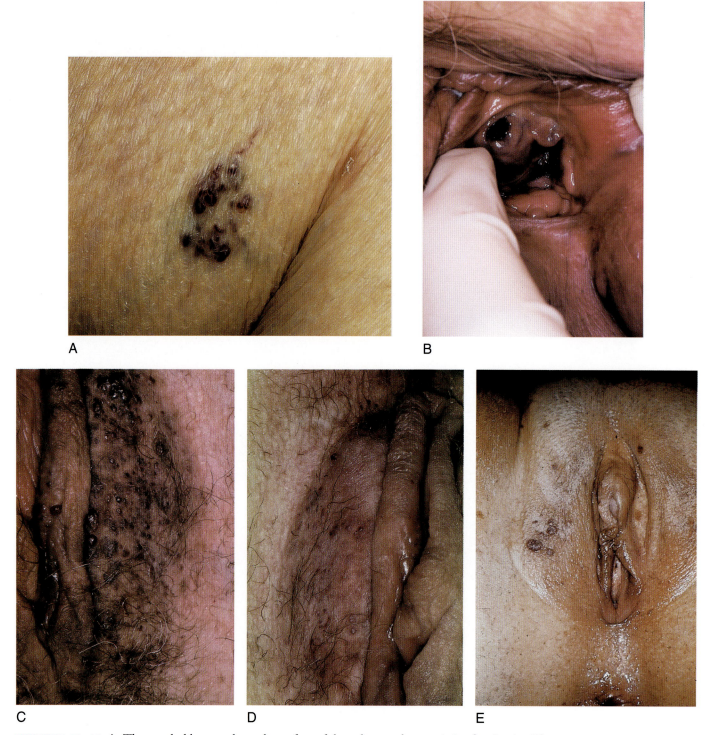

FIGURE 19-19 **A,** The purple-blue vessels on the surface of the vulva are characteristic of varicosity. The single lesion is not clinically significant. **B,** An elderly patient had intermittent vaginal and vulvar bleeding. These urethral, suburethral, vestibular, and vaginal lesions are characteristic of a vascular malformation. The entire lower anterior vaginal wall is distended and cyanotic. **C,** A patient was born with this lesion. In addition to disfigurement, the patient experienced rupture and bleeding of the fragile surface vessels. The diagnosis was vulvar hemangioma. **D,** The patient seen in *C* after three series of hexascan laser treatments. The varicose vessels are gone, and the native skin shows no scarring. **E,** These small surface vessels are angiokeratoma.

CHAPTER 20
Terminology

The terms used to describe vulvar lesions are significantly different from those used for the vagina and cervix. Vulvar terminology is more closely related to dermatology than to gynecology. In some cases, the descriptions are familiar (e.g., focal vs. diffuse, condylomatous, leukoplakia) whereas others may seem foreign.

Basic Terms

Macule: A macule is a flat, colored lesion that is not palpable.

Papule: A papule is a small, raised lesion that is less than 0.5 cm in diameter.

Nodule: A nodule is an elevated lesion that is greater than 0.5 cm in diameter.

Lichenification: Lichenification is thickening of the epidermis that may include plaques, or flat, elevated lesions.

Cornification: Another term for thickening of the stratum corneum. This may be referred to as *hyperkeratosis* when the cornified layer of epidermis is excessively thickened.

Scaling: Scaling is thickening and shedding of cornified tissue.

Crust: Crusts are plaques of dried blood, mucus, or other bloody fluids.

Bleb: A small blister that is usually fluid-filled.

Vesicle: Vesicles are blebs on the surface of the skin that are created by fluid-filled spaces within the epidermis.

Bulla: A bulla is a large bleb.

Ulcer: An ulcer is a defect or loss of epidermis that exposes the underlying connective tissue, or dermis.

Fissure: A fissure is a crack, or furrow, in the skin that exposes the underlying dermis.

Erosion: Erosion is loss of the surface epithelium that is less deep than an ulcer.

Ectasia: Ectasia is dilation of the superficial vessels, such as punctate vessels, that is seen with a colposcope, with or without the application of acetic acid.

Atrophy: Atrophy is thinning or loss of epithelium and stroma.

Eczematoid lesion: An eczematoid lesion is round, red, scaly, and crusted.

Targetoid lesion: A targetoid lesion has a concentric ring-like pattern, with central blanching.

Pustule: A pustule is a bump-like projection that is filled with purulent fluid.

Condylomatous lesion: A condylomatous lesion is raised, warty, and papillomatous, and may be white, fleshy, or pigmented.

Erythema: Erythema is red discoloration that suggests inflammation.

Ecchymosis: Ecchymosis is black and blue discoloration that occurs after subdermal blood collection.

Other Descriptive Language

Red lesions are characteristically associated with parakeratosis, whereas white lesions are seen with hyperkeratosis. In contrast to the cervix and vagina, pigmentation is a significant finding in a vulvar lesion. Blue-black lesions indicate melanoma, brown lesions indicate nevi, and brown-black-gray lesions indicate intraepithelial neoplasia. The colposcope provides magnification and high-intensity light that permits the examiner to view anatomic structures and lesions in greater detail. This enhanced viewing capability allows the examiner to detect nuances in contour, pigmentation, and vascularity.

CHAPTER 21
Sampling Techniques

As in the cervix and vagina, colposcopic magnification aids the gynecologist in performing biopsy of the vulva. The magnification provided by the colposcope aids the gynecologist in differentiating normal skin, particularly in contoured areas, from abnormal skin. Additionally, small lesions that cannot be seen by the unaided eye can be detected on colposcopic examination.

In the office or clinic setting, a variety of techniques are used to perform vulvar biopsy. Vulvar biopsy requires local anesthesia because the surface of the skin contains many pain nerve endings. More than one biopsy may be required, and specimens should include the transitional areas between normal skin and abnormal tissue.

Approximately 10 to 20 minutes before biopsy is performed, a generous amount of lidocaine and prilocaine cream (EMLA) is applied to provide surface anesthesia. The skin is prepared with povidone–iodine (Betadine). The abnormal tissue is infiltrated with 1% lidocaine (Xylocaine) with the use of a 10-mL syringe and a 1.5-inch-long, 25-gauge needle. The adequacy of anesthesia at the biopsy site is assessed by squeezing the skin with a toothed forceps.

As stated above, several techniques are available for sampling. With the first technique, the skin is elevated with a forceps. A Stevens scissors or a scalpel is used to sever the base of the stretched skin, and a disk-like sample of skin is obtained (Figs. 21-1A to C). The sample is placed in a formalin container, labeled, and sent for pathologic evaluation. The wound is sutured with 3-0 Vicryl or covered with Monsel's solution. The patient is instructed to cleanse the wound daily and to apply hydrogen peroxide with a cotton-tipped swab three times daily.

A second method uses a dermal punch (see Figs. 21-1A to C). The biopsy site is blocked and prepared as described earlier (Fig. 21-2A). The skin at the biopsy site is flattened and spread between the gynecologist's fingers,

and a punch is applied with pressure and twisted to the right and then to the left two to three times (Figs. 21-1A and 21-2B). When the punch is removed, it shows a disk of tissue cut from the surrounding skin. The disk is elevated with forceps, and the base of fat is cut (Figs. 21-1A and 21-2C). The specimen is placed in a jar of formalin. The skin edges are closed with two or three 3-0 Vicryl stitches (Fig. 21-2D).

The third method uses the same punch biopsy clamps that is used for cervical and vaginal sampling. The advantage of this method is the ready availability of the necessary instruments. The techniques for preparation and anesthesia are identical to those described earlier. This method does not require the use of tissue forceps. The biopsy clamp grasps the tissue and cuts simultaneously (Figs. 21-3A to E). After the specimen is obtained, it is placed in formalin. Additional specimens may be obtained at the same site and placed in formalin.

The only disadvantage of this technique compared with the use of scissors or a dermal punch is the potential for crushing tissue at the periphery of the cup bite. Crushing produces artifact in the subsequent microscopic section.

Multicentric lesions that occupy a large area of the vulvar surface require special management. To map the lesion and set treatment margins, multiple biopsy specimens must be obtained. The patient is taken to the operating room and anesthetized. The surgeon creates a numerical map of the lesions with respect to vulvar landmarks. Biopsy specimens are obtained with a knife or scissors and placed in containers that are numbered according to the surgeon's map (Fig. 21-4). A schematic and labeled map or photograph of the vulva, including the biopsy results, is constructed. This map provides a template for subsequent treatment.

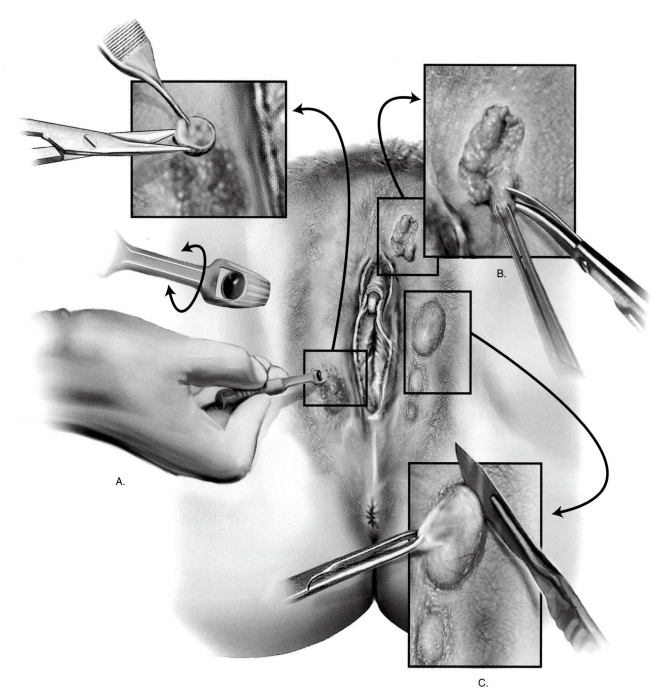

FIGURE 21-1 Several methods for sampling vulvar lesions are seen. **A,** A dermal punch is twisted (as in turning a door key) to cut the skin, and the disk of tissue is lifted away. **B,** Tissue is pulled up with an Allis clamp, and the base is cut off with dissection scissors. **C,** In a similar technique, a knife substitutes for the scissors.

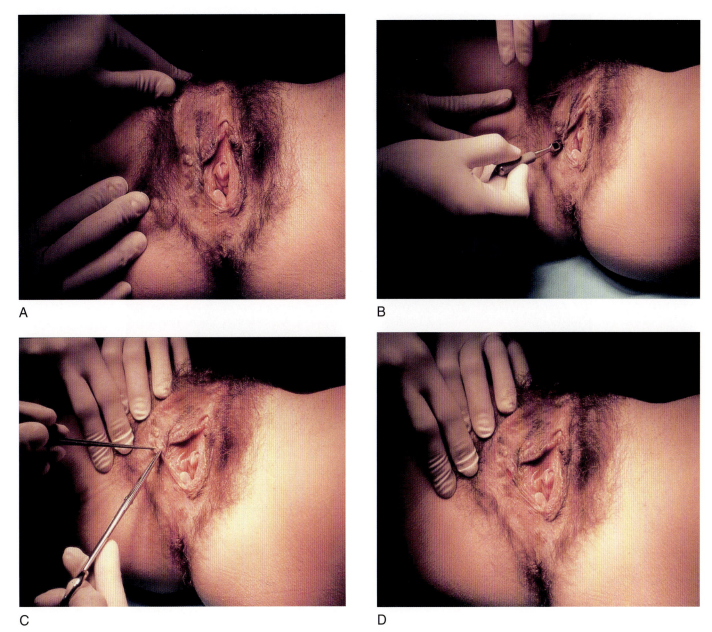

A

B

C

D

FIGURE 21-2 A, The vulva is exposed and flattened to show many pigmented, papillomatous lesions in the interlabial sulcus, labia minora, and perineum. **B,** A dermal punch is applied to the skin and twisted twice. **C,** The cut disk of tissue is elevated with a tissue forceps and cut free from the base with scissors. **D,** The small, circular wound is closed with 3-0 Vicryl sutures.

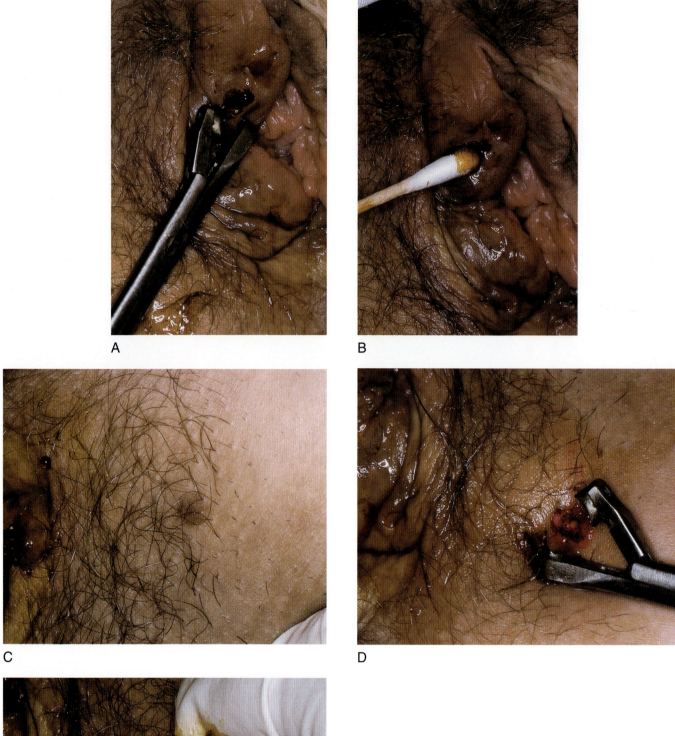

A

B

C

D

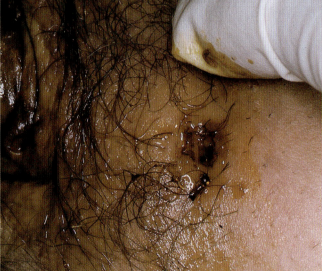

E

FIGURE 21-3 **A,** A biopsy clamp is closed on a lesion located on the labium minus. The labium minus is edematous after the injection of 1% lidocaine (Xylocaine). **B,** After a biopsy specimen is obtained, a cotton-tipped applicator soaked in Monsel's solution is placed in the wound crater. **C,** This perineal lesion may be a nevus, and biopsy is needed. **D,** Bleeding is seen after the biopsy is performed. **E,** Excellent hemostasis is obtained by applying Monsel's solution with a small, cotton-tipped applicator.

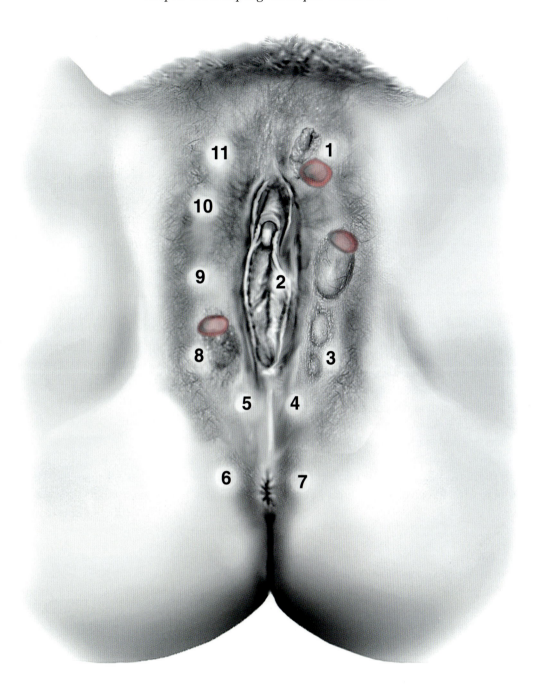

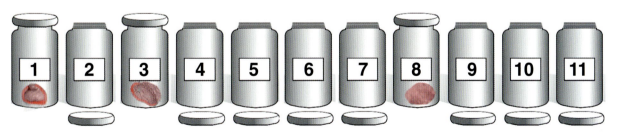

FIGURE 21-4 Mapping of the vulva is required for multicentric lesions that extend over a large surface area. Each site and specimen are numbered, and each specimen is placed in a numbered jar that contains formalin.

CHAPTER 22
Case Examples

Case 1

A 26-year-old pregnant woman who had itching and vulvar discomfort was treated twice with topical antifungal agents. The infant was delivered at 39 weeks' gestation and had a generalized rash and respiratory difficulty within 24 hours. *Candida stellatoidea* was cultured from the infant, who was treated with intravenous amphotericin B. Examination showed that the mother had fungal vulvitis and vaginitis. The infection resolved after 2 weeks of treatment with fluconazole (Diflucan) (Figs. 22-1A and D).

Case 2

A 30-year-old woman had a 5-year history of dyspareunia and vulvar pruritus. The itching had become worse during the last 12 months. She took antifungal medication continuously for more than 1 year because of what was believed to be a chronic yeast infection (Fig. 22-2).

Case 3

A 29-year-old woman had a 10-year history of lichen sclerosus. She underwent dexamethasone (Decadron) injections, but missed several appointments. After an absence of 8 months, she returned to the office with clitoral pain (Fig. 22-3).

Case 4

A 59-year-old woman had severe vulvar itching for 1 year. It did not respond to treatment. The patient was especially uncomfortable at night and tore at the vulva to relieve the itching. Eventually, she began to wear white cotton gloves to bed (Figs. 22-4A and C).

Case 5

A 60-year-old woman had constant burning of the vulva, stinging on urination, and occasional bleeding after wiping. She could not recall when the symptoms began, but stated that she had not engaged in sexual activity for at least 2 years. Her primary gynecologist prescribed testosterone ointment, but application of the ointment only made the burning worse (Figs. 22-5A to D).

Case 6

An 18-year old woman had clitoral discomfort and no sexual feeling. She stated that she injured her genitals as a child by falling on a bicycle. As a result of this injury, the clitoris became swollen and remained enlarged (Figs. 22-6A and B).

Case 7

A 42-year-old woman had severe vulvar itching. Several treatments, including oral and topical antifungal agents, did not resolve the problem (Fig. 22-7).

Case 8

A 25-year-old woman had vulvar itching that she thought was caused by a yeast infection. Seven days later, she had increasingly severe pain. When she arrived for evaluation, she could not stand even the touch of her underwear on her vulva (Fig. 22-8).

Case 9

A 28-year-old woman had a progressive increase in the number of what she considered vulvar warts. She was angry that she had warts because she and her husband had a long-standing, monogamous relationship (Figs. 22-9A to D).

Case 10

A 40-year-old woman had a chronic, red, granulating lesion on the left labium majus. She had a long history of Crohn's disease that was in remission (Fig. 22-10).

Case 11

A pregnant woman in her mid-thirties had extensive genital warts. The lesions persisted after delivery (Figs. 22-11*A* and *B*).

Case 12

An 86-year-old woman was referred from a nursing home because of a "sore bottom." She had constant burning of the vulvar area and stated that urination was particularly uncomfortable. Her primary care physician had performed a biopsy that showed condylomata acuminata. She was referred to a gynecologist, who performed a biopsy on a warty lesion. The biopsy report confirmed the diagnosis of benign condylomata acuminata (Figs. 22-12*A* and *B*).

Case 13

A 79-year-old woman had long-standing pruritus and vulvar discomfort. The extensive red lesion suggests Paget's disease of the vulva. Pathologic examination of multiple biopsy specimens confirmed the diagnosis (Figs. 22-13*A* and *B*).

Case 14

A young Ethiopian woman had a draining sinus at the lower margin of the right labium majus. The tract was investigated under fluoroscopy and was probed 8 cm deep but was just lateral to the rectum. Contrast placed into the rectum and into a cannula within the tract showed no connection to the bowel (Figs. 22-14*A* and *B*).

Case 15

A 50-year-old woman was treated for vulvar carcinoma in situ of the perineum and labia minora. Colposcopic examination showed extensive darkly pigmented perianal lesions that suggested vulvar intraepithelial neoplasia (Figs. 22-15*A* to *C*).

Case 16

A 64-year old woman underwent colposcopy because of chronic vulvar pruritus. Examination showed many multifocal, raised, pigmented lesions. Biopsy showed carcinoma in situ (Figs. 22-16*A* to *E*).

Case 17

A 33-year-old woman who underwent vulvar excision with skin grafting 5 years earlier was referred for colposcopy because of condylomatous lesions (Figs. 22-17*A* and *B*).

Case 18

A 44-year old woman had perianal itching and a "raw" feeling in the area below the vaginal opening (Fig. 22-18).

Case 19

A 41-year-old woman had a persistent gray, raised, flattened lesion that occupied approximately 25% of the right labium majus. Biopsy showed carcinoma in situ (Fig. 22-19).

Case 20

A 28-year-old woman had a persistent "warty lesion" that recurred after she was treated twice with trichloroacetic acid and once with electrosurgery. She had no symptoms and no history of sexually transmitted disease, but she wanted to have the lesions removed. Preoperative biopsy revealed carcinoma in situ (Figs. 22-20*A* and *B*).

Case 21

A 19-year old woman who was 13 weeks' pregnant had rapid growth of genital warts that occurred with the onset of pregnancy. She stated that the vulva was heavy, wet, and irritated, and that urination caused stinging. In consultation with the patient's obstetrician, the decision was made not to treat the warts during the pregnancy (Figs. 22-21*A* and *B*).

Case 22

A 38-year-old patient had warty lesions on the perineum that were detected during a routine physical examination. Although she was treated 11 times over the course of 1 year, first with podophyllum and then with trichloroacetic acid, the warty lesions persisted (Figs. 22-22*A* to *C*).

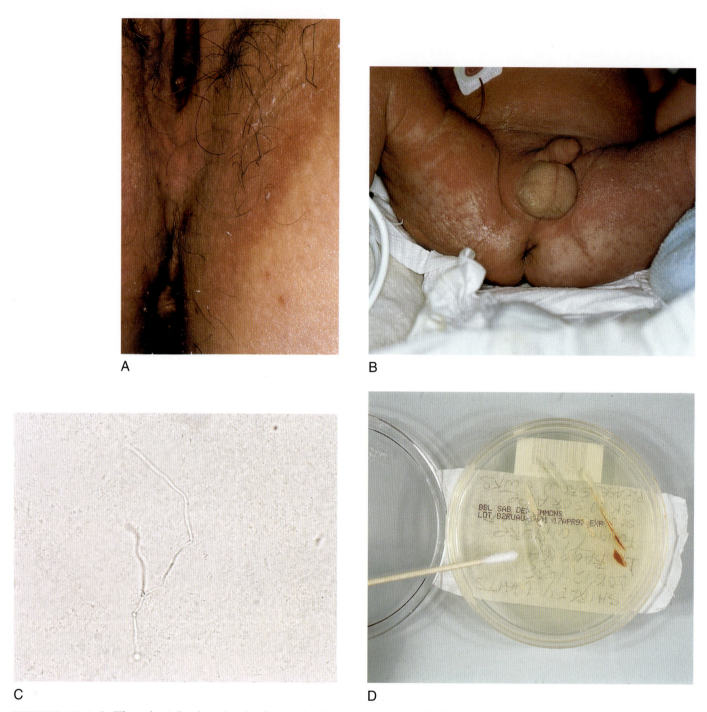

FIGURE 22-1 A, The vulva is bright red and inflamed. Scaling within the area of inflammation strongly suggests fungal infection. The skin was scraped with a scalpel onto fungal culture medium. **B,** The infant was covered with a red, papular rash that had some areas of scaling. Cultures obtained from the infant's skin, nose, mouth, respiratory tract, and gastrointestinal tract grew *Candida* species. **C,** The potassium hydroxide preparation from the mother's vagina shows branching mycelia and buds. **D,** Positive fungal identification was made by culturing maternal skin scrapings onto Sabouraud's agar.

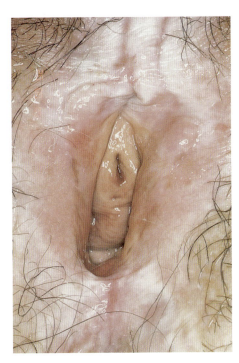

FIGURE 22-2 Colposcopic findings suggest lichen sclerosus. The interlabial, periclitoral, and perineal areas are white. Extensive agglutination is seen between the labia, the clitoral hood, and the skin of the anterior and posterior commissures. Fissure formation is evident near the commissure and perineum.

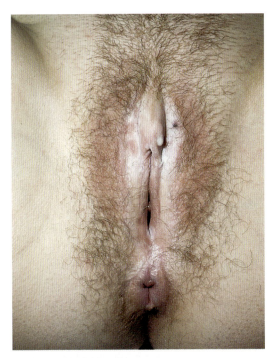

FIGURE 22-3 The clitoris is enlarged. The skin pallor and agglutination of the tissues are characteristic of lichen sclerosus. The clitoris was completely sealed off by the agglutinated hood. Surgery was performed to drain pus from within the sealed hood. Definitive surgery to remove scar tissue and relocate the clitoris was performed later.

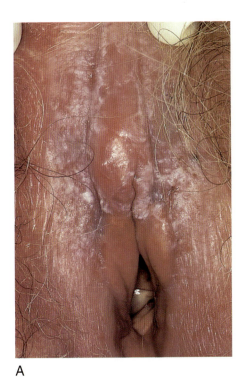

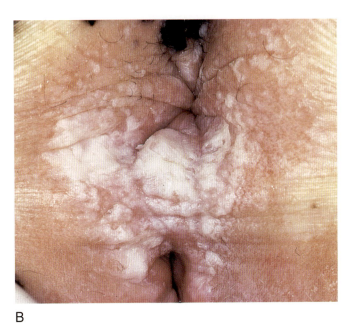

A   B

FIGURE 22-4 **A,** The vulva is red as a result of acute and subacute vulvitis. White plaques are seen on the labia and periclitoral tissues. Biopsy showed lichen simplex chronicus. Treatment included cleansing with Instant Ocean and hexachlorophene (pHisoHex) twice a day, and application of silver sulfadiazine cream (Silvadene) three times a day and at bedtime. After this phase of treatment was completed, fluticasone propionate (Cutivate) cream was applied twice a day for 2 weeks. This treatment was repeated for another 2 weeks. **B,** Thickened, white areas of hyperkeratosis are seen. The initial diagnosis was lichen simplex rather than vulvar squamous hyperplasia. (continued)

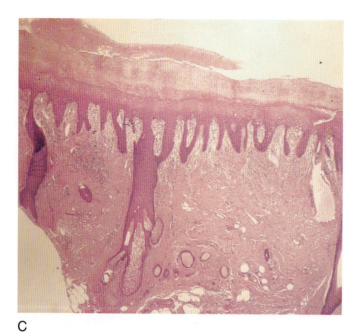

C

FIGURE 22-4 C, However, a microscopic section (×2) shows thickened epidermis and a thick layer of hyperkeratosis. The underlying cells are hyperplastic, and deep rete pegs are seen. The correct diagnosis was squamous hyperplasia.

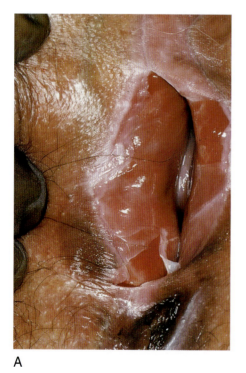

A

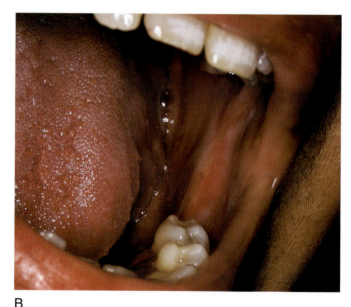

B

FIGURE 22-5 A, The vestibule has only a paper-thin covering of skin that has peeled away at the level of the posterior fourchette, exposing the raw dermis. These findings are consistent with erosive lichen planus. **B,** Examination of the buccal mucosa shows similar ulceration. (continued)

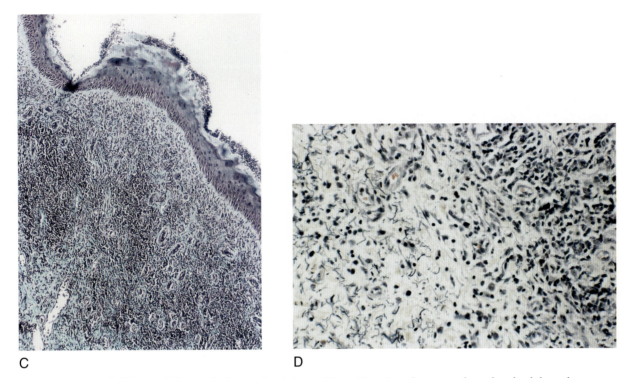

C   D

FIGURE 22-5 C, Biopsy of the vestibule seen in *A* shows thin epidermis and a severe dermal and subdermal inflammatory infiltrate. **D,** Reticulum staining shows interruption of the reticular network of stromal support as well as an extensive chronic inflammatory infiltrate.

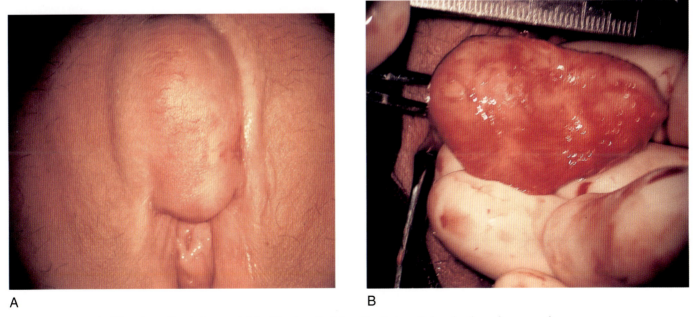

A   B

FIGURE 22-6 A, The glans clitoris is not visible. The hood of the clitoris is sealed and enlarged to several times its normal size. The mass was slightly tender to touch. **B,** At surgery, a large cystic mass was microscopically dissected free from the body and glans of the clitoris. The clitoris was normal. The cyst was an epidermal inclusion cyst.

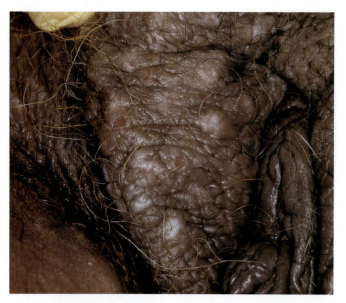

FIGURE 22-7 Many bumps are seen on the mons veneris and labia majora. This distribution is characteristic of Fox-Fordyce disease. Biopsy confirmed the diagnosis. The patient was treated with tretinoin (Retin-A) and systemic estrogen and became asymptomatic.

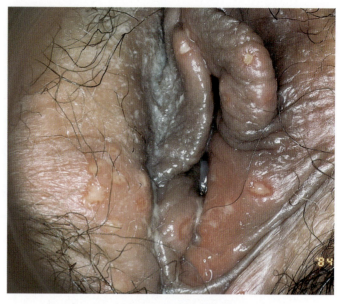

FIGURE 22-8 The vulva has several red-rimmed, punched-out ulcers. The ulcers are widespread and involve the labia, perineum, and vestibule. These lesions are characteristic of herpes simplex infection. Herpes simplex type 2 antibody titers were elevated, and culture findings were positive.

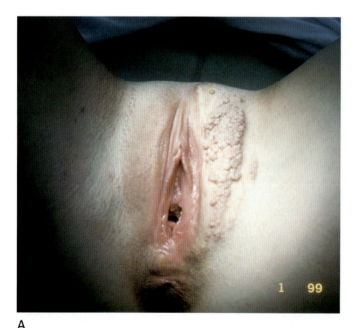

A

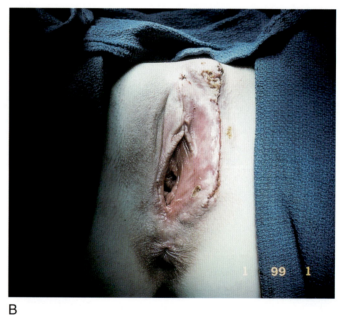

B

FIGURE 22-9 A, The entire right side of the vulva contains many homogenous, rounded, pebble-like lesions that resemble a cluster of grapes. These lesions clearly are not warts. **B,** The vulva is seen immediately after excision of the right labium majus. (continued)

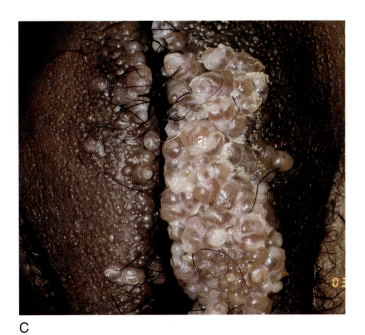

C

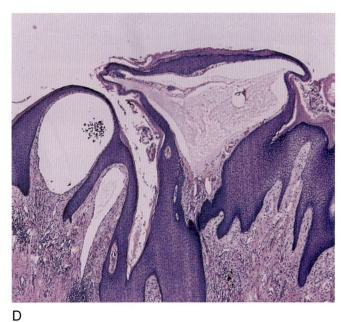

D

FIGURE 22-9 C, A close-up view of another patient who had a similar lesion that affected both labia. These lesions are consistent with lymphangioma of the vulva. **D,** A microscopic section of the lesions seen in *C* shows dilated subepidermal lymphatics. The diagnosis was lymphangioma, or lymphectasia.

FIGURE 22-10 Colposcopic examination of this lesion showed a small opening. A baby Hegar dilator was inserted, and the probe easily traced a path to the anus. This type of rectocutaneous fistula is commonly associated with Crohn's disease.

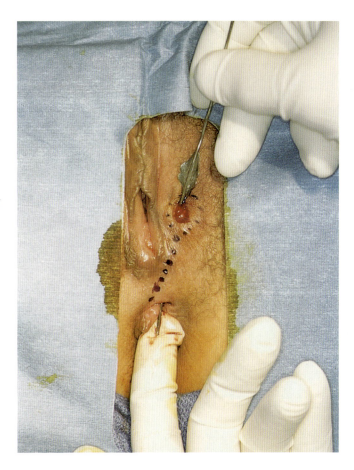

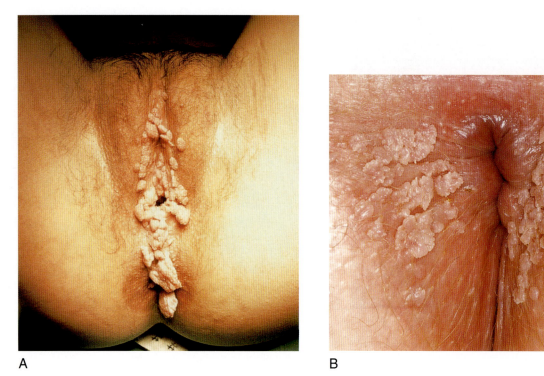

A

B

FIGURE 22-11 **A,** Condylomata acuminata lesions fill the vestibule and involve the labia majora, labia minora, and perianal skin. **B,** A close-up view of the perianal condylomata shows their regular pattern and symmetrical distribution. A butterfly-like pattern is created by autoinoculation by the human papillomavirus.

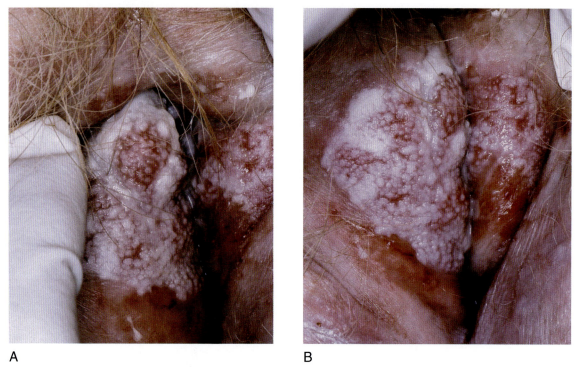

A

B

FIGURE 22-12 **A,** A white, condylomatous lesion occupies the greater part of the right labium majus and minus and extends across the vestibule to involve the left labia. The vulva is red and inflamed. **B,** A magnified view of the lesion seen in *A*. Deep excisional biopsy showed invasive squamous cell carcinoma.

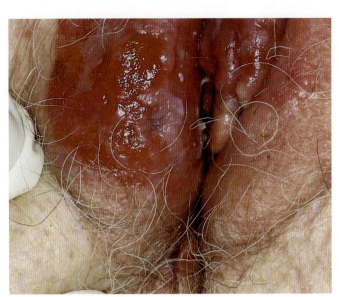
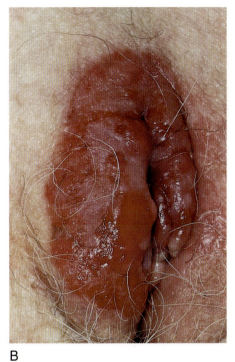

A

B

FIGURE 22-13 **A,** These labia are abnormal. A deep red lesion occupies the right and left labia, and the surface is slightly raised. **B,** A full frontal view of the labia seen in *A*. An extensive lesion covers the right labium majus and the left labium minus. Multiple biopsies confirmed the diagnosis of Paget's disease of the vulva.

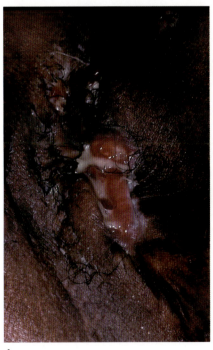
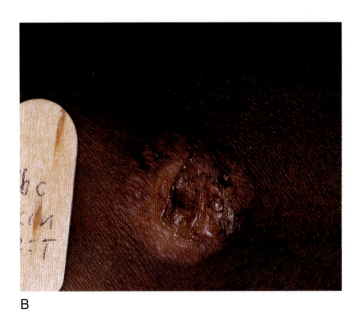

A

B

FIGURE 22-14 **A,** Culture of the pus-like material obtained from the tract showed acid-fast bacteria. Biopsy showed acute and chronic inflammation. **B,** Tuberculin skin test showed 2-cm induration and ulceration at 48 hours.

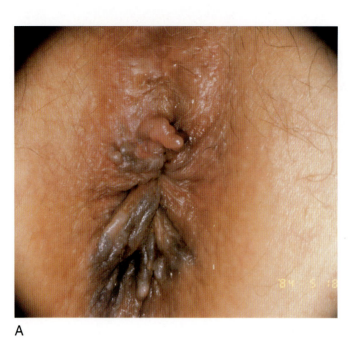

A

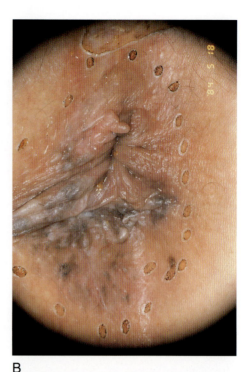

B

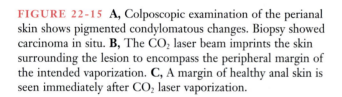

FIGURE 22-15 A, Colposcopic examination of the perianal skin shows pigmented condylomatous changes. Biopsy showed carcinoma in situ. **B,** The CO_2 laser beam imprints the skin surrounding the lesion to encompass the peripheral margin of the intended vaporization. **C,** A margin of healthy anal skin is seen immediately after CO_2 laser vaporization.

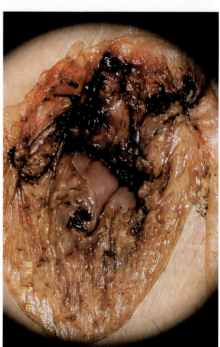

C

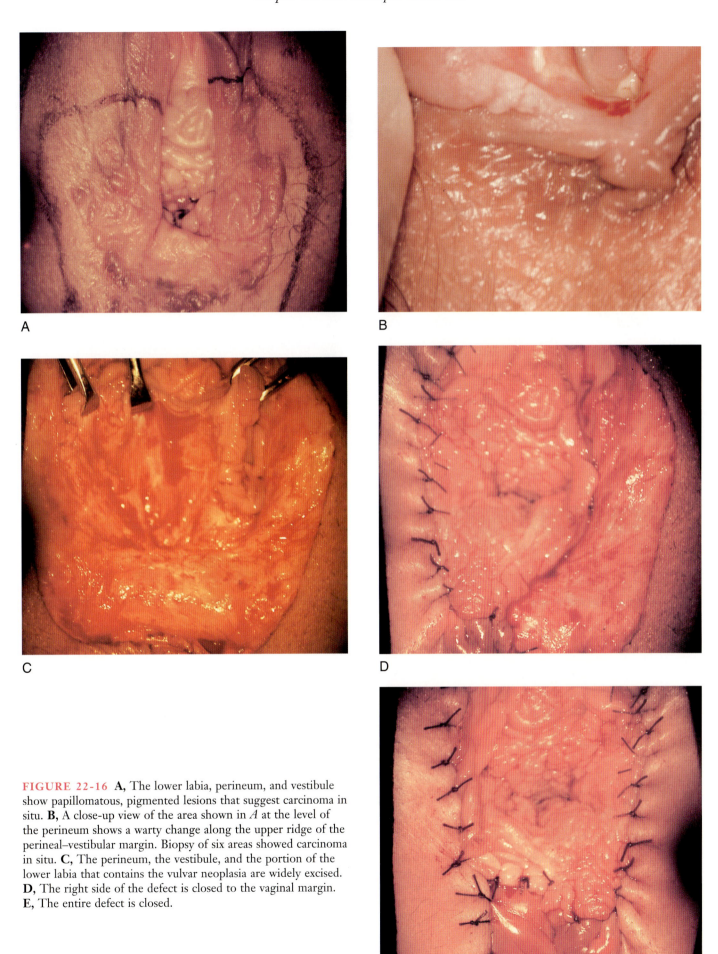

FIGURE 22-16 A, The lower labia, perineum, and vestibule show papillomatous, pigmented lesions that suggest carcinoma in situ. **B,** A close-up view of the area shown in *A* at the level of the perineum shows a warty change along the upper ridge of the perineal–vestibular margin. Biopsy of six areas showed carcinoma in situ. **C,** The perineum, the vestibule, and the portion of the lower labia that contains the vulvar neoplasia are widely excised. **D,** The right side of the defect is closed to the vaginal margin. **E,** The entire defect is closed.

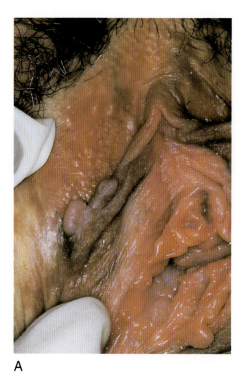

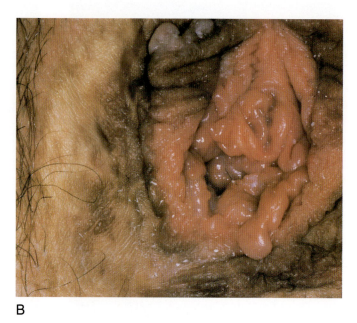

A   B

FIGURE 22-17 **A,** Colposcopic examination shows two pigmented, atypical warty lesions on the edge of the right labium minus. Excisional biopsy showed carcinoma in situ. **B,** The pigmented area of the labia majora, especially the interlabial sulcus, suggests neoplasia. Biopsy showed cellular atypia and hyperplasia.

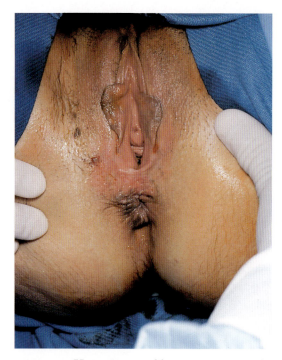

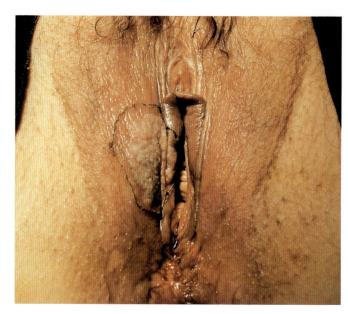

FIGURE 22-18 Hyperpigmented lesions are seen on the right labium majus and the perianal skin. The perineal skin also is deep pink, thickened, and slightly macerated. Biopsy of the perineum and perianal skin showed vulvar intraepithelial neoplasia grade 3, and biopsy of the lesion on the labium majus showed vulvar intraepithelial neoplasia grade 1.

FIGURE 22-19 The large, gray lesion of the right labium majus and labium minus has a flat, warty configuration. The pigmentary changes suggest neoplasia. Biopsy showed vulvar intraepithelial neoplasia grade 3 and confirmed the clinical impression.

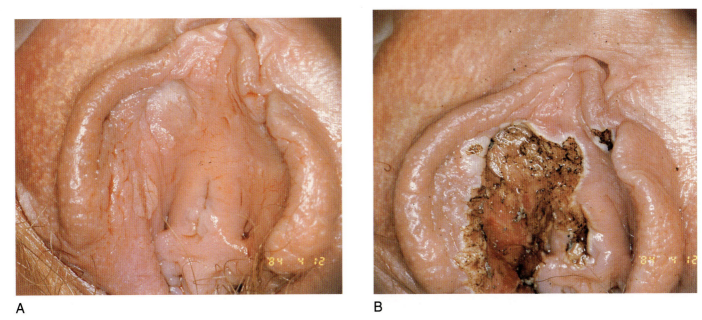

A

B

FIGURE 22-20 **A,** The white, flat papillomas that occupy the right vestibule do not have the characteristics of benign warts. Biopsy showed vulvar intraepithelial neoplasia. **B,** A CO_2 laser was used to vaporize the lesions seen in *A* to a depth of 2 to 3 mm, with wide margins.

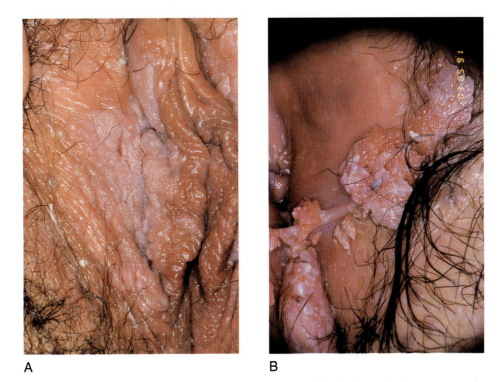

A

B

FIGURE 22-21 **A,** Confluent warts are seen in the interlabial sulcus. Fleshy warts extend to the labia majora, labia minora, and periclitoral tissues. Biopsy showed benign condylomata. **B,** Four weeks after delivery, the warts persisted and were treated with a CO_2 laser.

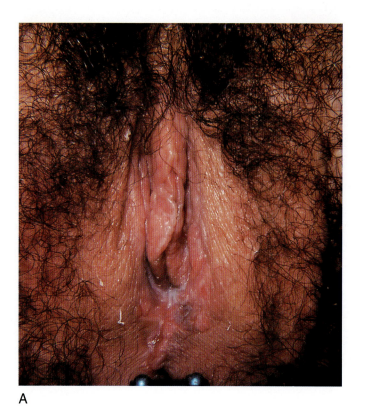

A

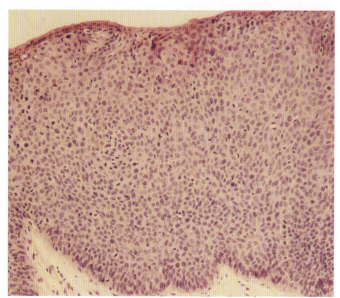

B

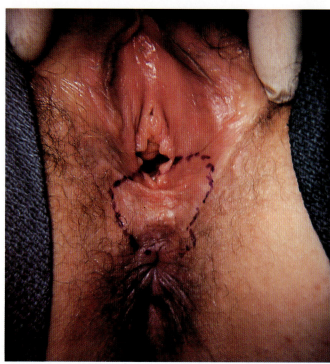

C

FIGURE 22-22 A, Condylomatous lesions are seen at the posterior commissure and on the perineum. A fissure is seen within an area of thickened, darkly pigmented skin. **B,** A section obtained from the pigmented perineal tissue shows thickening of the epidermis to 1.5 mm. No cellular organization is seen. Many epithelial cells show hyperchromatic, enlarged nuclei. The parakeratotic cells constitute the top three to four cellular layers. The diagnosis was squamous cell carcinoma in situ. **C,** The patient shown in *A* and *B* is seen before surgical treatment was performed. Surgical options include sharp resection, laser vaporization, and a combination of excision and vaporization.

SECTION III
Treatment of Intraepithelial Neoplasia

CHAPTER 23
Treatment of Cervical Intraepithelial Neoplasia

Several treatment options that range from conservative to radical are used to treat cervical intraepithelial neoplasia (CIN). The most conservative option includes careful monitoring of the cytologic findings, human papilloma virus typing, and colposcopy at regular intervals. This method is appropriate for patients who have low-grade disease (CIN grade 1, or condylomatous atypia) and no evidence of dysplasia within the endocervical canal. However, it is not appropriate for the management of intraepithelial glandular disease. Additionally, this approach requires a compliant patient who understands the need for follow-up every 6 months.

Hysterectomy is both the most radical therapy and the most illogical approach. Typically, CIN is confined to the cervical epithelium and rarely extends to the endometrial cavity. High-grade intraepithelial neoplasia rarely propagates more than 1.5 cm up the endocervical canal from the squamocolumnar junction. Finally, intraepithelial neoplasia is not a life-threatening condition. When performed to treat CIN, which typically affects only a finite portion of the cervix, hysterectomy unnecessarily sacrifices the uterus. Hysterectomy is an appropriate option for the treatment of CIN only when the patient has a coexisting pathologic condition in addition, e.g. symptomatic prolapse, pelvic congestion syndrome, or the desire for surgical sterilization.

Between these two extremes exist several good treatment options, including cryosurgery, laser conization, laser vaporization, electrical loop excision, and sharp scalpel conization.

Because CIN affects young, fertile women, many factors must be considered when making treatment decisions. The need for surgical intervention must be weighed against the sacrifice of cervical length and volume. Treatment of a condylomatous or minimally dysplastic disorder that is neither life-threatening nor

likely to progress does not justify the virtual amputation of a young woman's cervix.

Indications for Treatment

CIN is a continuum of disease that begins as a unifocal cellular aberration at the squamocolumnar junction. It spreads either into the endocervical canal or, less commonly, out onto the portio. The dysplastic cells tend to migrate from the junction and do not become multifocal. In other words, no skip areas of normal epithelium are seen between contiguous areas of dysplastic cells. The pattern of spread into the canal is affected by the configuration of the endocervical epithelium and clefts, or glands. The endocervical canal is lined by a single, continuous layer of columnar mucous epithelium. Its surface area is increased by folds and clefts that may make deep inroads, up to 1 cm, into the underlying stroma. In a study of many conization specimens, the mean depth of the clefts that were infiltrated by neoplastic cells was 3 mm from the surface (Fig. 23-1A).

To achieve negative upper (endocervical) margins, the surgeon must know the extent to which neoplastic cells ascend the endocervical canal from their origin at the squamocolumnar junction. Unfortunately, to determine the extent of neoplastic penetration, the tissue specimen must be cut, stained, and studied under a microscope. Studies show that extension of carcinoma in situ from the squamocolumnar junction into the endocervical canal rarely exceeds 1.5 cm (15 mm). Therefore, by obtaining a 1.5-cm-high cone specimen, the surgeon should remove 99% of the CIN that extends into the canal (Fig. 23-1B). To treat squamous intraepithelial neoplasia, only a small portion of the total cervical volume must be destroyed or removed.

Specifications for Treatment

The following treatment model is proposed:

Specification 1 To obtain an accurate view of the entire abnormal transformation zone, colposcopy is performed during the treatment phase.

Specification 2 The peripheral margins of the abnormal transformation zone are determined and marked. A 3-mm margin is obtained around the abnormal transformation zone to allow for glandular involvement.

Specification 3 For low-grade disorders, which are not likely to extend into the canal, an endocervical margin of 1 cm is adequate.

Specification 4 For high-grade lesions, an endocervical margin of 1.5 cm is required.

Specification 5 Excisional techniques are considered superior to ablative techniques because they provide a pathologic specimen.

Specification 6 Among excisional techniques, when compared to non-energy techniques, energy devices (e.g., electrosurgery, laser) provide acceptable histologic results at the endocervical, ectocervical, and peripheral (depth) margins.

Excisional Techniques

Sharp Conization

Sharp knife conization is one of the oldest techniques used to diagnose and treat CIN. Before the colposcope was introduced in the United States, conization was performed after Lugol's solution was applied to the cervix to aid the operator in identifying the peripheral margins. In the 1950s and 1960s, a cone specimen was a geometric cone that typically was at least 2 cm high. The goal of the cone procedure was to remove all possible dysplasia, and the vectored height was aimed at the internal cervical os. These procedures were bloody, and the use of large mass ligatures to control bleeding led to distortion and stenosis of the cervix (Fig. 23-2A). The modern (contemporary) cold knife procedure includes the use of vasoconstrictors and lateral sutures to decrease intraoperative and postoperative bleeding. The height and configuration of cones have changed to reflect a

more conservative approach, and the typical cone rarely exceeds 1.5 cm in height. The configuration of the specimen is based on the extent of disease as visualized colposcopically, and shapes vary from short, stubby cones to cylinders (Fig. 23-2B). The goal is to excise disease while preserving a functional volume of cervix. The margins of the cone are plotted colposcopically with the use of acetic acid or Lugol's solution. The endocervical margin is based on the findings of previous endocervical sampling.

The old mass ligature technique has been replaced by the use of marginal running, or reefing, Vicryl sutures or colposcopically guided Vicryl suture ligatures that are placed at specific bleeding sites at the end of the procedure (Figs. 23-3A to D).

The technique for handling the postoperative specimen should be discussed with the pathologist in advance of the procedure. The specimen should be minimally traumatized by forceps and minimally handled by the surgeon. Most pathologists prefer the specimen to be wrapped in a saline-soaked sponge and sent to the pathology laboratory immediately for gross inspection and sectioning (Figs. 23-3E and F). Alternatively, the specimen may be opened at the 12 o'clock position, pinned to a cork that is inverted into a formalin solution, and sent to the laboratory.

Laser Excisional Conization

The CO_2 laser is a precision instrument that may be directly coupled to the colposcope and controlled with a micromanipulator (Fig. 23-4A). Proper operation of this device requires advanced training and skill. The degree of thermal injury that occurs at the tissue margins varies inversely with the hand–eye coordination of the surgeon and the sophistication of the laser instruments. Some reports do not adequately consider these factors. However, unskilled surgeons who use outdated equipment will obtain mediocre results.

A well-trained laser surgeon who uses a superpulse CO_2 laser will obtain a more precise cone than the same surgeon would obtain with a scalpel. A laser causes little blood loss, but the specimen may have thermal artifact that measures a fraction of a millimeter. The minimal thermal artifact permits accurate identification of the endocervical, ectocervical, and peripheral margins within the excised specimen (Fig. 23-4B).

A straightforward technique is used for CO_2 laser conization. The abnormal transformation zone is identified colposcopically (Figs. 23-4C and D). This area of the cervix is injected circumferentially and distally with a 1:100 diluted solution of vasopressin (Pitressin). Approximately 10 to 15 mL of this solution is injected. The diluent is 1% lidocaine (Xylocaine) if the cone is performed under local anesthesia. The laser beam is used to trace the peripheral extent of the cone around the squamocolumnar junction (Fig. 23-4*E*). The diameter of the laser beam should be 1 mm or less, and the beam should be delivered by superpulse to minimize thermal injury. The trace cut is extended deeper into the cervical stroma, and a long-handled titanium hook is used to pull the stroma at one of the cut edges to allow the laser beam to cut and sculpt the cone so that it bevels inward toward the endocervical canal (Fig. 23-4*F*). This technique is performed at the 12 o'clock, 3 o'clock, 6 o'clock, and 9 o'clock positions to a depth of 1.5 cm. The endocervical canal is cut with a laser beam or a scalpel (Figs. 23-4*G* and *H*). The procedure is performed under colposcopic magnification, and the laser micromanipulator is directly attached to the body of the microscope. Because the laser and the microscope have identical focal distances, this technique provides the best possible view of the cervix (Fig. 23-4*A*). A single-hinged laser speculum with a built-in smoke evacuation capability is the best accessory to facilitate the performance of this operation (Fig. 23-4*I*).

Laser Combination Conization

Extensive abnormal transformation zones may envelop a large portion of the ectocervix (≥ 75% of its surface) and extend into the endocervical canal. A conventional excisional cone procedure would functionally remove the entire cervix. However, a combination cone procedure relies on the findings of previous colposcopically directed ectocervical biopsy to ensure that only intraepithelial disease is present on the visible portion of the cervix.

A 1.5-cm-high cylindrical conization is performed according to the technique described for the CO_2 laser. After a cone specimen is obtained, a superpulse laser beam is used to perform graded vaporization of the external disease. Far out on the portio, the depth of vaporization averages approximately 3 mm, whereas closer to the canal, it is 5 to 7 mm. Disease that extends into the vaginal fornices is vaporized in that location to a depth of 1 mm or less (Figs. 23-5*A* to *H*). The laser combination cone procedure preserves cervical volume and structure while eliminating intraepithelial neoplasia.

Electrical Loop Excision

Cartier described this technique and used it for many years before Prendiville described large loop excision of the abnormal transformation zone. Large loop excision was used in Europe before its "discovery" in the United States between 1989 and 1991. Advantages of electrical loop excision include its simplicity, relatively low expense, and short learning curve. Because electrical loop excision requires far less skill and hand–eye coordination than the use of a CO_2 laser, the technique is ideal for the average gynecologist. Additionally, family practitioners and pathologists can perform this simple operation. However, the simplicity of the procedure belies its inherent vulnerability because unnecessary and excessive cervical excision occurs in 10% or more of cases.

Loop electrodes are available in a variety of shapes and sizes. The best loops are constructed of 0.2-mm-diameter tungsten steel (Figs. 23-6*A* to *C*). The height of the loop should be set at 1 cm or less. Small loops for endocervical excision are no more than 5 mm high. The surgeon must exercise judgment when performing any cervical excision, especially electrical loop excision (Fig. 23-6*D*). For example, an 8- to 10-mm excision of the abnormal transformation zone may be appropriate for a mature woman whose cervix is 3 to 4 cm high, but the same excision will virtually amputate the cervix of an adolescent girl. The surgeon cannot simply excise a prescribed amount of cervix in every case of premalignant cervical disease. Further, loop excision should be performed under colposcopic guidance.

Several preliminary steps are necessary before excision is performed. After 3% to 4% acetic acid is applied to the cervix, colposcopic examination is performed to map the peripheral extent of the abnormal transformation zone. After the boundaries of the excision are determined, a mixture that contains a local anesthetic agent and a vasoconstrictor is injected into the cervix. Multiple injections of a 1:100 solution of vasopressin are made along the peripheral marginal line, thus marking this area with a series of pinpricks (Figs. 23-6*E* to *G*).

The diameter of the loop must be large enough to encompass the mapped lesion. The cutting current of the electrosurgical generator is set at 35 to 60 W. A setting of 50 W pure cut is recommended. The electrode is placed against the cervix, and the power is activated (Fig. 23-6*H*). The electrode is guided through the tissue as the entire transformation zone is excised to a depth of 8 to 10 mm (Figs. 23-6*I* and *J*).

When selective double excision is performed to treat high-grade disease, a loop that measures 5 × 6 mm or 5 × 7 mm is used to obtain a second excisional specimen of the endocervical canal (Figs. 23-6*K* to *Q*). After cervical excision is complete, the specimens are placed in formalin-containing jars. A ball electrode is substituted for the loop. The generator is set for spray coagulation, or fulguration, at 50 to 60 W. A dry swab is used to compress the bleeding vessels at the excisional site (Fig. 23-6*R*). As the swab is lifted from the cervix, a ball electrode is inserted and the coagulation current is activated. Non-touch coagulation seals vessels without penetrating deeply into the cervix (Fig. 23-6*S*). This technique limits coagulation necrosis to 1 to 2 mm. Prolonged coagulation, forced coagulation, and the application of large amounts of caustic solutions can cause additional necrotic injury. In contrast, the use of the correct technique, adequate power, and a short dwell time results in minimal thermal artifact and provides an accurate pathologic evaluation of the specimen (Figs. 23-6*T* to *V*).

Ablative Techniques

Several ablative procedures are used. The principal disadvantage of these techniques is that they do not provide a specimen for pathologic evaluation. In particular, with these techniques, the endocervical canal, which is the nonvisible portion of the cervix, cannot be studied effectively. Another disadvantage of ablative techniques is the ill-defined and ill-controlled tissue destruction that is caused by elimination of the intraepithelial neoplasia.

Ablative techniques range from fine to rugged, and are simpler, faster, and more hemostatic than excisional techniques. However, ablative techniques are less precise, and the degree of stromal damage is greater and may be unpredictable. Further, stromal damage may vary widely from case to case. The rate of late complications, such as reduced cervical length and volume and cervical stenosis, is greater than with contemporary and measured excisional procedures.

Cryosurgery

The popularity of this technique peaked in the late 1960s and early 1970s (Fig. 23-7*A*). A probe is inserted into the cervix, and the passage and compression of gas is used to freeze the cervical tissue around the probe in a three-dimensional fashion (Fig. 23-7*B*). This process is sometimes described as the formation of an ice ball as the water in the cell crystallizes in response to the subfreezing temperature of the tissue (Fig. 23-7*C*). Initially, Freon gas was used in commercial models. Later models used N_2O or CO_2. Typically, the cervix is frozen to between −30°C and −50°C. The size of the ice ball is monitored by watching the frost line expand on the outer edge of the cryoprobe tip (Fig. 23-7*D*).

Various techniques have been described based on a minimum of scientific evidence. The two most common techniques include a single freeze followed by a gradual thaw and a freeze-thaw–freeze-thaw technique. Cryosurgery causes a large area of cervical necrosis and substantial vascular injury (Fig. 23-7*E*).

CO₂ Laser Vaporization

This technique directs laser beams to tissue and causes rapid boiling of intracellular water, conversion to steam,

and explosive evaporation. The technique is performed under colposcopic guidance with a micromanipulator. Compared with cryosurgery, this technique is more precise in terms of the volume of tissue vaporized. Precise depth and peripheral control is possible because the amount of surrounding thermal artifact, or heat injury, is limited to 500 μm beyond the zone of vaporization. Further, the CO_2 laser beam is well absorbed by water. Because water absorbs laser energy, it limits thermal propagation, and decreases necrosis.

Before the procedure is performed, the patient must undergo biopsy and endocervical curettage to exclude invasive disease or disease within the endocervical canal. Colposcopic examination is performed, and a laser beam that has a 1.5- to 2-mm spot diameter is used to trace the peripheral limit of vaporization onto the cervix (Figs. 23-8*A* and *B*). If the patient is sensitive to the action of the laser on the cervix, 1% Xylocaine may be injected directly into the cervix to produce anesthesia. The laser energy is set at 60 and 80 W continuous or 12 to 20 W superpulse. Vaporization is performed systematically, quadrant by quadrant, to a depth of 7 to 10 mm, with a 3-mm peripheral margin that circumscribes the abnormal transformation zone (Figs. 23-8*C* and *D*).

Electrocoagulation

This technique uses a monopolar generator and a variety of electrodes to coagulate rather than excise tissue. Tissue temperatures are less than 100°C. Implements such as needle electrodes, ball electrodes, and true electrocautery probes are used (Fig. 23-9*A*). Electrocoagulation probably is the oldest procedure designed to destroy cervical tissue locally. This technique also is the least sophisticated and least selective in terms of controlling tissue damage (Figs. 23-9*B* to *D*). However, the technique is simple, inexpensive, and adapted for office use. It can cure intraepithelial neoplasia, but also may eradicate a functional cervix by destroying a large volume of normal tissue.

A cold coagulator heats an element that subsequently transfers the heat to surrounding tissues through simple conduction. This instrument is a cautery in the sense that a hot poker is a cautery. Cold coagulation is a misnomer. This device clearly does not work cryogenically, and in fact, it burns tissue. The difference between this simple device and an electrosurgical unit is that electrical current is not conducted through the tissue by the "cold" coagulator, but spreads randomly outward from the heating element through radiant conduction.

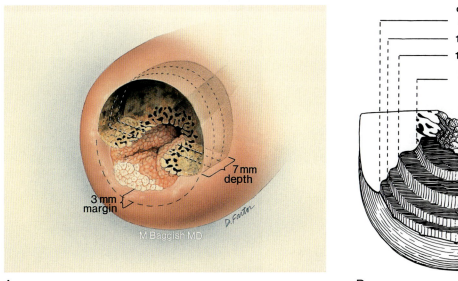
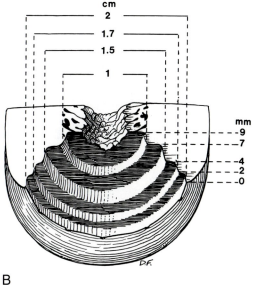

A   **B**

FIGURE 23-1 **A,** A three-dimensional view shows penetration of cervical intraepithelial neoplasia into the endocervical canal. The endocervical clefts, or glands, penetrate the underlying stroma to a mean depth of 3 mm. The lesion extends less than 0.5 cm. High-grade lesions rarely extend more than 10 mm to 15 mm up the canal. **B,** This treatment schema is based on the differential depth from the ectocervix to the squamocolumnar junction and includes peripheral excision or vaporization to encompass a margin of at least 3 mm circumferentially around the canal. High-grade lesions typically are removed with a 5-mm endocervical margin, or to a height of 1.5 cm.

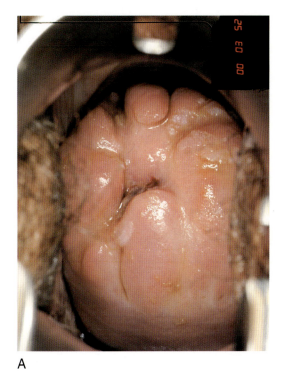
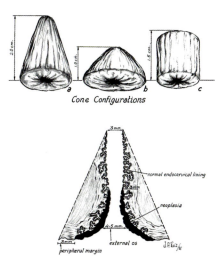

A   **B**

FIGURE 23-2 **A,** After conization, the anatomy can be distorted. The mass ligatures have created a deformed, stenotic cervix. **B,** Excisional cones may have different shapes depending on the geometry of the transformation zone and the characteristics of the neoplastic lesion. For example, a cylindrical cone would be most appropriate for a narrow lesion that is located at the transformation zone and extends into the canal. This shape would encompass the lesion and conserve cervical volume.

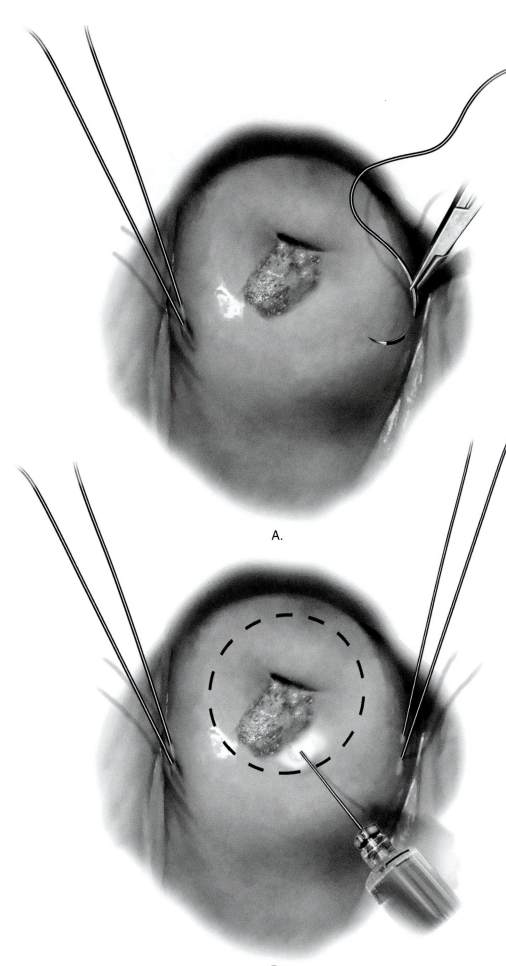

A.

B.

FIGURE 23-3 **A,** Stay sutures of 0 Vicryl are placed at the 3 o'clock and 9 o'clock positions. **B,** A 1:100 solution of vasopressin is injected into the cervix to blanch the area surrounding (and including) the abnormal transformation zone. (continued)

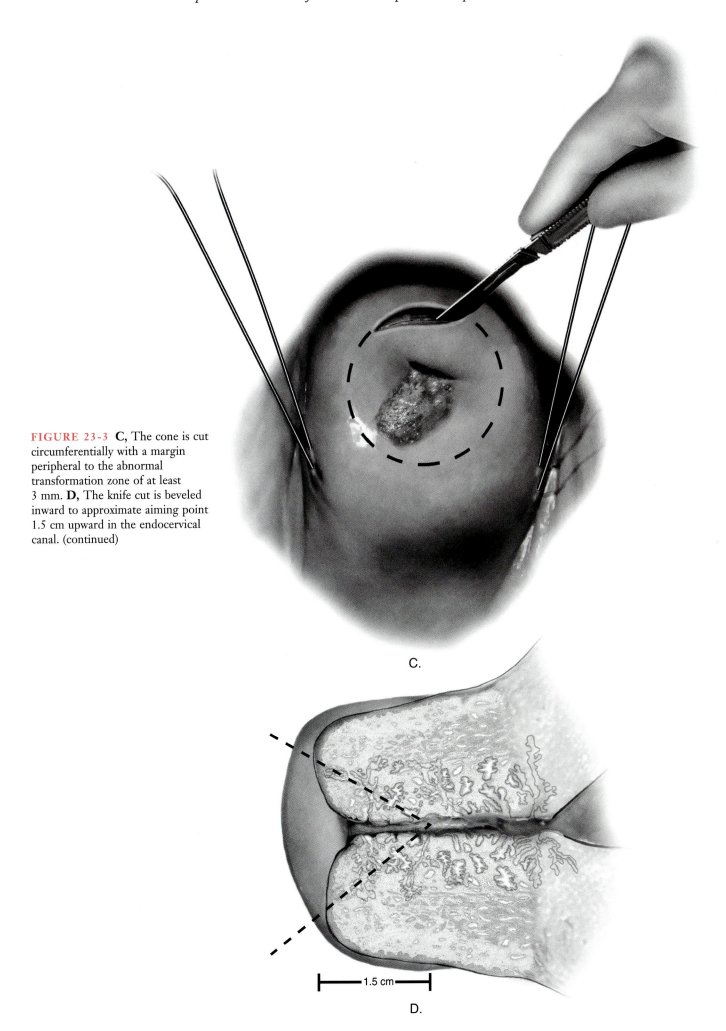

FIGURE 23-3 **C,** The cone is cut circumferentially with a margin peripheral to the abnormal transformation zone of at least 3 mm. **D,** The knife cut is beveled inward to approximate aiming point 1.5 cm upward in the endocervical canal. (continued)

C.

1.5 cm

D.

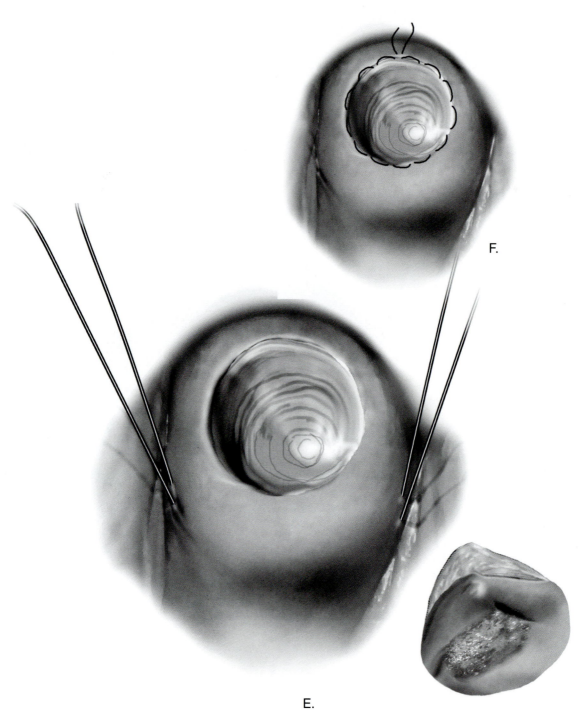

E.

F.

FIGURE 23-3 **E,** The specimen is removed and sent fresh for pathologic examination in a saline-soaked sponge. A suture marks the 12 o'clock position. **F,** The ectocervical margin of the cone is sutured with a running 3-0 Vicryl suture. Bleeding sites are sutured with 3-0 Vicryl.

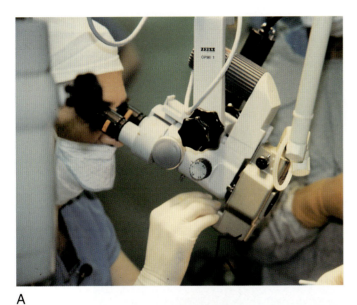

A

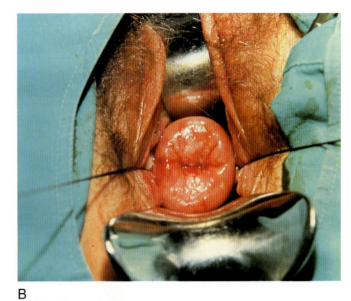

B

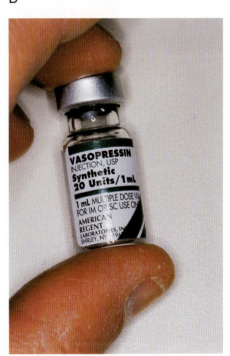

C

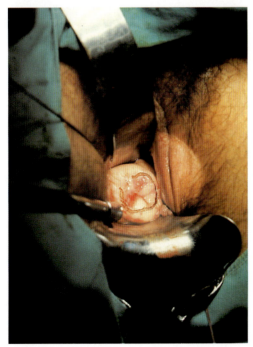

D

E

FIGURE 23-4 A, The CO_2 laser is coupled to the lens system of the colposcope, and the laser beam is controlled with a micromanipulator (*arrow*). **B,** In preparation for laser excisional conization, stay sutures are placed at the 3 o'clock and 9 o'clock positions. **C,** A 1:100 diluted solution of vasopressin is injected at multiple points into the cervix. **D,** This ampule of vasopressin contains 20 units/1 mL. **E,** A trace incision is made into the cervix, outlining the peripheral margin of the anticipated conization. (continued)

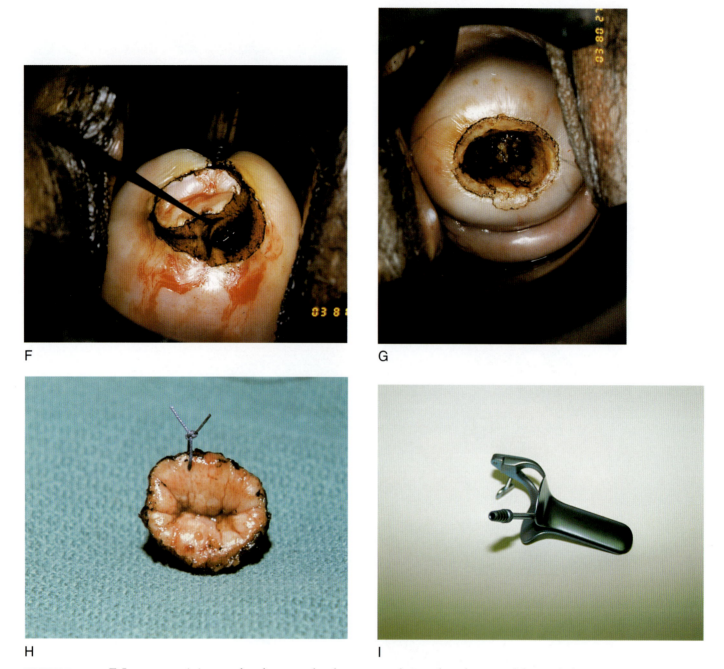

F

G

H

I

FIGURE 23-4 **F,** Laser power is increased as deep, angulated cuts are made into the substance of the cervical stroma. The cone is sculpted by differential traction with a long-handled, fine laser hook. **G,** The endocervical margin is cut with a knife to avoid thermal artifact. The cone bed is clean and bloodless, and a vaporization zone is seen on the ectocervical margin. This zone is created by defocusing the beam to a 2-mm spot size. **H,** A geometrically perfect specimen is marked with a suture at the 12 o'clock position and sent to the pathology laboratory for sectioning. **I,** An alternative to the exposure shown in *B* to *D* is seen. The laser speculum contains a built-in smoke evacuator and is hinged on one side for better access.

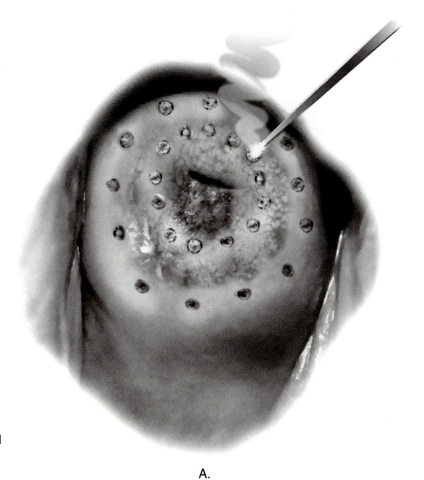

A.

FIGURE 23-5 A, Laser trace spots are placed at the far periphery of the cervix to encompass the ectocervical portion of the extensive abnormal transformation zone. Inner trace spots outline the site for the cone portion of the procedure. **B,** A focused laser beam is used to connect the trace spots. (continued)

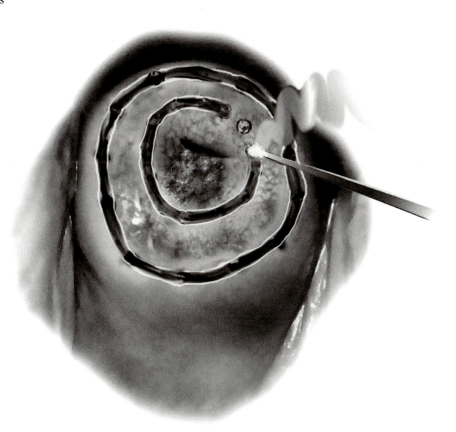

B.

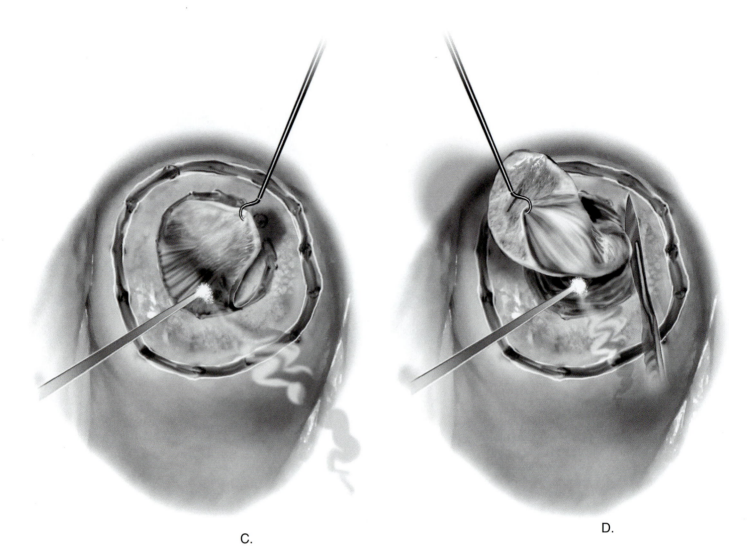

C.

D.

E.

FIGURE 23-5 **C,** A cylindrical excision is made using a laser hook to manipulate the specimen. **D,** Typically, the 1.5-cm high cone is cut out with a knife at the endocervical margin. **E,** The ectocervical portion of the lesion is vaporized according to the schema shown in Figures 23-1*B* and 23-8. (continued)

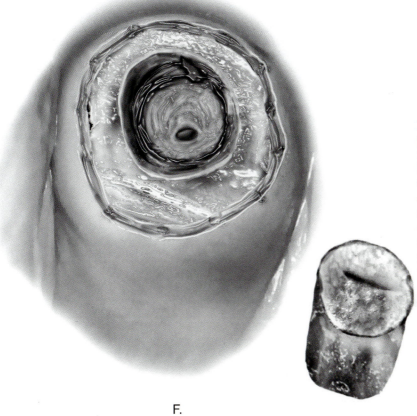

F.

FIGURE 23-5 **F,** After the combination procedure is completed, the specimen is sent to the pathology laboratory for evaluation. **G,** A hemisection of the cervix shows the geography of the combination cone. The blue area shows ectocervical vaporization, and the orange area shows the endocervical canal excision. **H,** This combination procedure was performed as shown in *A* to *G.* Because the lesion extended into the posterior vaginal fornix, less than 1 mm depth vaporization was performed in the vagina.

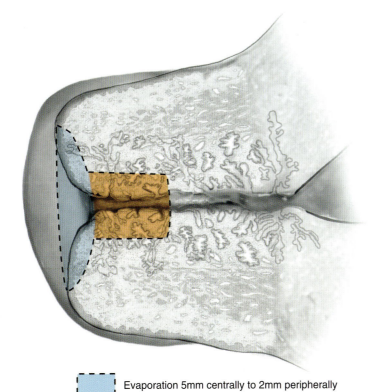

H

▨ Evaporation 5mm centrally to 2mm peripherally

▨ Laser excision 1.5 cm

G.

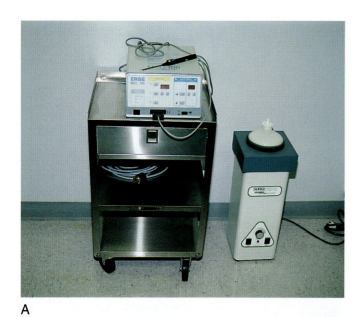

A

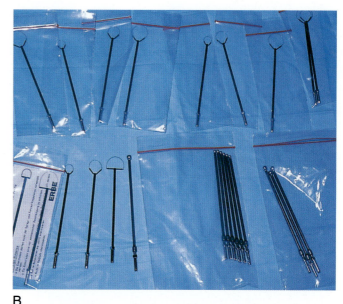

B

C

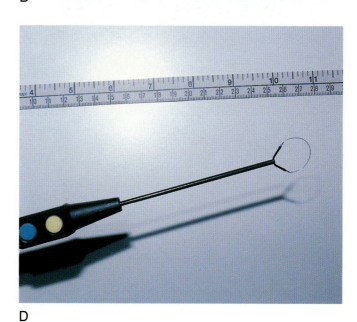

D

FIGURE 23-6 **A,** Cervical resection performed with a loop electrode requires a contemporary electrosurgical unit that has an adequate range of power (≥ 100 W), a computerized control system, and several integrated safety systems. **B,** Many electrodes are available, including two types of cutting electrodes and several coagulating balls. **C,** A ball electrode (*left*), an 8-mm loop (*center*), and a 5-mm loop (*right*) are shown. **D,** The electrodes plug into a hand control unit. By convention, the blue button delivers coagulation current and the yellow button delivers cutting current. (continued)

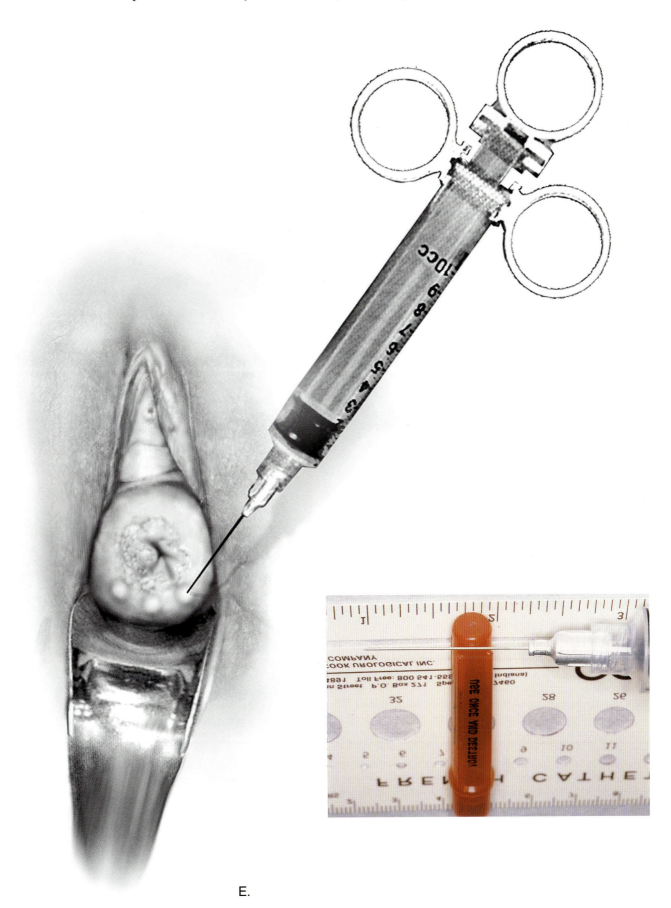

E.

FIGURE 23-6 **E,** A 1:100 diluted solution of vasopressin is injected into the cervix with a 1.5-inch, 25-gauge needle coupled to a 10-mL syringe. **Inset.** A 1.5-inch, 25-gauge needle. (continued)

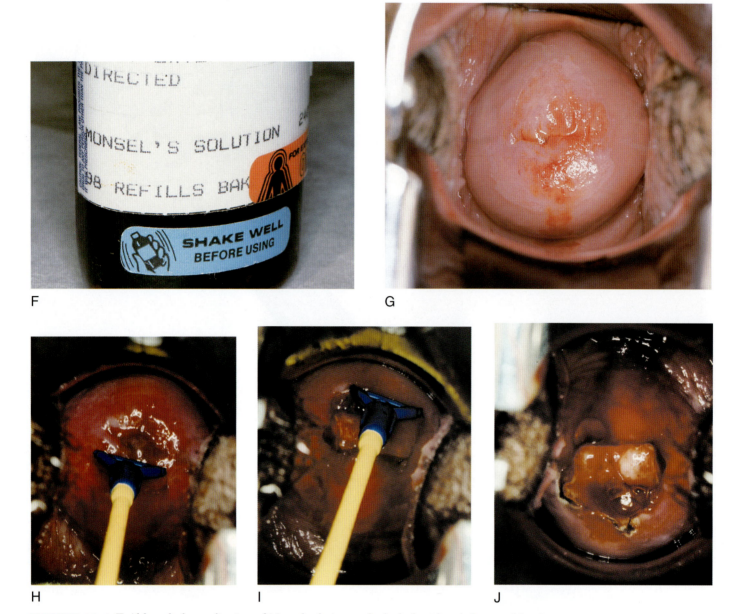

FIGURE 23-6 **F,** Although the application of Monsel solution to the bed after electric loop excision is not recommended, some clinicians routinely use this solution for hemostasis. Monsel solution must be used sparingly because it is caustic and causes further tissue devitalization. **G,** This cervix has an extensive abnormal transformation zone. Pap smear and biopsy showed cervical intraepithelial neoplasia grade 2. A vasopressin injection will be performed next. **H,** An electrode of proper size has been selected. The leading edge of the 8-mm-high cutting loop makes contact with the posterior cervical lip 3 mm below the posterior margin of the abnormal transformation zone. **I,** Power is activated by pressing the yellow control button on the handheld (pencil) unit. The electrode is guided through the substance of the cervix and upward to the margin of the anterior cervical lip in a single sweep. If the gynecologist interrupts the flow of electrical current, the electrode usually must be removed and the cut reinitiated at the cervical surface. **J,** After the cutting loop is removed, the cut disk of cervix will be removed with tissue forceps and placed in fixative. (continued)

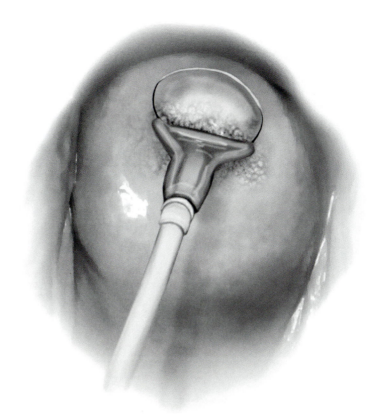

K.

FIGURE 23-6 K, For a selective double excision, the electrical loop engages the cervix peripheral (3 mm) to the margin of the abnormal transformation zone. **L,** The loop is guided through the cervical substance, encompassing the entire abnormal transformation zone. (continued)

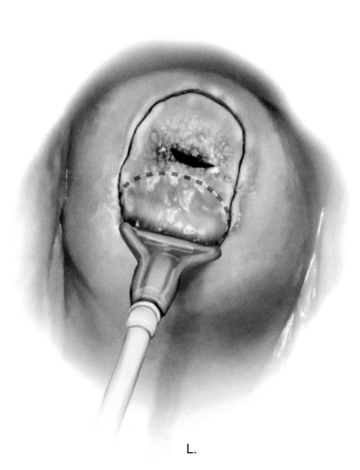

L.

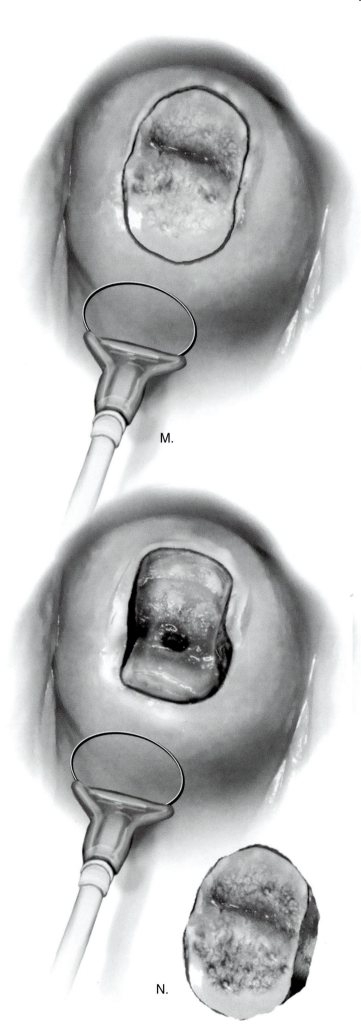

FIGURE 23-6 **M,** The loop is extracted from the cervix. **N,** The specimen, a 10-mm disk of the abnormal transformation zone, is removed. **O,** A 5-mm small loop electrode is placed in the pencil, and the tissue immediately surrounding the endocervical canal is excised to a further 5 mm depth. (continued)

M.

N.

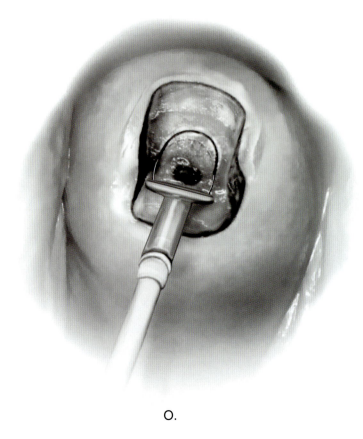

O.

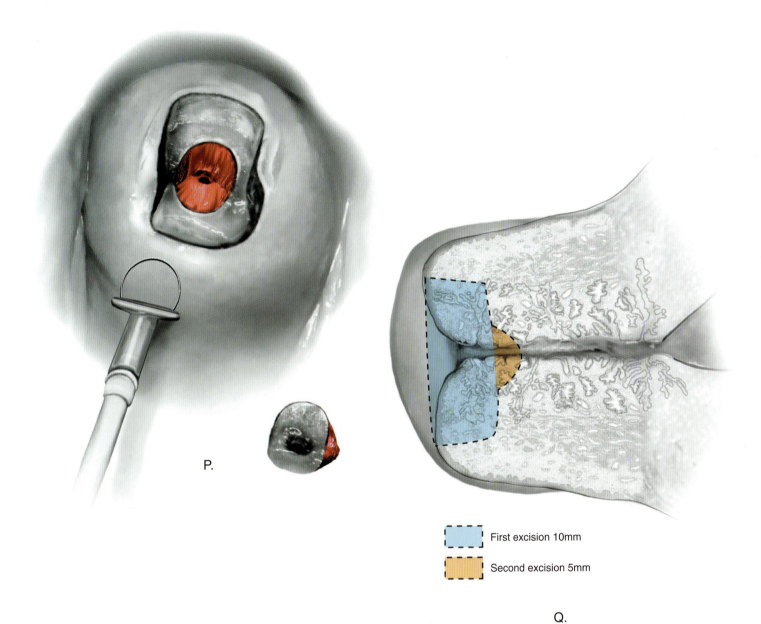

P.

First excision 10mm

Second excision 5mm

Q.

FIGURE 23-6 P, The additional specimen is sent to the pathology laboratory. **Q,** The volume of tissue typically removed by the selective double incision, or top hat, technique is seen. **R,** Some bleeding often occurs after electrical loop excision. A large, cotton-tipped swab (Proctoswab) is placed into the crater for tamponade. **S,** A ball electrode is substituted for the cutting loop. The blue button on the handpiece is depressed, and coagulation current flows. Spray (non-touch) coagulation is the best choice for surface coagulation. Because little tissue coagulation occurs, as bleeding vessels are sealed, the field becomes progressively easier to see. (continued)

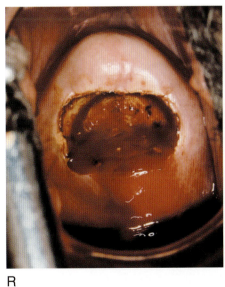

R

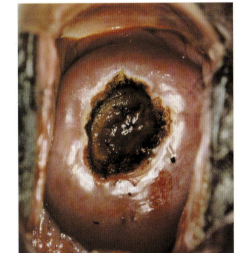

S

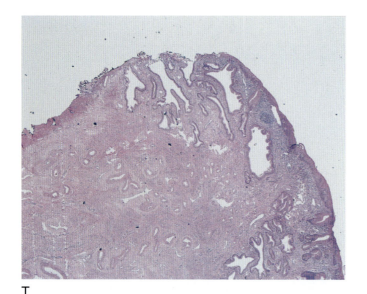

T

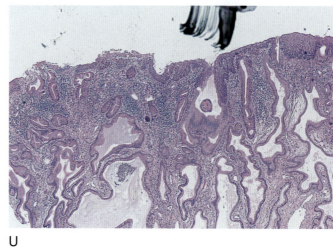

U

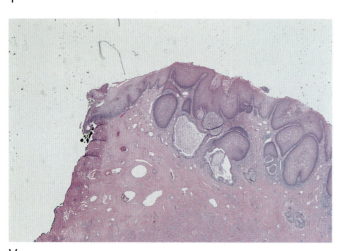

V

FIGURE 23-6 **T,** The endocervical margin is clearly visible. When performed correctly, electric loop excision produces a specimen that has readable margins. **U,** A higher-power view of the endocervical margin seen in *I*. **V,** The ectocervical margin of the specimen excises in *M* and *N*. Slight thermal artifact. The margin is readable and negative.

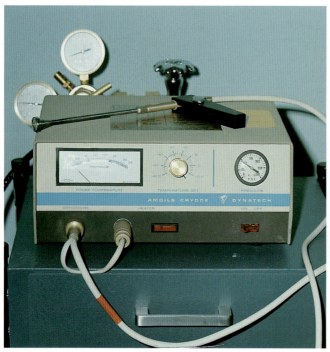

A

FIGURE 23-7 **A,** Cryosurgery equipment consists of a generator that controls (reduces) flow from the tank of CO_2 or N_2O gas. The cryosurgical probe includes the handle, shaft, and tip. The tip is applied to the cervix. The dials on the generator allow the temperature to be set, the temperature to be read, and the pressure. This unit includes a heater that serves as a defrosting device. (continued)

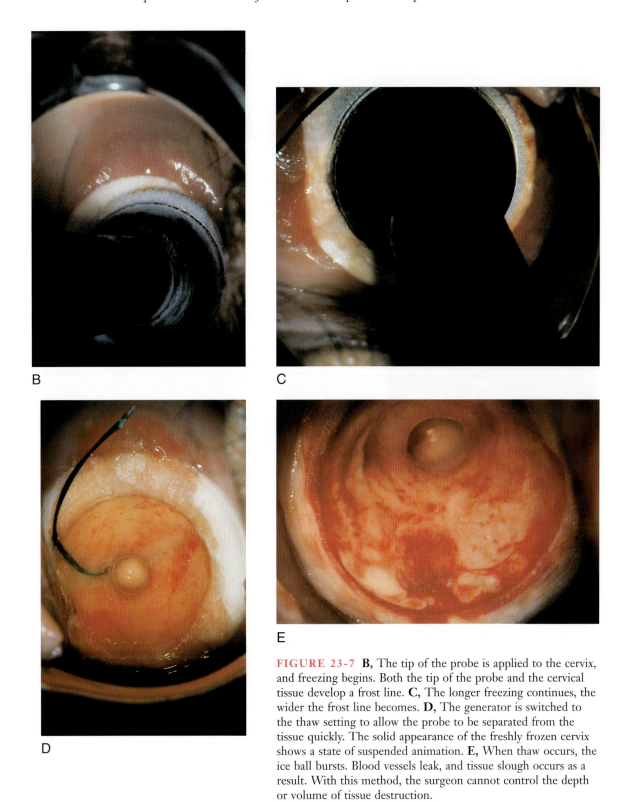

FIGURE 23-7 **B,** The tip of the probe is applied to the cervix, and freezing begins. Both the tip of the probe and the cervical tissue develop a frost line. **C,** The longer freezing continues, the wider the frost line becomes. **D,** The generator is switched to the thaw setting to allow the probe to be separated from the tissue quickly. The solid appearance of the freshly frozen cervix shows a state of suspended animation. **E,** When thaw occurs, the ice ball bursts. Blood vessels leak, and tissue slough occurs as a result. With this method, the surgeon cannot control the depth or volume of tissue destruction.

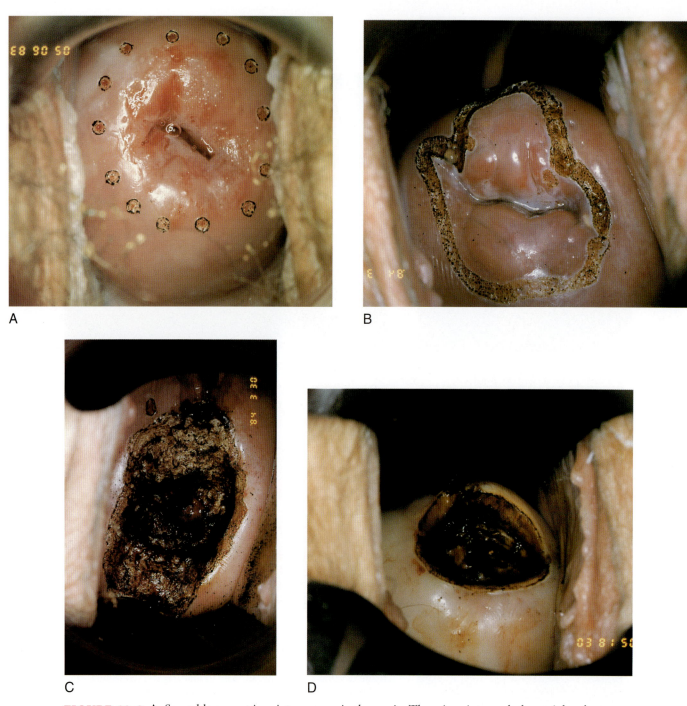

FIGURE 23-8 A, Several laser spot imprints are seen in the cervix. These imprints mark the peripheral margin for vaporization. **B,** A solid laser trace line is cut into the cervix to outline the zone to be vaporized. **C,** After 10-mm-deep vaporization, the formation of carbon creates char that must be irrigated away. **D,** A smaller abnormal transformation zone results in a smaller zone of vaporized tissue.

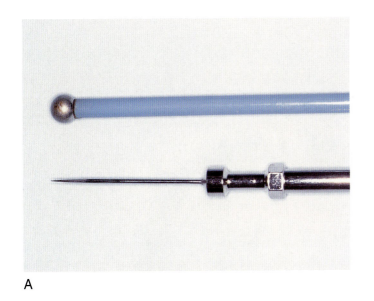

A

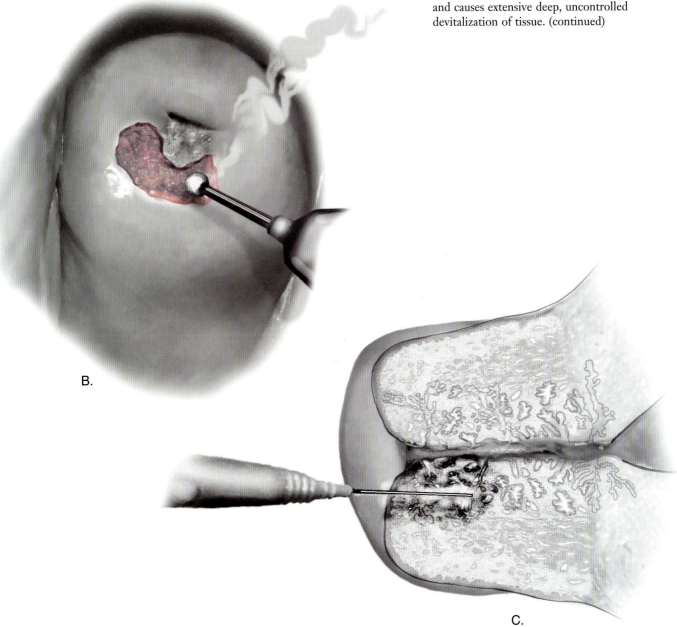

B.

C.

FIGURE 23-9 A, Needle and ball electrodes are seen. **B,** A ball electrode is used to coagulate the surface. Forced coagulation, or application of the electrode to the tissue, creates deeper penetration and damage than spray coagulation, or fulguration, which causes superficial coagulation. **C,** A needle electrode penetrates deeply into the cervical tissue and causes extensive deep, uncontrolled devitalization of tissue. (continued)

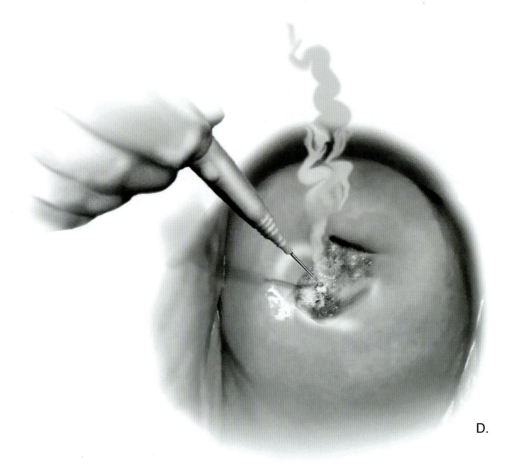

D.

FIGURE 23-9 **D,** As the needle is withdrawn, poorly controlled tissue vaporization occurs.

CHAPTER 24

Treatment of Vaginal Intraepithelial Neoplasia

As noted earlier, the vagina is structurally different from the cervix and consists entirely of stratified squamous epithelium and a fibromuscular stroma that is rich in elastic tissue fibers. Normally, no glandular tissue is seen within the vagina. The entire thickness of the vaginal epithelium is 0.45 to 0.60 mm.

In contrast to cervical intraepithelial neoplasia, which begins at the squamocolumnar junction after the mutation of a single cell, vaginal intraepithelial neoplasia (VAIN) begins within a zone of the vagina. Multiple cells at many sites simultaneously undergo neoplastic transformation. Therefore, one or more regions of the vagina may have multicentric foci of intraepithelial neoplasia between intervening areas of normal tissue.

Specifications for Treatment

The following treatment model is proposed:

Specification 1   After the diagnosis is made and the lesions are mapped, the vagina is swabbed with acetic acid and the areas for treatment are verified colposcopically.

Specification 2   Depth of treatment is limited to 1 mm or less. This specification exceeds the mucosal epithelium thickness by a factor of 2.

Specification 3   Very wide peripheral margins are required to eliminate existing disease and prevent persistent disease. Treating the vagina in thirds is recommended. For disorders in the vault and fornices, the entire upper third is treated. When disease extends into the middle third, the upper two thirds are treated. If the disease

affects only the lower third, the lower third is treated. If the disorder involves scattered areas in the upper, middle, and lower thirds, the entire vagina is treated, preferably in stages.

Specification 4   Treating VAIN deeply slows healing and increases the risk of injury to the bladder, rectum, and intraperitoneal structures.

Specification 5   Preoperative and intraoperative sampling is essential to exclude coexisting invasive squamous cell carcinoma or adenocarcinoma (arising in adenosis).

Specification 6   Atrophic vaginas are treated with topical estrogen for at least 4 weeks preoperatively. Vaginal infections are cultured and treated preoperatively.

Excisional Techniques

Knife Excision

Vaginectomy is performed, with or without magnification, using a sharp scalpel and scissors. A microscope or headlight with optical loops is recommended. Vaginectomy can be radical if the entire vagina is removed. When a large area of vagina is removed, split-thickness skin grafts are used to preserve normal function. Vaginectomy usually is bloody, and hemostasis must be maintained throughout the procedure. Because the vagina is thin and is in close proximity to the bladder, rectum, and ureters, care must be exercised during surgery. The injection of dilute vasopressin offers two advantages: it creates a more hemostatic operative field and it balloons the vaginal mucosa, thereby facilitating a better plane for dissection. The most difficult area to dissect is the vaginal vault, particularly in patients who have undergone hysterectomy. The lateral wall may be dissected by making incisions lateral to the hymenal ring, into the vestibule, and then sharply opening the space on the lateral aspect of the vagina. Dissection includes the bulb of the vestibule, a major source of bleeding that must be controlled with fine suture ligatures. The anterior and posterior walls of the vagina are separated from the urethra, bladder, and rectum in a procedure similar to anterior or posterior colporrhaphy. Finally, the vaginal vault is dissected (Figs. 24-1*A* to *E*).

After the surgeon ensures that bleeding is controlled throughout the vaginal connective tissue, a split-thickness graft is placed into the vagina over a form and secured (Figs. 24-1*F* and *G*). The graft is left undisturbed for at least 2 weeks. To avoid disturbing or dislodging the vaginal form (Fig. 24-1*H*), the patient's activities are limited. The donor site is covered with "op site" or another suitable dressing that is left in place until it falls off.

Limited Knife or Laser Excision

With this procedure, only a portion of the vagina is resected. For example, lesions that are identified colposcopically in the right upper third of the lateral vaginal wall and in the lateral fornix must be excised (Figs. 24-2*A* to *C*). The rest of the upper third of the vagina, which contains no visible lesions, is vaporized with a CO_2 laser. Depending on the location of the excised tissue, closure may be accomplished without tension and without constricting the vagina. Closure may be performed with interrupted 3-0 Vicryl sutures. If adequate primary closure cannot be accomplished, a split, or defatted, full-thickness graft is placed over the defect and sutured to the surrounding vaginal mucosa (Figs. 24-2*D* to *G*). Clindamycin (Cleocin) cream is applied to keep the vaginal walls from adhering. A nonadherent dressing may be tacked over the graft, but must be removed in 24 hours.

An UltraPulse CO_2 laser is an alternative cutting device. A laser is more precise than a knife because the 1-mm beam is directed colposcopically and controlled with a micromanipulator. The tissue is manipulated with long titanium hooks. To limit the depth of penetration of the laser beam, a 1:100 diluted solution of vasopressin may be administered subepidermally. The beam penetrates the mucosa and is absorbed by the submucosal water. The superpulse laser causes little thermal injury and no conduction artifact. Whether the wound is primarily closed or grafted, healing is identical to healing after knife excision.

Monopolar electrosurgical devices are not used for vaginal surgery because the zone of thermal injury is difficult to control and impossible to predict. Injectable water is not a barrier to electrosurgery as with the CO_2 laser. Cryosurgical devices are more difficult to control than electrosurgery and should not be used in the vagina.

Ablative Techniques

CO_2 Laser Vaporization

As noted in the discussion of cervical intraepithelial neoplasia, excisional procedures are preferred for use in the cervix. Laser vaporization of the vagina is much simpler and causes significantly fewer complications than knife or laser excision. Because VAIN involves an epithelial thickness of less than 1 mm, skillful application of superficial vaporization is safe and causes few complications. The risk of injury to the bladder or rectum should be nearly zero, and most patients experience only modest postoperative pain. The operation is nearly bloodless, and the risk of hemorrhage is low. The only substantial risk is infection because tissue is destroyed and the vagina is an area that is infested with microorganisms (Figs. 24-3*A* to *C*).

During laser vaporization, a long, fine titanium hook is used to expose the recessed and folded mucosa (Fig. 24-3*B*). The laser operates in the superpulse mode at approximately 12 to 15 W, and the diameter of the spot is 1.5 to 2.5 mm. The key is to superficially vaporize the mucosa only in the affected third of the vagina (Fig. 24-3*E*). A laser speculum fitted with a smoke evacuation channel is required for this type of surgery. The micromanipulator stick is moved slowly in a fine, circular motion, either clockwise or counterclockwise, to allow the surgeon to control depth precisely. When the procedure is complete, the area is swabbed clean with sterile water or saline (Figs. 24-3*F* to *M*).

Before an ablative technique is performed, the patient must undergo preoperative sampling to exclude more extensive disease. This sampling is particularly important in the vagina, which has an extensive surface area and can have multicentric intraepithelial neoplasia (Figs. 24-3*N* to *P*). Several colposcopically directed and mapped biopsy specimens are obtained to allow the surgeon to plan the treatment strategy.

5-Fluorouracil Cream

Topical preparations of 2% or 5% 5-fluorouracil (Efudex) interfere with the synthesis of DNA and therefore inhibit cell division (Fig. 24-4*A*). Rapidly dividing cells, such as epithelial cells of the skin or mucous membrane, are especially vulnerable to the drug. The drug should not be administered to a pregnant patient. Because the cream is specifically indicated for use on external skin surfaces, vaginal application is an off-label use.

One-half vaginal applicator full of 5% 5-fluorouracil cream is placed into the vagina at bedtime (Fig. 24-4*B*) daily for 7 days. The course of therapy may be repeated monthly for 3 or 4 consecutive months. Problems associated with this treatment include the following: First, distribution of the cream is imprecise, and patient skill determines whether the cream is delivered to the vaginal vault. Appropriate delivery of the cream cannot be assumed because many variables are involved. Second, the depth of action of the cream for a specific region of the vagina is unknown. Third, residue of the cream spills into the vestibule and onto the perineum, causing a painful chemical burn. If significant discomfort occurs, the patient may become reluctant to use the cream as directed or to even continue the treatment. Finally, the long treatment period decreases the likelihood of even marginal compliance.

Electrosurgery and Cryosurgery

Because of the risk of injury to the urinary tract or intestines, these techniques should not be used to treat VAIN.

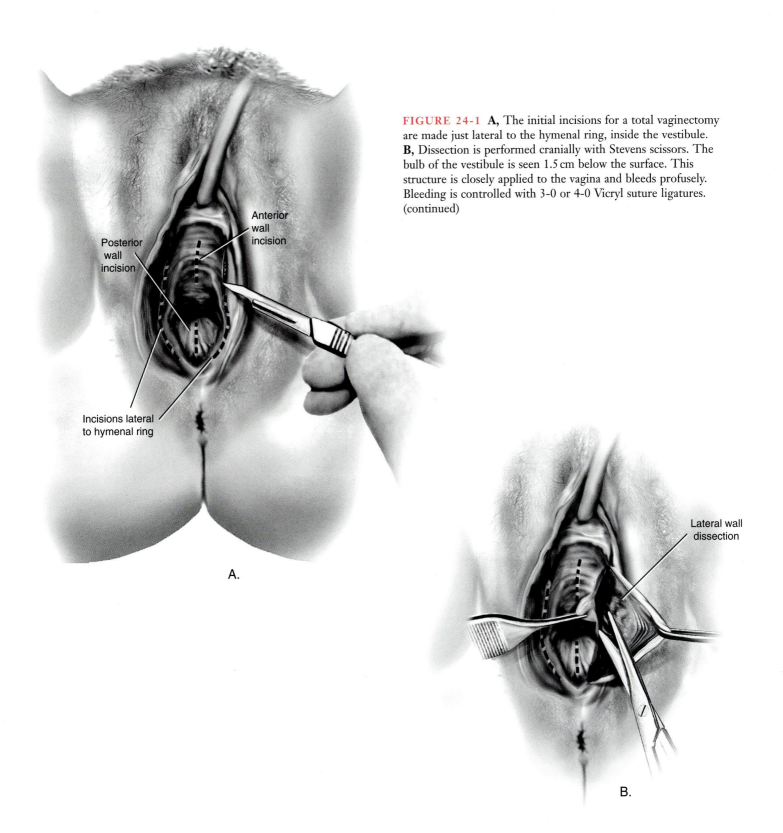

FIGURE 24-1 **A,** The initial incisions for a total vaginectomy are made just lateral to the hymenal ring, inside the vestibule. **B,** Dissection is performed cranially with Stevens scissors. The bulb of the vestibule is seen 1.5 cm below the surface. This structure is closely applied to the vagina and bleeds profusely. Bleeding is controlled with 3-0 or 4-0 Vicryl suture ligatures. (continued)

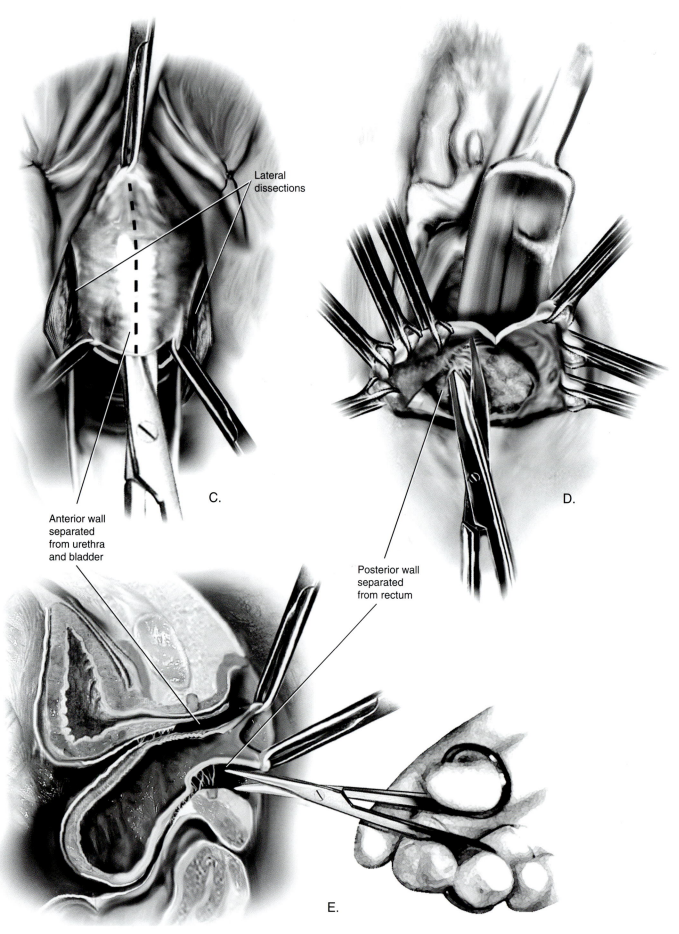

Lateral dissections

C.

D.

Anterior wall separated from urethra and bladder

Posterior wall separated from rectum

E.

FIGURE 24-1

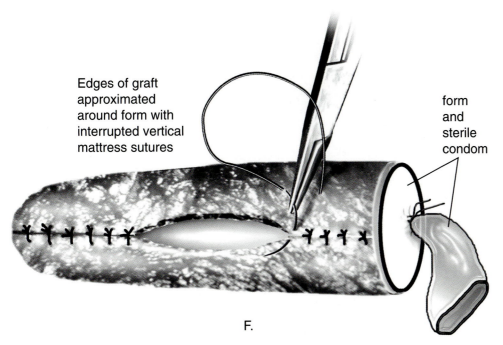

Edges of graft
approximated
around form with
interrupted vertical
mattress sutures

form
and
sterile
condom

F.

FIGURE 24-1 C, The anterior wall
is distended with a 1:100 solution of
vasopressin and incised in the midline,
as is done during anterior repair. The
anterior incision (*dotted lines*) is cut,
creating two anterior flaps that are
dissected to the lateral dissection
margins. **D,** The posterior vaginal
wall is injected, cut, and dissected, as
described for the anterior vaginal wall
(Figure C). **E,** Because the vagina
shares a common wall with the urethra,
bladder, and rectum, dissection must be
performed carefully to avoid injury to
these structures. The surgeon should
check these structures for injury
throughout and at the end of the
procedure. **F,** After the vaginal mucosa
is cut away and hemostasis is secured, a
split-thickness skin graft is positioned
over a vaginal form that is covered with
a sterile rubber condom. **G,** The form
is secured in the space previously
occupied by the vagina. The edges of
the graft are sutured to the vestibular
skin margin. **H,** A pressure dressing
secures the form and graft in the
neovagina.

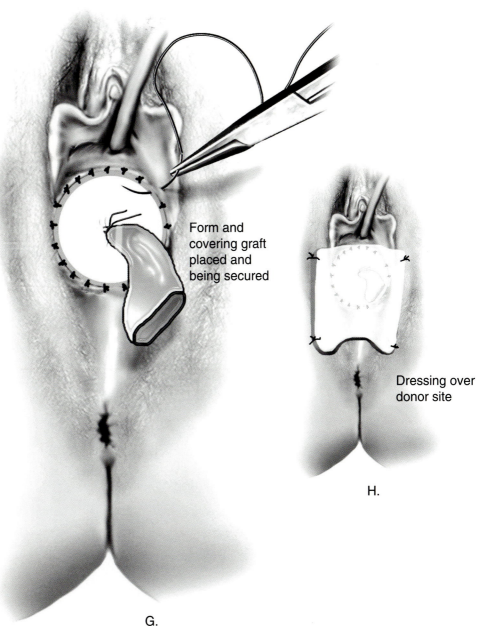

Form and
covering graft
placed and
being secured

Dressing over
donor site

H.

G.

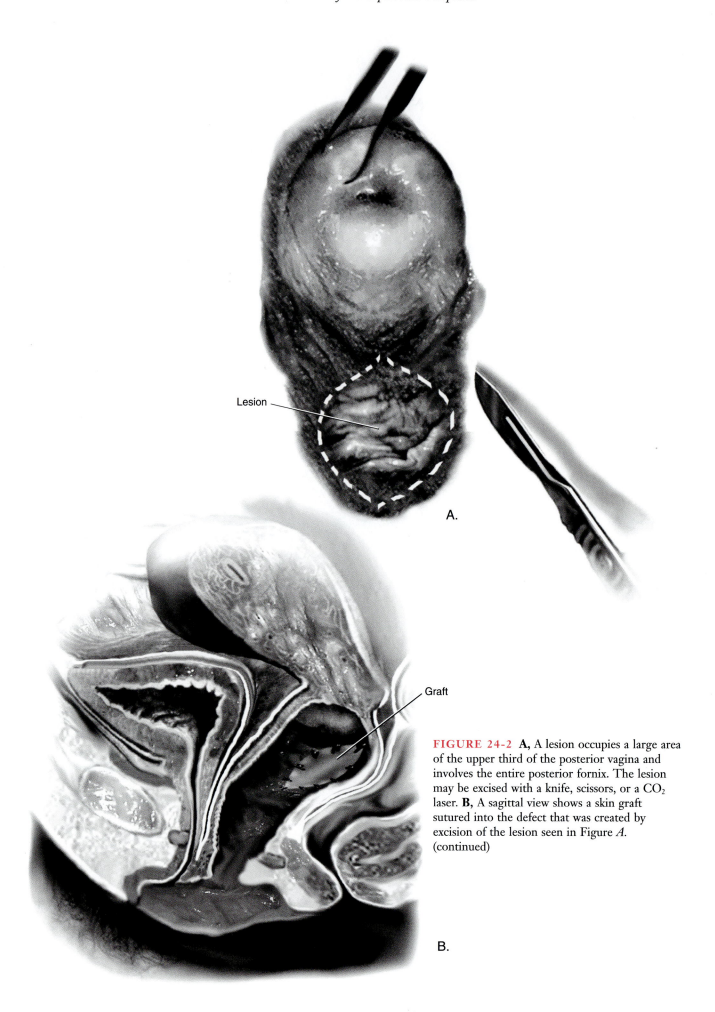

Lesion

A.

Graft

FIGURE 24-2 A, A lesion occupies a large area of the upper third of the posterior vagina and involves the entire posterior fornix. The lesion may be excised with a knife, scissors, or a CO_2 laser. **B,** A sagittal view shows a skin graft sutured into the defect that was created by excision of the lesion seen in Figure *A.* (continued)

B.

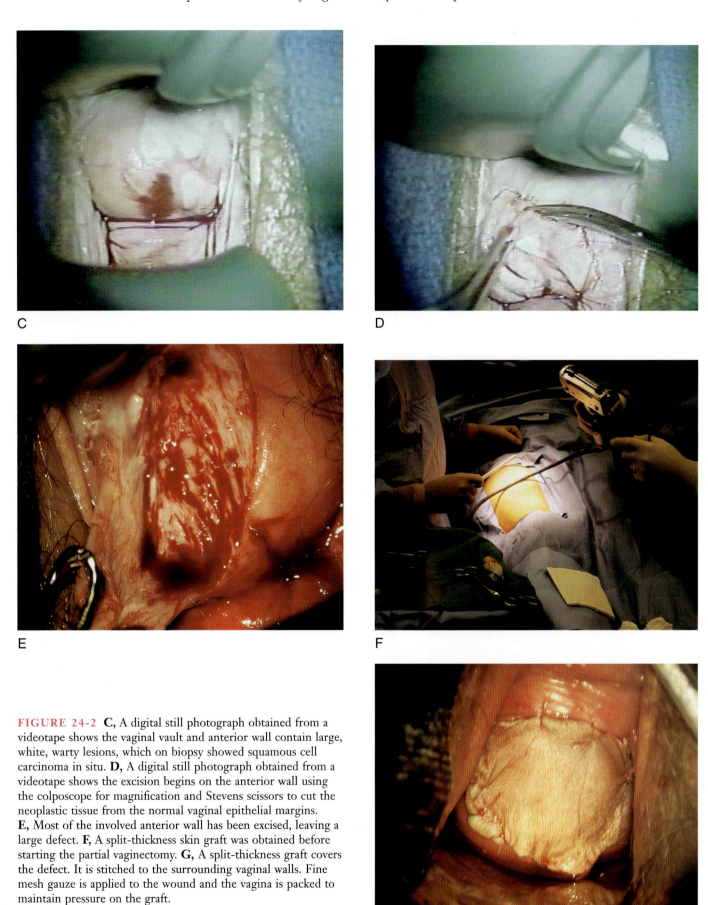

FIGURE 24-2 C, A digital still photograph obtained from a videotape shows the vaginal vault and anterior wall contain large, white, warty lesions, which on biopsy showed squamous cell carcinoma in situ. **D,** A digital still photograph obtained from a videotape shows the excision begins on the anterior wall using the colposcope for magnification and Stevens scissors to cut the neoplastic tissue from the normal vaginal epithelial margins. **E,** Most of the involved anterior wall has been excised, leaving a large defect. **F,** A split-thickness skin graft was obtained before starting the partial vaginectomy. **G,** A split-thickness graft covers the defect. It is stitched to the surrounding vaginal walls. Fine mesh gauze is applied to the wound and the vagina is packed to maintain pressure on the graft.

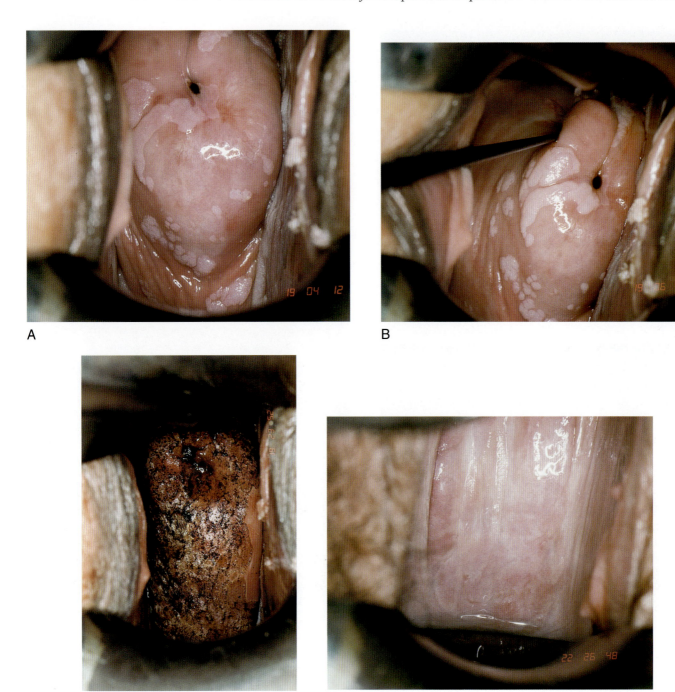

FIGURE 24-3 A, This patient has multifocal vaginal epithelial neoplasia (VAIN). Viral typing of the warty lesions showed human papillomavirus types 16, 18, 31, and 33 (hybrid capture panel). **B,** A long-handled, fine skin hook is used to retract the cervix to expose several more foci of VAIN in the vaginal fornix. **C,** Extensive vaporization of the cervix and upper vagina was performed to a maximum depth of 1 mm. Postoperatively, the patient received interferon alpha 1 million units three times per week. **D,** Another patient had extensive VAIN on the anterior vaginal wall and within the vaginal fornices. (continued)

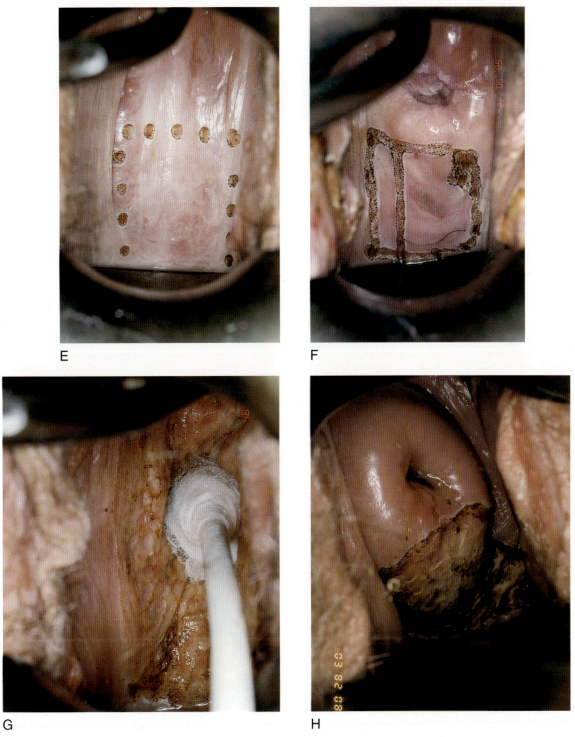

E

F

G

H

FIGURE 24-3 **E,** The anterior vaginal wall is trace marked with a CO_2 laser beam. **F,** Laser vaporization is initiated within the boundaries previously marked in the vagina. **G,** Vaporization extends to the lateral vaginal wall. **H,** The posterior fornix was vaporized. (continued)

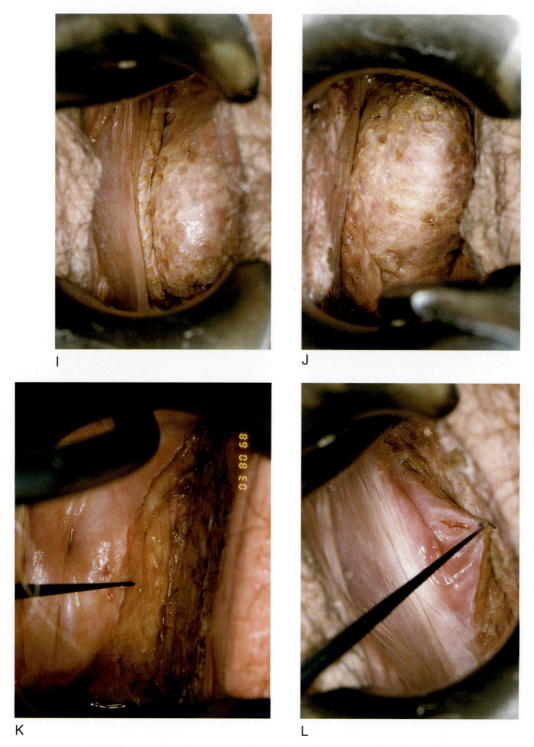

FIGURE 24-3 **I,** The margin of the vaporized anterior and anterolateral walls and the normal posterolateral wall is seen. **J,** The entire anterior wall was vaporized. No char is present because vaginal vaporization was performed with a superpulse laser system. **K,** A vaginal hook is used to expose hard-to-reach areas, such as the vaginal fornices. **L,** This patient underwent a hysterectomy 10 years before VAIN was discovered. Pap smear and biopsy showed VAIN. A skin hook is used to expose the vaginal tunnel before the epithelium is vaporized with a CO_2 laser. (continued)

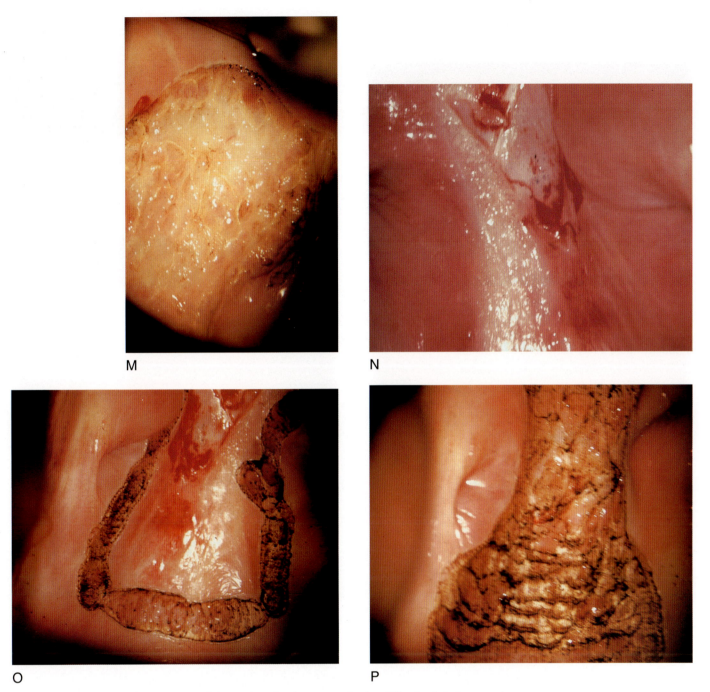

M

N

O

P

FIGURE 24-3 **M,** A close-up view of the vagina after laser vaporization. The depth is 1 mm or less.
N, Three biopsy specimens of the vault showed VAIN grades 2 and 3. **O,** The lesion is outlined carefully
with a power density of less than 1000 W/cm^2 and a spot size of 2 to 3 mm. Care is taken to avoid transmural
penetration of the thin vaginal vault. **P,** Vaporization is complete. No bleeding is seen. The water injected into
the subepidermal tissue served as a heat sink and protected against deep penetration by the laser beam.

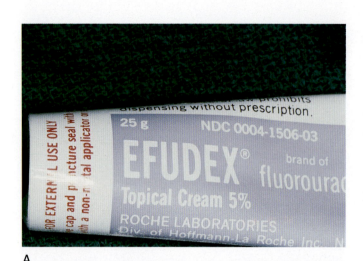

A

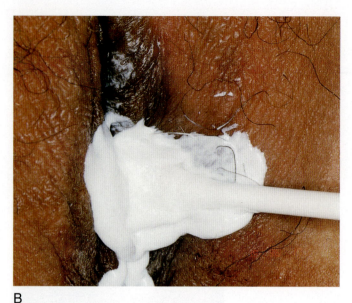

B

FIGURE 24-4 A, Topical 5% 5-fluorouracil cream (Efudex) may be applied to the vagina to treat VAIN. **B,** After vaginal application, some of the cream invariably makes its way onto the vulva and into the vulvar vestibule, where it may cause severe excoriation.

CHAPTER 25
Treatment of Vulvar Intraepithelial Neoplasia

Vulvar intraepithelial neoplasia (VIN) is easier to treat than cervical or vaginal intraepithelial neoplasia because the vulva is easily viewed and is readily accessible for surgery. However, the vulva is much larger than the cervix or the vagina and has several microanatomic components.

Specifications for Treatment

Multicentric disease is seen in 68% of cases. The epidermis thickens by a factor of 2 to 5 as the cells transform from normal to neoplastic. In a patient who has VIN grade 3, the mean thickness of the epidermis is approximately 0.9 mm. Skin appendages within normal vulvar hair-bearing skin may extend into the underlying subcutaneous fat to a depth of 4 mm. In 38% of women who have VIN grade 3, the neoplastic process extends into skin appendages, including hair shafts and sebaceous and sweat glands. In older women (50 to 60 years of age) who have VIN grade 3, the rate of appendage involvement approaches 60%. The depth of neoplastic extension into skin appendages ranges from 0.43 to 3.60 mm, with a mean depth of 1.53 ± 0.77 mm (0.76 to 2.3 mm, 95% confidence). In non-hair-bearing areas, the mean depth of neoplastic extension into sebaceous glands is 1 mm.

Treatment of VIN includes tissue excision or ablation to a depth of 2 to 2.5 mm in hair-bearing areas and to a depth of 1 mm in non-hair-bearing areas. The peripheral margins must be at least 3 mm. In Paget's disease, the treatment depth is 3 to 4 mm and the peripheral margins are 6 to 10 mm.

The clitoris has a very thin epidermis and plays an important role in sexual response. Therefore, treatment of VIN should be performed cautiously and under magnification, with care taken to preserve function and conserve tissue. In addition, care must be taken to avoid adhesions between the clitoral hood and glans.

Excisional Techniques

Knife Excision

The most direct method used to treat VIN is knife excision. As with all therapeutic measures, preservation of function is an important goal. In the vulva, function includes cosmetic preservation of the anatomy. For this reason, total vulvectomy should be avoided if possible. If vulvectomy is required to treat extensive multicentric disease, the patient should undergo skilled skin grafting and plastic reconstruction of the area (Figs. 25-1*A* to *I*).

After knife excision is performed, the skin edges of the wound may be closed without tension (Figs. 25-2*A* to *E*). Alternatively, if primary closure cannot be achieved without deformity, a pedicle graft can be used to repair the defect (Figs. 25-3*A* to *D*). Because the internal pudendal artery and its branches provide the principal blood supply to the vulva, the base of the graft should be approximately twice its height (Figs. 25-3*E* to *H*). Occasionally, combinations of closures are indicated, such as a combination skin graft and primary closure (Figs. 25-4*A* to *I*).

When the neoplasia is widely distributed (e.g., affecting the labia majora, labia minora, vestibule, and perineum), skinning vulvectomy is indicated. Before this procedure is performed, a split-thickness graft is obtained from the thigh or buttock. To perform skinning vulvectomy, transdermal skin excision is carried out to the level of the junction between fat and dermis. The contouring fat is spared. The labia minora and clitoral frenulum may be removed because they are too thin to partially excise. The graft is sewn over the contouring fat to create a reconstructed, functional vulva (Figs. 25-5*A* to *D*).

CO₂ Laser Excision

An UltraPulse (superpulse) CO_2 laser coupled to a colposcope (microscope) is used in a fashion similar to a sharp scalpel (Fig. 25-5E). A tightly focused laser beam with a spot, or beam diameter, of less than 1 mm can be used to cut through tissue precisely, with no char formation (Figs. 25-5F and G). Subdermal injection of a 1:100 solution of vasopressin creates a vasoconstrictive heat sink that prevents distal penetration of the laser and supplements its hemostatic properties. The laser beam also can be used to perform an intradermal, or split-thickness, excision (Figs. 25-6A to H). The laser thin section does not require grafting for primary healing. This technique requires skillful manipulation of tissue to obtain a parallel cut. The laser thin section must be performed with an UltraPulse laser to avoid irreversible thermal injury to tissue (Figs. 25-7A to C). Laser thin section offers two advantages over knife excision. It provides a relatively large tissue sample for pathologic examination and determination of margin status. It also allows the surgeon to cut only within the reticular dermis, thereby avoiding the need for skin grafting. When the laser thin section is completed, the wound is covered with silver sulfadiazine (Silvadene). The patient is instructed to take two baths each day with synthetic sea salt (Instant Ocean) and to apply Silvadene to the wound three times a day and at bedtime.

Ablative Techniques

Laser vaporization, or CO_2 laser ablation, may be used to treat VIN. However, ablative techniques should be performed only after the patient undergoes extensive sampling and mapping to exclude invasive squamous cell carcinoma. Vaporization should be performed according to the specifications described for hair-bearing and non-hair-bearing areas. Since the late 1990s, the standard for laser vaporization has included the use of a superpulse laser to limit collateral thermal injury (Figs. 25-8A to C). Vaporization must be performed carefully to avoid third-degree thermal skin injury, which can cause scarring (Figs. 25-8D to I).

Typically, laser vaporization is combined with excision. Vaporization is used primarily at the skin margins (Figs.

25-9A to C). The clitoris is an ideal site for superpulse laser vaporization because this technique preserves normal tissue while eliminating VIN. After laser vaporization, the postoperative routine is the same as for CO_2 laser-thin section.

Other Techniques

Cryosurgery and topical 5-fluorouracil cream have doubtful efficacy and are not used in the management of VIN. These techniques offer no advantages over the methods discussed earlier, and they have many inherent deficiencies. The only potential advantage of these techniques is that they are relatively simple to perform and do not require a high level of skill. However, clinicians who cannot treat VIN adequately with excision or laser treatment should not attempt to manage the disorder.

Special Considerations

Paget's disease of the vulva is a variant of VIN. It differs from squamous cell carcinoma in situ in that the cell of origin arises either from the specialized sweat glands in the vulva (apocrine glands) or directly from a totipotential sub-basilar reserve cell. Occasionally, Paget's disease of the vulva becomes invasive. Because Paget's disease likely originates in the sweat glands, it often recurs at multifocal sites. The natural course of this disorder is an endless cycle of excision and recurrence (Fig. 25-10A). The key to therapy is full-thickness excision and wide peripheral excision. Even when negative margins are obtained, however, Paget's disease of the vulva often recurs. Therefore, close follow-up is needed. Colposcopic examination is helpful, and biopsy of suspicious lesions, particularly those that border the excision margins, is imperative. Also, the perianal skin should be examined closely. Excisional procedures provide the best treatment of Paget's disease because pathologic analysis is a priority in the management of this disorder (Figs. 25-10B and C).

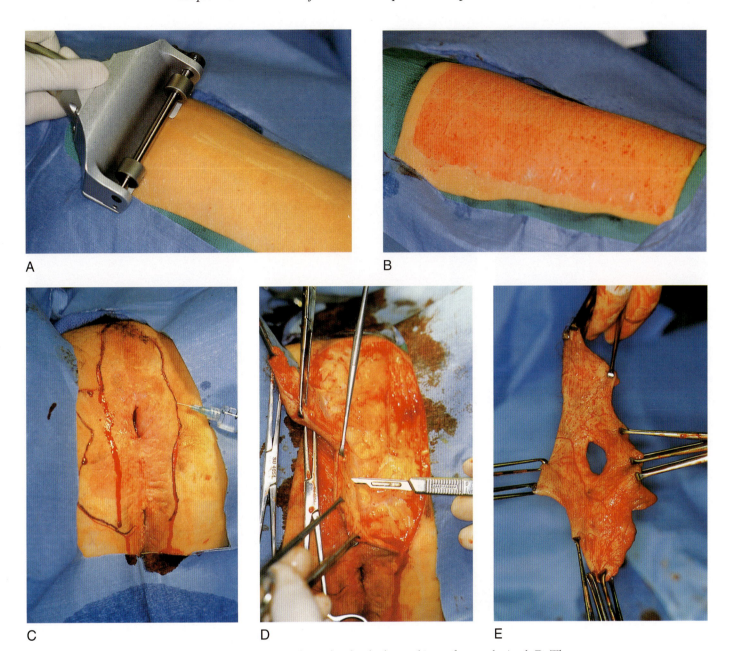

FIGURE 25-1 **A,** Before a simple vulvectomy is performed, split-thickness skin grafts are obtained. **B,** The donor site on the thigh is covered with op-site, and the dressing remains in place until it falls off. **C,** The margins of excision are marked, and a 1:100 solution of vasopressin is injected subcutaneously. **D,** The full thickness of vulvar skin is cut away. The surgeon attempts to conserve as much contouring fat as possible. **E,** After the specimen is removed, it is marked to permit accurate pathologic assessment of the margins. (continued)

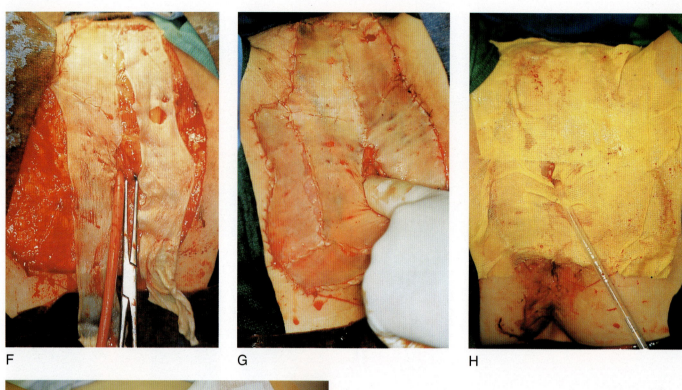

F

G

H

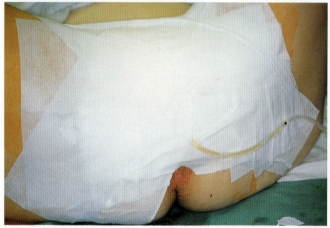

I

FIGURE 25-1 F, Split-thickness skin grafts are placed on the wound for closure. **G,** The grafts are sewn together to cover the defect that is created by extensive excision. **H,** The patient is catheterized, and fine mesh gauze is applied directly to the graft. **I,** A Curlex uniform pressure dressing is applied above the fine mesh gauze.

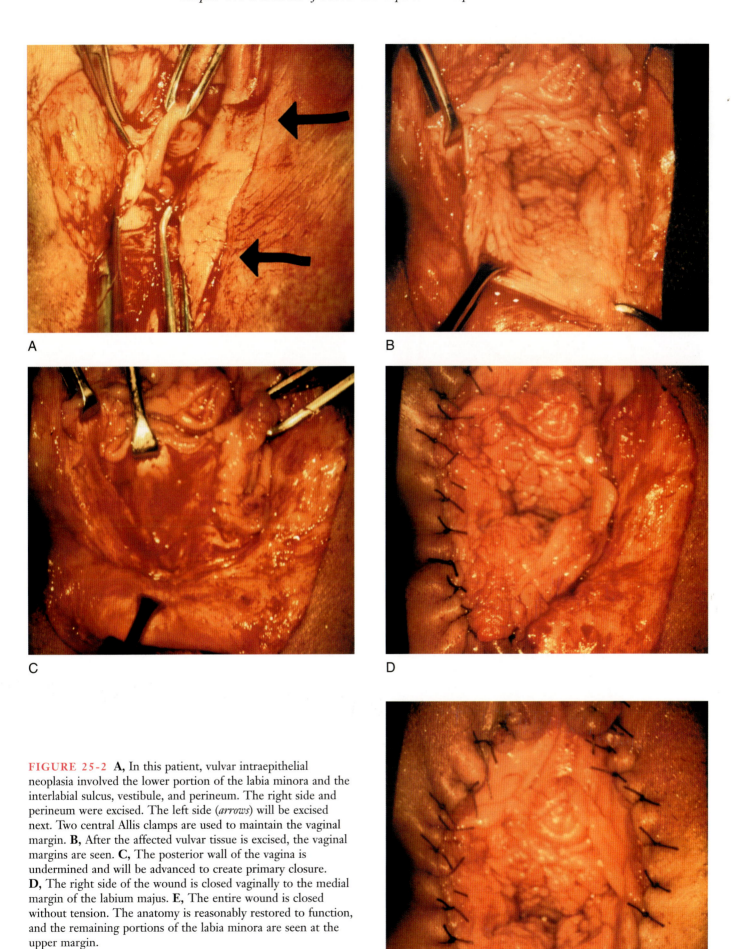

FIGURE 25-2 A, In this patient, vulvar intraepithelial neoplasia involved the lower portion of the labia minora and the interlabial sulcus, vestibule, and perineum. The right side and perineum were excised. The left side (*arrows*) will be excised next. Two central Allis clamps are used to maintain the vaginal margin. **B,** After the affected vulvar tissue is excised, the vaginal margins are seen. **C,** The posterior wall of the vagina is undermined and will be advanced to create primary closure. **D,** The right side of the wound is closed vaginally to the medial margin of the labium majus. **E,** The entire wound is closed without tension. The anatomy is reasonably restored to function, and the remaining portions of the labia minora are seen at the upper margin.

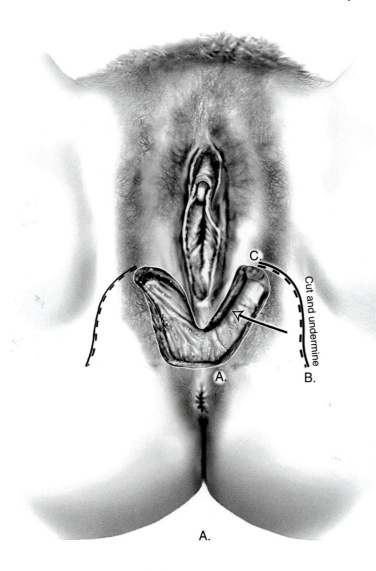

A.

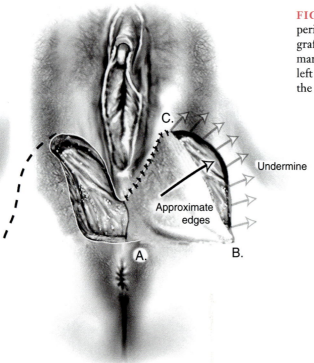

B.

FIGURE 25-3 **A,** This patient underwent resection of the perineum and lower labia because of carcinoma in situ. Pedicle grafts with bases that are two to three times their height are marked. The direction of rotation is shown (*arrow*). **B,** After the left pedicle is rotated, it is sutured into place. Undermining at the lateral margin facilitates mobility (*arrows*). (continued)

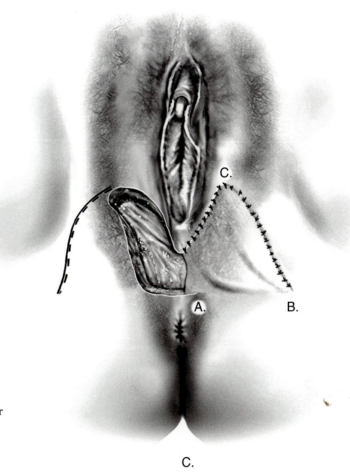

C.

FIGURE 25-3 **C,** The right pedicle is mobilized in a similar fashion. **D,** Grafting is complete, and the wounds are closed. The lower, or most distal, portions of the pedicles may be attached with tissue cement rather than sutured. (continued)

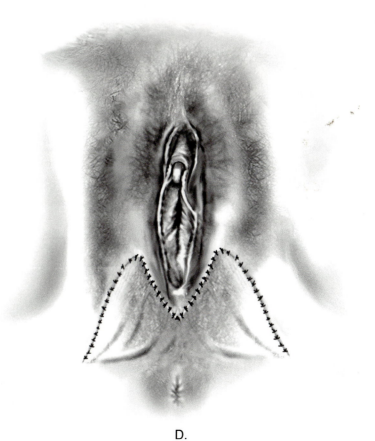

D.

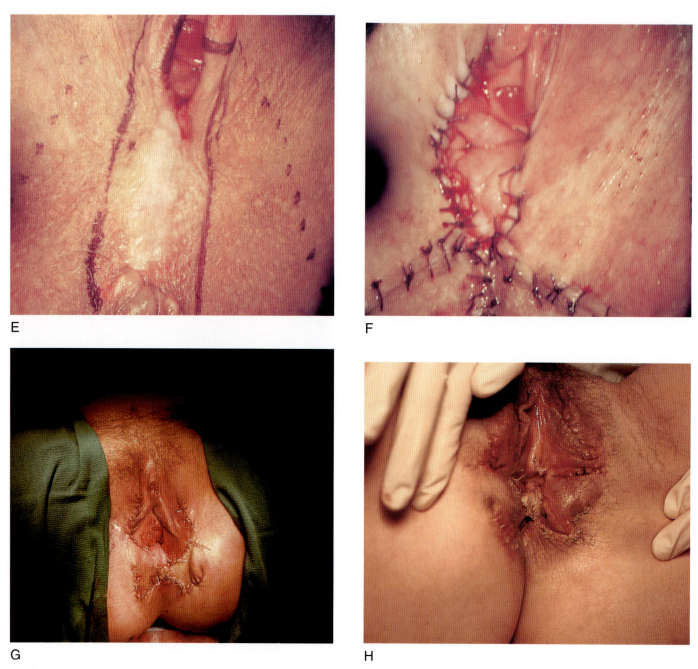

E

F

G

H

FIGURE 25-3 **E,** Pedicle grafting will be necessary to close the wound after this large area of vulvar tissue is excised. **F,** The peri-introital margins were closed primarily, and the grafts closed the perineal and perianal tissue deficits. **G,** Extensive vulvar carcinoma in situ was excised and closed with a combination of primary apposition and swinging-in pedicle grafts. The bulge on the patient's left disappeared by 2 months postoperatively. **H,** A view of G obtained 2 weeks postoperatively shows the good color of the grafts.

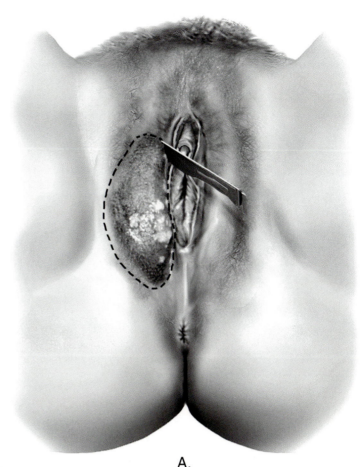

A.

FIGURE 25-4 A, Simple excision is performed on an extensive area of the labium majus. **B,** The excised area cannot be primarily closed without excessive tension. (continued)

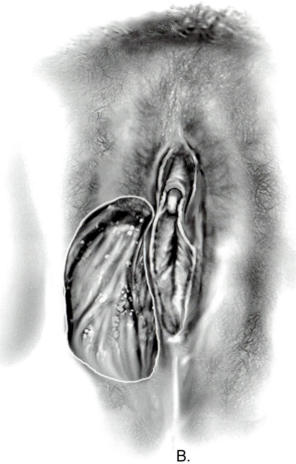

B.

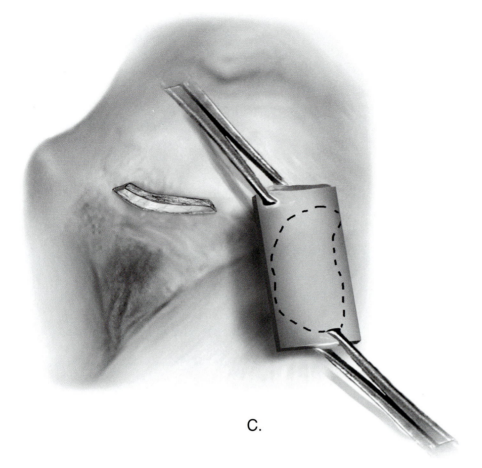

C.

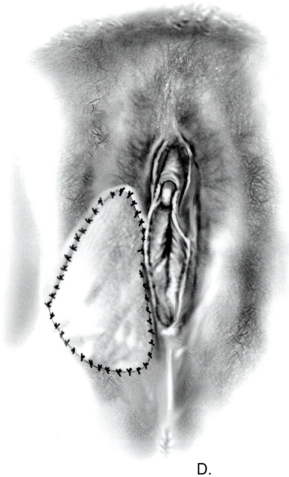

D.

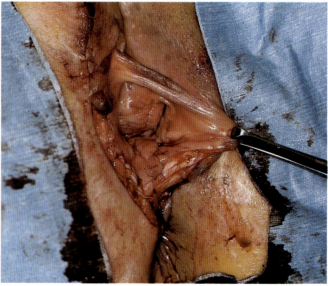

E

FIGURE 25-4 **C,** A full-thickness strip of abdominal skin is excised, and the fat is cut away. **D,** The graft is trimmed and sutured into place. **E,** This patient required excision of the right side of the vulva because of vulvar intraepithelial neoplasia grade 3 affecting the labium majus, labium minus, vestibule, and perineum. (continued)

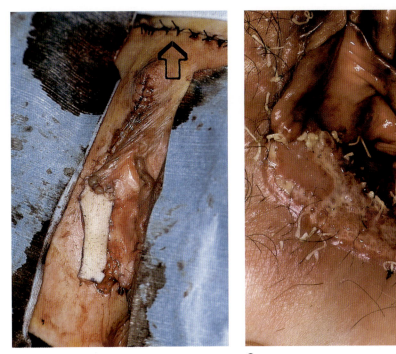

F

G

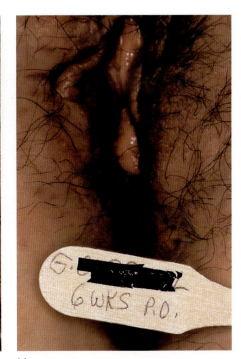

H

FIGURE 25-4 **F,** A free, full-thickness graft was performed to provide tension-free closure. The tissue for the graft was obtained from the lower abdomen (*arrow*). **G,** Ten days after surgery, the graft shows sloughing of the epidermis. The underlying dermis has a healthy, pink appearance. **H,** Six weeks postoperatively, the graft site cannot be differentiated from the surrounding normal tissue. **I,** The graft site is seen 1 year postoperatively.

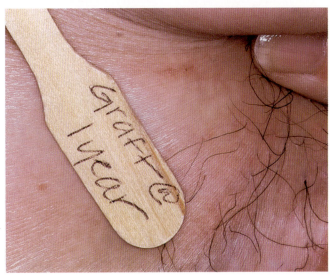

I

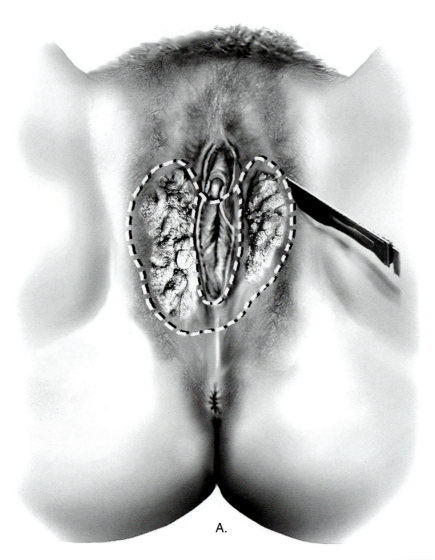

A.

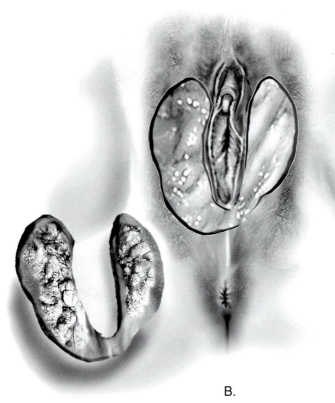

B.

FIGURE 25-5 A, Excision of the labia majora and the lateral portions of the labia minora, or skinning vulvectomy, is shown. **B,** After the skin is excised to the level of the fat layer, hemostasis is obtained. (continued)

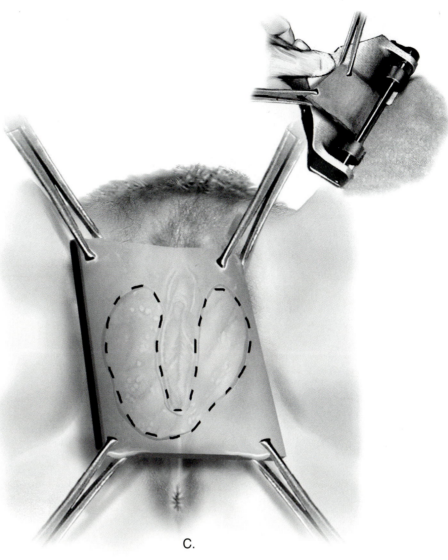

C.

FIGURE 25-5 C, A full-drum, split-thickness graft is placed over the defect and cut in a pattern to cover the wound precisely. **D,** The sutured graft is covered with a pressure dressing and left undisturbed for at least 1 week. The dressing is removed and replaced weekly. (continued)

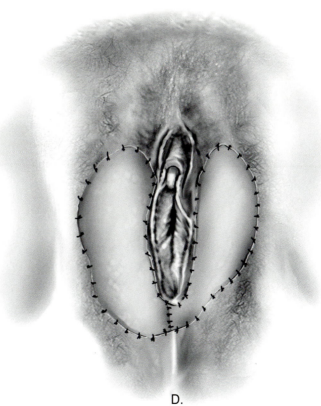

D.

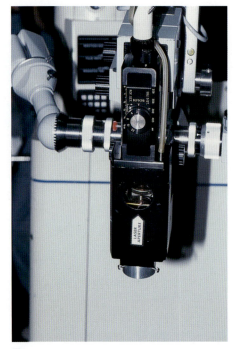

E

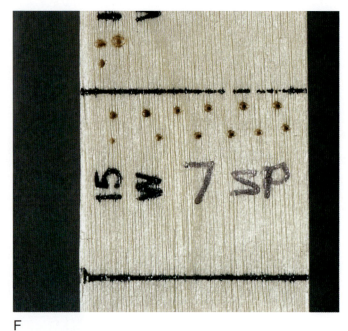

F

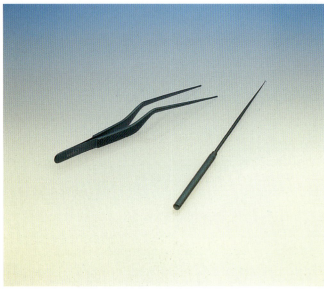

G

FIGURE 25-5 **E,** The best contemporary CO_2 laser for the treatment of neoplasia of the lower genital tract is the UltraPulse (superpulse). Advantages of this instrument include precise control through the use of a microscope and a micromanipulator and minimal thermal injury. These wounds are equivalent to knife wounds in terms of healing and the creation of devitalized tissue. **F,** Laser imprints, or spots, are tested on a dry, sterile, wooden tongue blade. The spots range from 0.5 mm to 1 mm in diameter. These spots are used for cutting, but not for vaporization. **G,** Accessory instruments used for a CO_2 laser thin section are a long-handled, fine skin hook and long forceps with Brown-type teeth.

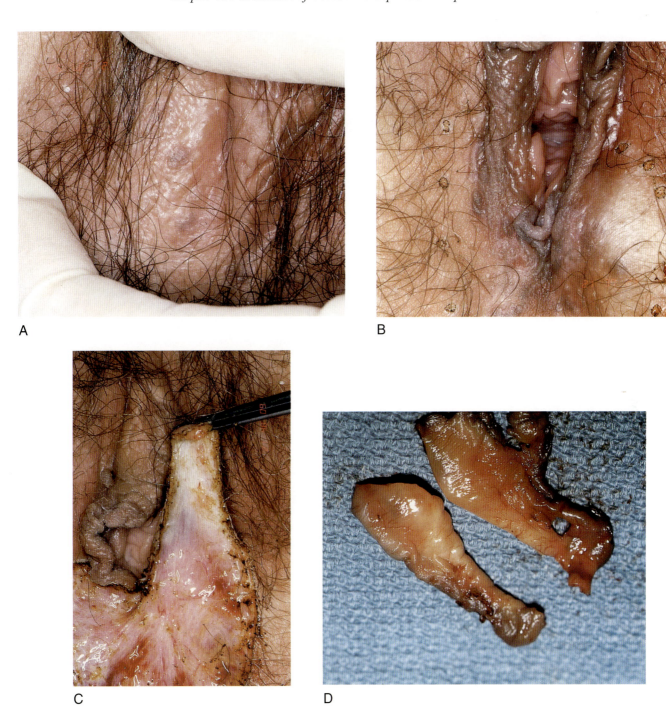

FIGURE 25-6 A, In this 28-year old woman, the classic lesions associated with vulvar intraepithelial neoplasia are seen on the labia majora and perineum. **B,** The area of excision is infiltrated with a 1:100 solution of vasopressin and traced with laser imprints. **C,** A well-developed thin section shows the underlying pink dermis. **D,** Two segments of vulvar skin are excised and sent for pathologic examination. (continued)

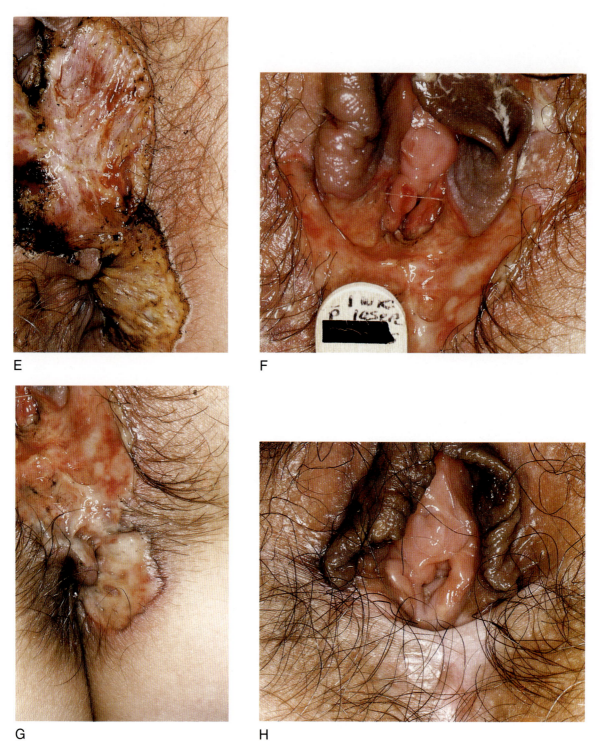

E

F

G

H

FIGURE 25-6 **E,** After the excision was completed, an area of perianal skin (*left*) was vaporized. The results of vaporization and sharp laser excision can be compared. The vaporized tissue shows thermal artifact (yellow color and a dark char line). **F,** The thin section wound is seen 1 week postoperatively (×4). **G,** A colposcopic view (×10) of the wound 2 weeks postoperatively shows the differences in healing between vaporization and thin section excision. **H,** Six weeks postoperatively, the wound is completely healed.

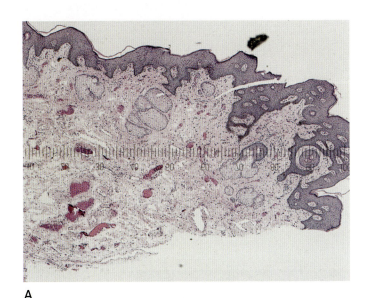

A

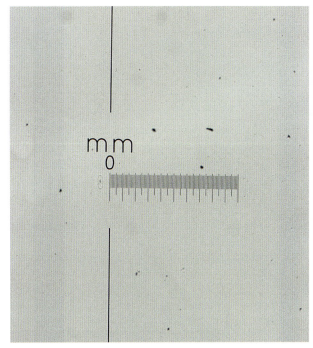

B

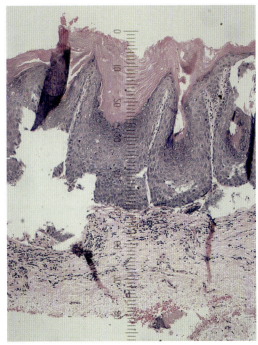

C

FIGURE 25-7 A, Thin section excision is very sharp, and the pathologic findings are easily interpreted. The stage micrometer scale on a microscope can be used to measure tissue precisely. **B,** A Zeiss millimeter standard is used to calibrate the micrometer. **C,** The thickness of the neoplastic epithelium is measured on a thin section.

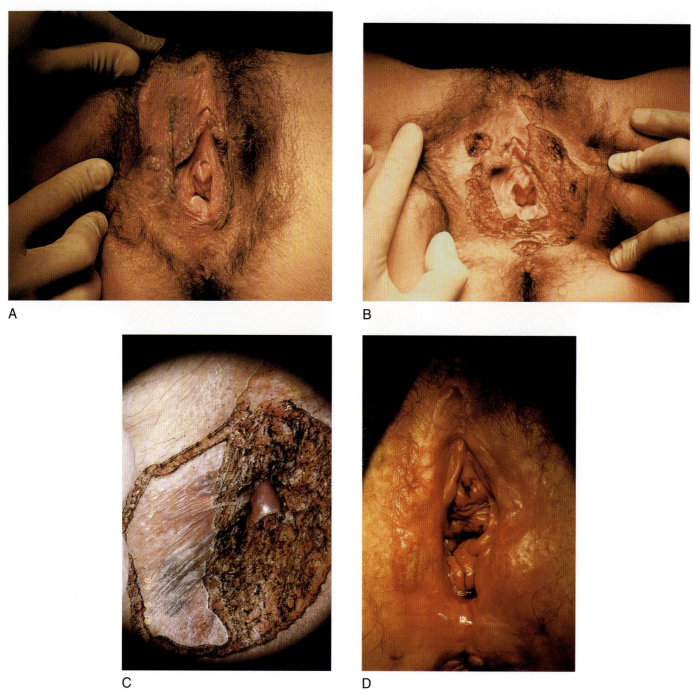

FIGURE 25-8 A, These multifocal, pigmented, warty lesions are characteristic of vulvar intraepithelial neoplasia (VIN). Human papilloma virus typing showed type 16 DNA. **B,** Immediately after the procedure, complete vaporization of all visible lesions is seen. **C,** A magnified view obtained after perianal vaporization of VIN grade 3 shows the sharp detail and controlled depth of the wound. **D,** This 38-year old woman has biopsy-proven VIN of the left and right labia majora. (continued)

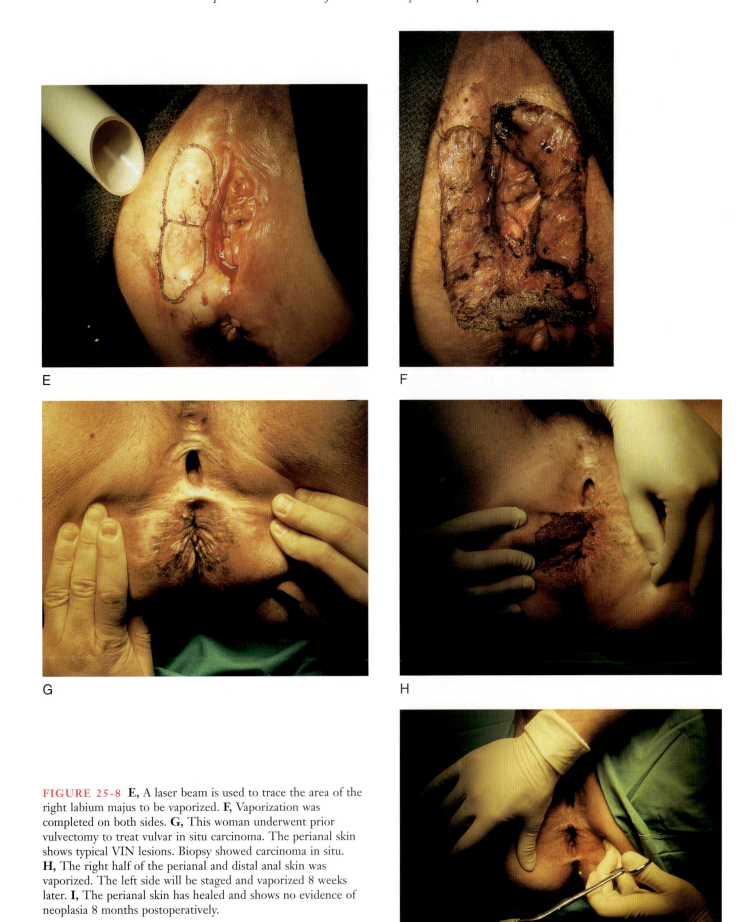

FIGURE 25-8 E, A laser beam is used to trace the area of the right labium majus to be vaporized. **F,** Vaporization was completed on both sides. **G,** This woman underwent prior vulvectomy to treat vulvar in situ carcinoma. The perianal skin shows typical VIN lesions. Biopsy showed carcinoma in situ. **H,** The right half of the perianal and distal anal skin was vaporized. The left side will be staged and vaporized 8 weeks later. **I,** The perianal skin has healed and shows no evidence of neoplasia 8 months postoperatively.

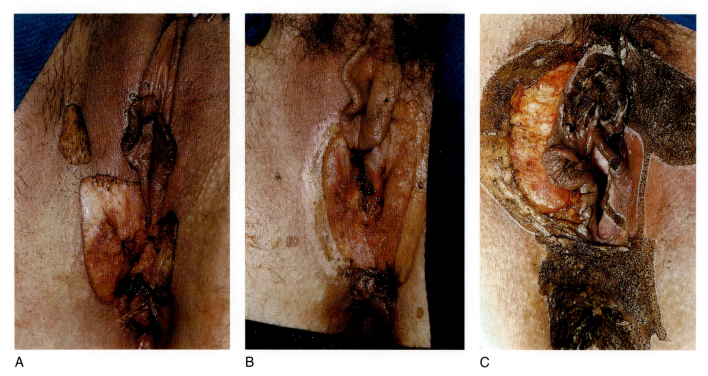

A B C

FIGURE 25-9 **A,** This vulva was treated for vulvar intraepithelial neoplasia with a combination of excision and CO_2 laser vaporization. **B,** Most of this extensive vulvar intraepithelial neoplasia grade 3 lesion was excised, and the peripheral margin was extended with laser vaporization. **C,** The inner portion of the right labium majus was excised, and the rest of the vulva was vaporized with 5-mm peripheral margins.

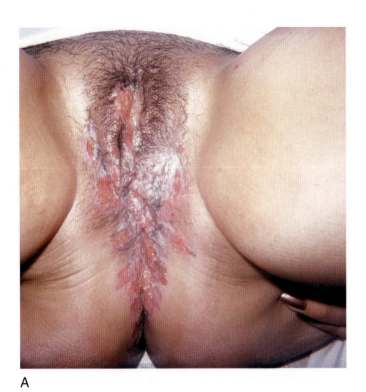

A

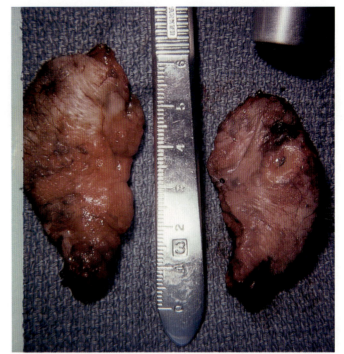

B

FIGURE 25-10 **A,** This patient has extensive Paget's disease of the vulva. Red, affected areas and the characteristic multicentric distribution of this disorder are shown. **B,** Two months after the initial visit, the patient seen in *A* underwent extensive excision of the vulva. **C,** This colposcopic photograph of the vulva of the patient seen in *A* and *B* was obtained 6 years later. The perineum and perianal skin show suspicious areas that require biopsy.

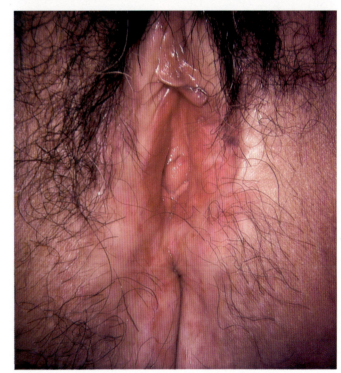

C

SECTION IV
Special Considerations

CHAPTER 26
Human Papillomavirus DNA Typing and Vaccination

Human papillomavirus (HPV) typing has and will become an exceedingly important screening test, not only for women with ASCUS cytology, but also for the future selection of candidates for HPV vaccination. Recently, a controlled trial of a vaccine to create antibodies against HPV-16 has been reported. 2392 women between the ages of 16–23 years of age were divided into 2 groups, consisting of 1194 women receiving vaccine and 1198 of women receiving placebo. The women in the study were negative for HPV-16 DNA and HPV-16 antibodies at enrollment and at month 7 in the study. Additionally, these women reported no prior abnormal pap smears and had ≤5 male sex partners during their lifetime. HPV testing can be performed on material obtained for cytologic testing, e.g., thin-layer Papanicolaou smears, as well as from biopsy material. The most sensitive test for HPV DNA typing is the polymerase chain reaction (PCR). Hybrid capture is currently the method utilized in most clinical testing. The results of the vaccination study included the following data:

1. The mean **antibody titer (HPV-16)** for women who received the vaccine was 1510 m MU per mL and less than 6 m MU per mL for controls.

2. The incidence for persistent HPV-16 infection was 3.8 per 100 women years in the placebo group and 0 per 100 women years in the vaccine group.

3. 41 cases of HPV-16 infection in the placebo group were distributed accordingly: thirty-one without CIN, 5 with CIN1, 4 with CIN2, 1 DNA positive lost to follow-up.

4. 44 additional cases of CIN were identified **not related to HPV-16**. Twenty-two were in the placebo group and 22 in the vaccinated group.

Since HPV-16 is associated with >50% of invasive cervical cancer as well as vaginal and vulvar neoplasia, testing for and prevention of HPV-16 infection, including nuclear transformation, is vital for the prevention of lower genital tract neoplasia in the female population. The cost implications relative to defensive vaccination worldwide versus the costs of management as well as the human depredations of invasive cancer are significantly positive in favor of vaccination.

CHAPTER 27

Pregnancy

Colposcopy is done on a regular basis for pregnant women. During the first and second trimesters, the examination is similar to that of a non-pregnant woman. In fact, the examination should be technically easier because the endocervical canal is relatively more accessible to view.

The most important aspects of examination during pregnancy are to avoid rubbing the acetic acid swab across the exposed glandular epithelium at the T-zone. Invariably, a rubbing versus blotting action creates bleeding.

Biopsies may be performed as they would be in non-pregnant women and Monsel's solution may be applied, as in non-pregnant women, for hemostasis. No endocervical curettage should be done during pregnancy.

Once a pre-malignant disorder has been diagnosed during pregnancy, the patient may be followed-up at the 28-weeks gestation visit for a repeat colposcopy. If no worsening of the lesion is observed and no suspicion of invasive disease exists, the patient may be instructed to return at 6–8 weeks postpartum for a repeat colposcopy and possible biopsy.

If invasive disease is suspected or cannot be ruled out, a directed biopsy should be obtained under colposcopic guidance regardless of the length of the gestation. The technique that is best suited for late pregnancy has been described. Briefly, a long shank biopsy forceps is directed under colposcopic magnification to the site of the suspected abnormality. The gynecologist's other hand holds a Monsel's soaked swab immediately adjacent to the positioned biopsy forceps. As the biopsy forceps jaws close on the sample site and are withdrawn, the Monsel's swab immediately is thrust into the defect created by the biopsy.

Conization during late pregnancy may be performed but exposure is difficult and blood loss is excessive; therefore, beyond the second trimester conization is best avoided until the pregnancy terminates. If conization must be performed, the author recommends placing 2 lateral hemostatic stitches of O-chromic catgut at 3 and 9 o'clock positions. The latter suture ends are cut short. Next, 4 stabilizing O-vicryl sutures are placed at 12, 3, 6, and 9. Next, 1 : 100 Vasopressin is injected into the cervix. The small 1-cm height cone specimen is obtained with a knife or via electrical loop. Next, hemostasis is obtained by a reefing suture of O-vicryl. The stay sutures are cut out and the patient is sent home for 24–48 hours bed rest. I prophylactically treat the patient with 1 gm of intravenous Cefotan prior to starting the procedure. No packs or sponges are placed into the vagina. Optionally, the surgeon may squirt an applicatorful of Cleocin vaginal cream into the vagina at the end of the operation.

CHAPTER 28
The Young Patient

A colposcope may be used to view the vagina and cervix in young girls. Neoplasia is unlikely to occur in this age group; however, trauma, foreign bodies, and venereal infections as well as viral, fungal, or bacterial infections may be seen. A pediatric speculum and a colposcope aid the examiner in obtaining an accurate view of the vagina and obtaining specimens. Foreign bodies, such as beans, marbles, pencils, and jewelry, may be extracted under direct vision.

Adolescent patients may have human papillomavirus (HPV) infections of the vulva, vagina, or cervix. Susceptible patients also may have intraepithelial neoplasia. Evaluation of these patients, including biopsy, is identical to that of adult patients. However, injectable local and topical anesthesia typically is administered to eliminate discomfort in young patients, who may be anxious or frightened. Before cervical biopsy is performed, the injection of 1% lidocaine (Xylocaine)

into the cervix is recommended. Before ECC, application of viscous 2% Xylocaine into the endocervical canal with a cotton-tipped applicator is recommended.

A patient who has condylomatous atypia or cervical intraepithelial neoplasia (CIN) grade 1 may simply be followed. HPV typing may be performed as well. However, if CIN grade 2 or 3 is diagnosed, electrical loop excision or CO_2 superpulse laser excision is performed. Surgical judgment is crucial to the success of the surgery. A 5-mm loop is used to treat a small, immature cervix, and the surgeon should be careful to remove the smallest possible volume of tissue. The 1- to 1.5-cm rule does not apply to the immature cervix because it is smaller than the adult cervix. Finally, the surgeon must advise the patient to avoid smoking because of the link between tobacco use and persistence or recurrence of cervical lesions.

CHAPTER 29
Advanced Age and Elderly

Abnormal pap smears in this cohort of women are particularly worrisome because invasive squamous cancer affecting both cervix and vagina occurs most commonly in this age category. Additionally, adenocarcinoma of the uterus is most frequently diagnosed in this age group. Finally, the cervical transformation zone may be hard to view because of the relocation of the squamo-columnar junction upwards and within the endocervical canal. Data has been published that the duration of the intraepithelial neoplasia phase in women >60 years of age as compared to women <40 years of age may be diminished by a factor of 1 to 16.

If the T-zone cannot be seen in the face of abnormal cytology, then a loop excision may be the only practical means of obtaining a specimen. It may also be the only manner by which access via an endocervical curette or brush to the cervical canal may be gained. Here, as in children, the use of topical and injectable local anesthesia may pay dividends by eliminating pain thereby maximizing patient cooperation. A report describing mildly dysplastic cells emanating from an atrophic vagina should trigger the utilization of 4 weeks of topical estrogen followed by repetition of the Pap smear and the performance of colposcopy. The finding of a vaginal abnormality on biopsy is more meaningful following vaginal pre-treatment with topical estrogen than prior to the initiation of local hormonal therapy.

As compared to women below the age of 40, vulvar intraepithelial neoplasia diagnosed in the >50-year age group has a greater propensity to progress to invasive disease and is less likely to spontaneously revert from pre-malignancy to benignancy.

CHAPTER 30
DES
(Diethylstilbestrol-Exposed Women)

The congenital abnormalities produced by the "in utero" administration of stilbestrol have been discussed and illustrated in the sections dealing with the cervix and vagina. Associated factors should also be considered when managing these women. The upper vagina may be congenitally constricted as compared to non-DES exposed women. Care must be taken when opening the speculum so as to avoid tearing the lateral vaginal wall or forniceal walls. If the tissues are overstretched, the resulting vaginal tear will bleed profusely.

In the case of DES-exposed women, the findings of mosaic and punctation patterns set in ground leukoplakia, which would otherwise invoke a serious concern in the non-DES-exposed patient may not show any significant pathology beyond atypical squamous metaplasia. The author can bear witness to the fact that some of the most blatant mosaic patterns have been observed on the rims of congenital DES-induced cervical hoods. In fact, I have questioned the accuracy of the pathology report after biopsying through such areas of mosaic. Two subsequent biopsies finally convinced me that no neoplasia existed.

The uterine cavities of DES-exposed women may be deformed and reduced. The "T"-shaped cavity seen on hysterogram is illustrative of such volume reduction.

Finally, DES-exposed women may complain of dyspareunia related to vaginal adenosis. The most common complaint is burning discomfort during coitus. The medical therapy consists of attempting to convert the adenosis to squamous metaplasia hormonally or to surgically eliminate the adenosis.

CHAPTER 31
Non-Compliant Patients

A patient who, by conscious choice, decides not to pay attention to her doctor's advice represents a problem for the responsible gynecologist. Not only does this type of person present a potential medical liability risk but additionally she will precipitate therapeutic dilemmas.

The decision to follow low-grade cervical, vaginal, or vulvar neoplastic lesions depends on the assumption that the patient will cooperate to the extent of returning for follow-up visits at specified dates and times. If that assumption is incorrect, the patient will be at risk for undiagnosed, and therefore untreated, progression of disease. Clinical decisions will be adjusted depending on the patient's historical record of missed visits as well as the doctor's objective appraisal about the patient's reliability. The decision to perform an all-in-one electrical loop excision of the cervix to serve as biopsy as well as treatment following abnormal cytology is an excellent practical example of this type of deliberation.

Because vaginal and vulvar neoplasia is multicentric, follow-up after treatment is essential to identify recurrent disease. The latter requires cytology in the vagina and colposcopy and biopsy for both vagina and vulva. Women who do not show up for follow-up examinations should be notified first in writing by First Class Mail service that it is important for their well-being to keep appointments. If the patient still does not attend to appointments, a certified letter (return receipt) should be sent, noting the risk of cancer and noting that the clinic, doctor, or office has made repeated attempts to notify the patient of the need for follow-up and the fact that all such entreaties have been ignored. The letter should specifically mention that this notification will serve to finish the attempts to arrange visits for the patient and that the relationship between the patient and the entity will be terminated if the patient does not respond.

Women who are to receive supplemental treatment, e.g., interferon, for the treatment of resistant warts, should be apprised that smoking and oral contraceptive medication must be stopped prior to the initiation of interferon therapy. If the patient will not terminate her smoking indulgence, then it is senseless to administer interferon.

As a general statement, the treating physician is responsible for ensuring that the patient has a complete understanding about the pathology of her disease and the facts about the proposed treatment. The latter should include details relative to potential complications and how those complications might affect outcome. Disfiguring surgery, such as vulvectomy, must be discussed in great detail, particularly regarding the ultimate cosmetic appearance of the vulva. Surgery likely to affect basic function, e.g., vaginectomy, must likewise be discussed from the standpoint of the risk of dyspareunia and future childbearing. Similarly, cervical surgery must be described relative to outcome, particularly focusing on fertility and pregnancy outcomes. The triad of cosmetic appearance, effect on sexual intercourse, and risk relative to future childbearing, are questions of concern in every woman's mind.

CHAPTER 32
Immunosuppressed Patients

Women who are immunologically deficient secondary to HIV (human immunodeficiency virus) infection or because of drug therapy, e.g., cyclosporin administered to prevent organ transplantation rejection, are clearly susceptible to a variety of HPV (human papillomavirus) and HSV (herpes simplex virus) infections. As a result of the latter, they are likely targets for lower genital tract neoplasia. Once CIN, VAIN, or VIN become established, the eradication of the disorder in this subset of patients may be difficult to achieve. In these cases, ablative techniques are particularly vulnerable to failure. The status of margins is very important; therefore, excisional techniques are recommended. Follow-up is exceedingly important and should combine methodology for greater accuracy, e.g., cytology, HPV-typing, colposcopy. Biopsy should be performed for any suspicious lesion. Serial photographic records utilizing cervicography or colpophotography provide an excellent and comparable documentary record. These patients require repetitive treatment and may end up with the most radical therapy, e.g., hysterectomy with wide vaginal cuff for cervical intraepithelial neoplasia; vaginectomy with grafting for vaginal intraepithelial neoplasia or vulvectomy with grafting for vulvar intraepithelial neoplasia. Obviously, drugs such as interferon cannot be used in such circumstances.

Relative immunodeficiency may be observed in cases of resistant warts as well as CIN, VAIN, and VIN. A graphic example of relative immunodeficiency may be observed relative to the behavior of condylomata accuminata associated with pregnancy and the recession of the warts upon the termination of the pregnancy. Diabetes mellitus is still another example of an impaired immune state. Less obvious immunocompromising states are associated with corticosteroid intake (asthma treatment, multiple sclerosis therapy, lupus control). Even more subtle deleterious effects on immunocompetence may be observed with oral contraceptive intake and cigarette smoking. Factors that exert relative immunodeficiency should be eliminated whenever possible before initiating treatment for HPV-related infections or lower genital tract intraepithelial neoplasia since persistence or recurrence of disease will be affected. In some cases, this will be rather easy to accomplish, e.g., stopping smoking and/or oral contraceptive intake. In other instances, a period of time may elapse, e.g., pregnancy, multiple sclerosis steroid therapy. In other cases, tight control of diabetes in conjunction with the treatment of the Lower genital tract disorder will produce more favorable outcomes.

CHAPTER 33
Cancer Phobia and Emotionally Disturbed Patients

The reception of an abnormal cytology or biopsy report will create anxiety for most women. Fear of cancer because of a similar or related affliction in family member(s), friends, or acquaintances may result in an irrational mental response. In such instances, the patient may need psychologic counseling or psychiatric referral. Patients may desire the abnormality, which they may mistakenly equate with cancer, to be gone regardless of the price for such therapy and may request hysterectomy to eliminate dysplastic disease. Patients similarly equate an abnormal biopsy with future inability to attain pregnancy.

The gynecologist's obligations to his/her patient relate to imparting accurate information about pre-malignant disease. Clarification may be required to properly inform as well as convince the patient that no person dies from a pre-malignant disorder; that progression within stages of dysplasia does not put them at imminent risk for invasive cancer; that treatment need not be immediate but may be safely planned; that successful elimination of dysplasia does not require radical treatment.

The most important aspect to meet an acceptable standard of care requires the gynecologist to make a timely and accurate diagnosis. Without knowing the true nature of the patient's disorder, the physician cannot in good conscience render reasonable advice relative to treatment. Diagnosis, as stated in previous sections, relies on cytologic screening, colposcopy, endocervical curettage, directed biopsies, and a variety of excisional procedures. The sine qua non in the above process remains the histopathologic biopsy and its appropriate interpretation in synchrony with cytologic findings.

CHAPTER 34
ASCUS*

ASCUS (atypical squamous cells of undetermined significance) is a term that was coined when the Bethesda System for reporting cytologic diagnoses was generated in 1988. It falls into the larger section of squamous cell epithelial abnormalities. Therefore, this is *not* a normal cytologic finding. In plain terms, it means the cytologist cannot say how significant the abnormal cells that have been identified are. In other words, the ASCUS reading may reflect reparative (reactive) changes or a serious high-grade pre-malignant lesion or even an invasive carcinoma. According to the most recent modification of the Bethesda System (2001), approximately 10–20% of women with ASCUS have an underlying CIN2 or 3 lesion and 1 in 1000 may have invasive cancer. The 2001 Bethesda System has bifurcated the former ASCUS into ASC-US and ASC-H (atypical squamous cells cannot exclude HSIL). The authors clarify that ASC is *not* a diagnosis of exclusion but rather "is considered to be suggestive of SIL." The new system has eliminated "ASCUS, favor reactive." The new ASC-H is predicted to encompass 5–10% of all atypical squamous cell (not specifically SIL categorized) cases. Within the ASC-H category, 24% to 94% will show biopsy proven CIN2, 3.

Any woman with ASC-US or ASH-H requires an additional work-up to make a definitive diagnosis. Those falling into the ASC-H cohort should have timely colposcopy, directed biopsy, and ECC. If the ATZ is not seen or incompletely seen, an electrical loop excision should be performed. Women with ASC-US may be followed by repeat cytological examination until 2 consecutive negative Pap smears are obtained. If the patient has 2 consecutive ASCUS (3–6 month interval), a colposcopy, directed biopsy, and ECC should be performed in a timely fashion.

Recently, HPV-DNA typing has been suggested as an alternative management program for ASC-US patients. Women who are negative for high-risk HPV-DNA can then be followed by repeated cytology at 12-month intervals. The presence of high-risk HPV-DNA should signal a timely colposcopic examination coupled with directed biopsy and ECC.

---

* A laboratory should not have an ASCUS diagnosis rate exceeding 2–3 times the reporting rate of SIL.

CHAPTER 35
AGUS

Atypical glandular cells of undetermined significance (AGUS) requires action to determine the source and characteristics of these cells. Adenocarcinoma of the endocervix has increased in incidence from 5% to 20% during the past 30 years. The major increase of cases has occurred in a younger subset of women and is associated with the presence of HPV 16 and 18 DNA. Adenocarcinoma is more insidious and unpredictable than is squamous cell carcinoma of the cervix. Typically, adenocarcinoma in situ (AIS) is multifocal in origin and a significant number of cases are associated with concurrent squamous cell carcinoma in situ. AGC (atypical glandular cells) on cytological examination is associated with a greater precentage of underlying high-grade disease (10%–39%). The 2001 Bethesda Classification now classifies AGC, AGC favor neoplastic, AIS, adenocarcinoma, other (endometrial cells >40 years of age) as separate categories. The question arises as to where AGC arise, i.e., endometrial or endocervical. The gynecologist's responsibility does *not* end with a colposcopy, endocervical curettage, and ectocervical biopsy, particularly if these studies are benign and not in concert with the cytological examination. According to the 2001 consensus study, the AGC category may be associated with CIN in 9%–54% of women, AIS in 0–8% of women, 1%–9% of invasive carcinoma. Clearly, the cytologic finding of AGC favor neoplasia category is associated with a higher risk of neoplasia with 27%–96% having CIN2, 3, AIS or cancer versus 9%–41% in the AGC-NOS group (NOS = not otherwise specified). Thus, further examination is mandated. These examinations include: cold knife conization, hysteroscopy with sampling, endometrial biopsy, and endometrial ultrasonography (transvaginal ultrasound utilizing a 3 mm endometrial thickness cutoff). Several studies have suggested that AGC cytology is associated with greater risks of high-grade CIN and adenocarcinoma in situ in pre-menopausal women and endometrial hyperplasia and endocervical/endometrial cancer in post-menopausal women.

CHAPTER 36
Unsatisfactory Colposcopy

An unsatisfactory colposcopic examination means that the examiner cannot see all or part of the squamous-columnar transformation zone. Thus, the gynecologist cannot determine whether a neoplastic lesion exists, cannot know the severity of a neoplastic lesion, and cannot give any assurance to the patient. Obviously, the colposcopic examination was indicated in the first place because of cytologic abnormalities or other stated reasons.

If the colposcopy is unsatisfactory and cannot be relied upon, other means to make a diagnosis must be embarked upon. Continuing to obtain repeated cytological samples is not an appropriate methodology to attain the diagnostic goal. If the cervical canal is stenotic or if the transformation zone lies in the endocervical canal, a small cone performed by knife, laser, or electrical loop will confirm or refute the diagnosis of CIN (or invasion). If an ECC or endocervical endoscopy can be performed and a suitable sample of tissue obtained, the patient may avoid conization. The major drawback to ECC is the inability to accurately grade the lesion because orientation is a problem when only tissue fragments are obtained. A negative ECC coupled with an unsatisfactory colposcopy in the face of abnormal cytology should trigger a promptly performed loop electrical excision in order to adequately provide a sample of the T-zone.

CHAPTER 37
Follow-Up

Follow-up appointments and subsequent diagnostic procedures are essential when the responsible physician or a surrogate, e.g., nurse practitioner or midwife, is dealing with a disorder that is not and cannot be cured so as to unequivocally guarantee absolutely no chance of persistence or recurrence (Flow Charts 1 and 2).

The follow-up guidelines utilized by most gynecologists are arbitrary and few published data can objectively support one protocol over another. Data published many years ago detailed that repeat cytology following documentation of an inflammatory condition of the cervix created by a variety of infectious agents was likely to repetitively show residual inflammation for 8–10 weeks posttreatment. Cellular abnormalities following pelvic radiation may last for years or may persist for a lifetime. Reparative abnormalities following conization may be present for approximately 3 months. Follow-up for ASCUS cytologic smears has been arbitrarily set for 3–6 months.

To avoid reparative cellular atypia, follow-up after colposcopy and biopsy (including ECC) following repetitive ASCUS or an LSIL Pap smear should take place within a period of approximately 3 months with the proviso that the colposcopy and biopsy findings were concordant with the cytology. The follow-up should consist of a colposcopy to check the biopsy site and a consultation to determine whether to treat or continue to follow the disorder with the hope of regression. If the follow-up pathway is chosen, the patient should be seen at 6-month intervals and have a Pap smear plus a colposcopy at each visit.

However, if the biopsy diagnosis is CIN2 or CIN3, the patient should return within 3 months for treatment. Follow-up for Pap smears showing high-grade squamous cellular abnormalities should be scheduled in a timely fashion, i.e., within a period of approximately 1 month. The patient should be informed that a colposcopy and biopsy (including an ECC) will be performed at that visit. If the biopsy and Pap smear are conforming, the patient should be scheduled for treatment by loop excision. If the ECC is positive and the biopsy does not show CIN2 or CIN3, a conization procedure should be performed. The latter is likely to dually serve as diagnostic and therapeutic.

Any Pap smear suggestive for or diagnostic of invasive carcinoma should trigger a priority appointment within 1 week or less for directed biopsies. If the biopsy shows less than invasion, a sharp knife conization should be promptly performed. Patients with normal and adequate Pap smears may be followed on a yearly basis with repeat Pap smears. Any patient in whom dysplasia has been diagnosed and in whom the disorder has regressed or has been therapeutically eliminated should be followed annually with a Pap smear after accruing 2 consecutive normal smears (4–6-month interval).

Any patient with abnormal bleeding associated with a mass lesion of the cervix, vagina, or vulva should be seen immediately and examined disregarding any delay because of bleeding. Biopsies should be performed. Pap smears in these circumstances would be superfluous.

FLOW CHART GUIDE

Initial cytology

Initial follow-up

First procedure

Result A

Second follow-up

Second procedure

Third follow-up

Third procedure

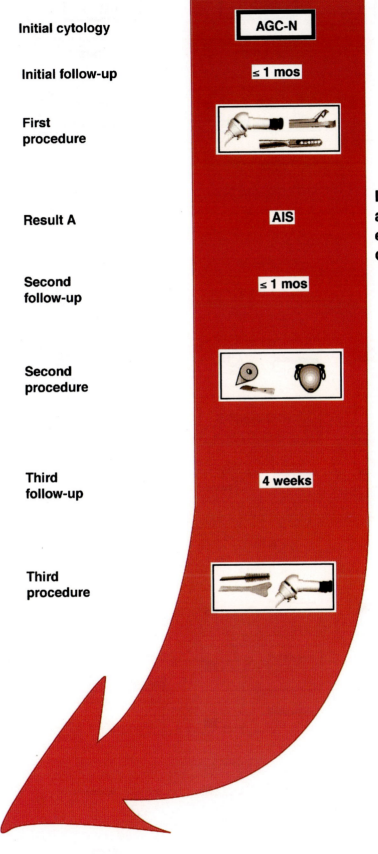

AGC-N

≤ 1 mos

AIS

≤ 1 mos

4 weeks

Look at chart and follow each color down

FLOW CHART # 1

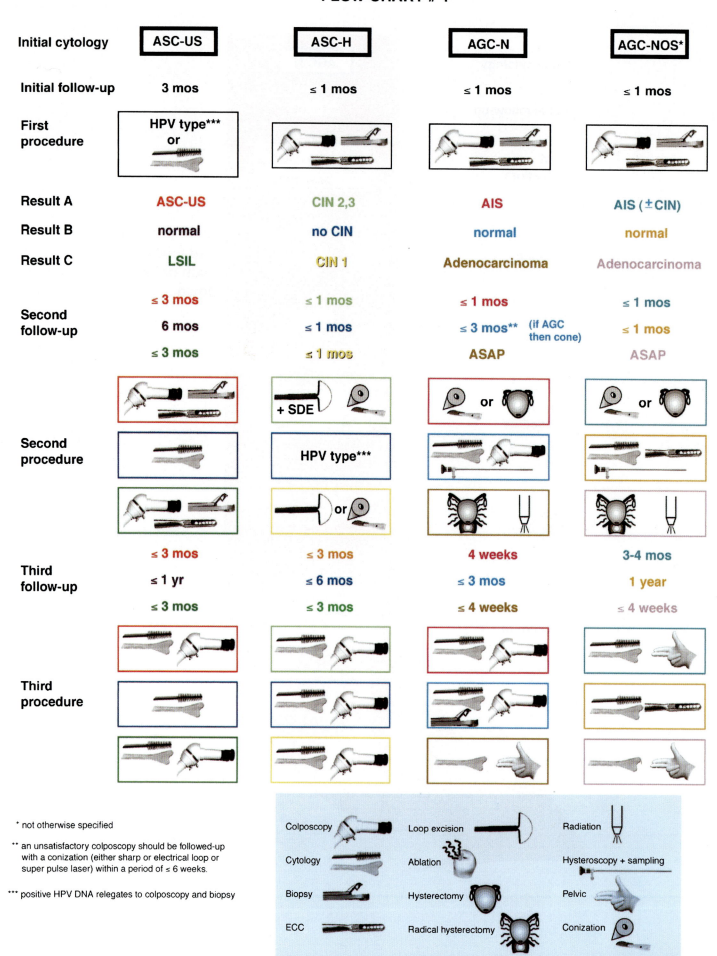

Initial cytology	**ASC-US**	**ASC-H**	**AGC-N**	**AGC-NOS***
Initial follow-up	3 mos	≤ 1 mos	≤ 1 mos	≤ 1 mos
First procedure	HPV type*** or			
Result A	ASC-US	CIN 2,3	AIS	AIS (±CIN)
Result B	normal	no CIN	normal	normal
Result C	LSIL	CIN 1	Adenocarcinoma	Adenocarcinoma
Second follow-up	≤ 3 mos 6 mos ≤ 3 mos	≤ 1 mos ≤ 1 mos ≤ 1 mos	≤ 1 mos ≤ 3 mos** (if AGC then cone) ASAP	≤ 1 mos ≤ 1 mos ASAP
Second procedure		+ SDE HPV type***		
Third follow-up	≤ 3 mos ≤ 1 yr ≤ 3 mos	≤ 3 mos ≤ 6 mos ≤ 3 mos	4 weeks ≤ 3 mos ≤ 4 weeks	3-4 mos 1 year ≤ 4 weeks
Third procedure				

* not otherwise specified

** an unsatisfactory colposcopy should be followed-up with a conization (either sharp or electrical loop or super pulse laser) within a period of ≤ 6 weeks.

*** positive HPV DNA relegates to colposcopy and biopsy

Colposcopy		Loop excision		Radiation	
Cytology		Ablation		Hysteroscopy + sampling	
Biopsy		Hysterectomy		Pelvic	
ECC		Radical hysterectomy		Conization	

FLOW CHART # 2

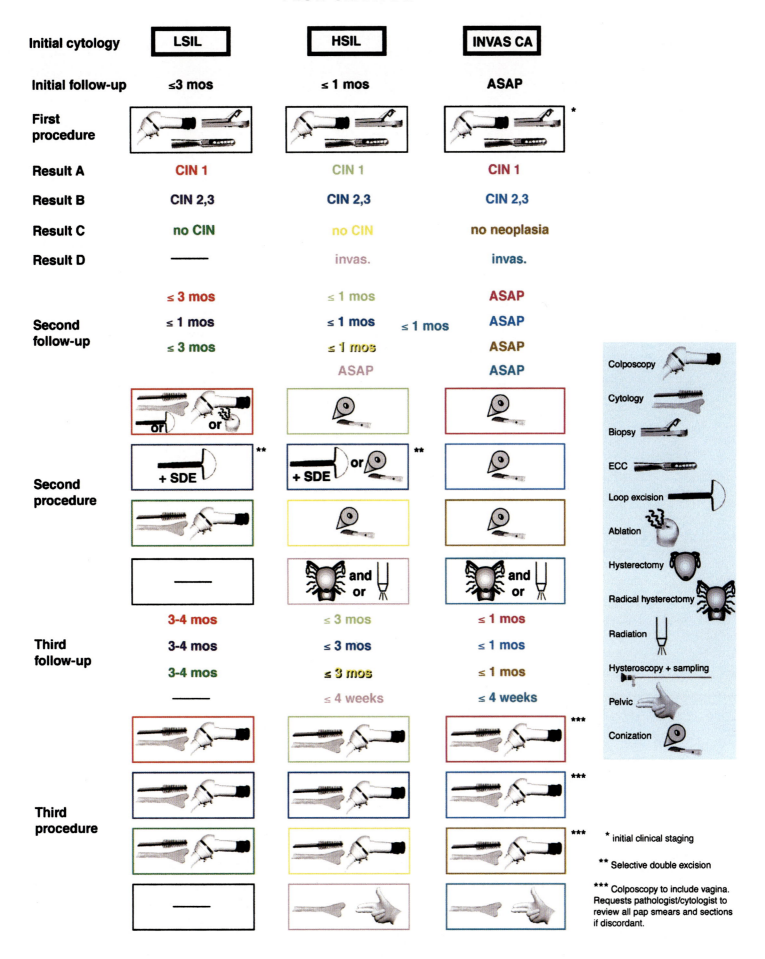

Initial cytology	**LSIL**	**HSIL**	**INVAS CA**
Initial follow-up	≤3 mos	≤ 1 mos	ASAP
First procedure			*
Result A	CIN 1	CIN 1	CIN 1
Result B	CIN 2,3	CIN 2,3	CIN 2,3
Result C	no CIN	no CIN	no neoplasia
Result D	——	invas.	invas.
Second follow-up	≤ 3 mos	≤ 1 mos	ASAP
	≤ 1 mos	≤ 1 mos ≤ 1 mos	ASAP
	≤ 3 mos	≤ 1 mos	ASAP
		ASAP	ASAP
Second procedure	or / or		
	+ SDE **	or / + SDE **	
	——	and / or	and / or
Third follow-up	3-4 mos	≤ 3 mos	≤ 1 mos
	3-4 mos	≤ 3 mos	≤ 1 mos
	3-4 mos	≤ 3 mos	≤ 1 mos
	——	≤ 4 weeks	≤ 4 weeks
Third procedure			***
			***
			***
	——		

Colposcopy
Cytology
Biopsy
ECC
Loop excision
Ablation
Hysterectomy
Radical hysterectomy
Radiation
Hysteroscopy + sampling
Pelvic
Conization

* initial clinical staging

** Selective double excision

*** Colposcopy to include vagina. Requests pathologist/cytologist to review all pap smears and sections if discordant.

SECTION V
Bibliography

Bibliography

Adad SJ, Souza MA, Etchebehere RM, et al: Cytohistological correlation of 219 patients submitted to surgical treatment due to diagnosis of cervical intraepithelial neoplasia. Sao Paulo Med J 1999;117(2):81–84.

Adam E, Decker DG, Herbst AL, et al: Exposure in utero to diethylstilbestrol and related synthetic hormones. JAMA 1976;236:1107.

Adelson MD, Semo R, Baggish MS, Osborne NG: Laser vaporization of genital condylomata in pregnancy. J Gynecol Surg 1990;6:257–262.

Ahlgren M, Ingemarsson I, Lindberg LG, Nordquist SRB: Conization as treatment of carcinoma in situ of the uterine cervix. Obstet Gynecol 1975;46:135.

Alvarez-Santin C, Sica A, Rodriguez M, et al: Microglandular hyperplasia of the uterine cervix: Cytologic diagnosis in cervical smears. Acta Cytol 1999;43:110–113.

Anclaux D, Lawrence WD, Gregoire L: Glandular lesions of the uterine cervix: Prognostic implications of human papillomavirus status. Int J Gynecol Pathol 1997;16:103–110.

Andersen ES, Pedersen B: Combination laser conization: Early and late complications. J Gynecol Surg 1997;13:51–56.

Andersen ES, Pedersen B, Boris J: Pregnancy outcome after combination laser conization: A case-controlled study. J Gynecol Surg 1999;15:7–12.

Andersen WA, Franquemont DW, Williams J, et al: Vulvar squamous cell carcinoma and papillomaviruses: Two separate entities? Am J Obstet Gynecol 1991;165:329–336.

Anderson B, Warting WG, Edinger DD Jr, et al: Development of DES-associated clear cell carcinoma: The importance of regular screening. Obstet Gynecol 1979;53:293.

Anderson MC: Should conization by hot loop or laser replace cervical biopsy? J Gynecol Surg 1991;7:191–194.

Anderson MC, Harteley RB: Cervical crypt involvement by intraepithelial neoplasia. Obstet Gynecol 1980;55:546.

Anderson MC, Jordan J, Morse A, Sharp F: Integrated Colposcopy. St. Louis, Mosby, 1991.

Antoine T, Grunberger V: Atlas der Kolpomikroskopie. Stuttgart, Thieme, 1956.

Aziz DC, Ferré F, Robitaille J, Ferenczy A: Human papillomavirus testing in the clinical laboratory: Part I. Squamous lesions of the cervix. J Gynecol Surg 1993;9:1–7.

Aziz DC, Ferré F, Robitaille J, Ferenczy A: Human papillomavirus testing in the clinical laboratory: Part II. Vaginal, vulvar, perineal, and penile squamous lesions. J Gynecol Surg 1993;9:9–15.

Baggish MS: The DES enigma "present précis." Conn State Med J 1978;42:395.

Baggish MS: High-power density carbon dioxide laser therapy for early cervical neoplasia. Am J Obstet Gynecol 1980;136:117–125.

Baggish MS: Evaluation and staging of endometrial and endocervical adenocarcinoma by contact hysteroscopy. Gynecol Oncol 1980;9:182.

Baggish MS: The CO_2 laser for treatment of condyloma acuminata infections. Obstet Gynecol 1980;55:711.

Baggish MS: Laser therapy of cervical intraepithelial neoplasia. Am J Obstet Gynecol 1980;138:838.

Baggish MS: Complications associated with carbon dioxide laser surgery in gynecology. Am J Obstet Gynecol 1981;139:568.

Baggish MS: CO_2 laser for CIN gynecologic laser surgery. New York, Plenum, 1981:173.

Baggish MS: CO_2 laser surgery for benign and malignant lesions of the vagina. In Bellina, JH. Gynecologic Laser Surgery. New York, Plenum, 1981:253–277.

Baggish MS: Management of cervical intraepithelial neoplasia by carbon dioxide laser. Obstet Gynecol 1982;60:378–384.

Baggish MS: Treating viral venereal infections with the CO_2 laser. J Reprod Med 1982;27:737–742.

Baggish MS: Laser management of cervical intraepithelial neoplasia. Clinical Obstet Gynecol 1983;26:980.

Baggish MS: Application of the CO_2 laser for cervical intraepithelial neoplasia. In Atsumi K (ed): New Frontiers in Laser Medicine and Surgery. Amsterdam. The Netherlands, Excerpta Medica, 1983:355.

Baggish MS: Improved laser techniques for the elimination of genital and extragenital warts. Am J Obstet Gynecol 1985;153:545.

Baggish MS: A comparison between laser excisional conization and laser vaporization for the treatment of CIN. Am J Obstet Gynecol 1986;155:39.

Baggish MS: The state of the art of laser surgery in gynecology. Lasers Surg Med 1986;6:390–395.

Baggish MS: Laser therapy for genital warts in clinical practice of gynecology. In Winkler B, Richart RM: Clinical Practice of Gynecology. New York, Elsevier, 1989:187–213.

Baggish MS: Lower genital tract laser surgery in gynecologic and obstetric surgery. In Nichols DH and Clarke-Pearson DL: Gynecologic, Obstetric and Related Surgery, 2nd ed., 2nd ed. Mosby, St. Louis 1999.

Baggish MS, Adelson MD, Semo R, Osborne NG: Laser vaporization of genital condylomata in pregnancy. J Gynecol Surg 1996;6:257.

Baggish MS, Baltoyannis P: Carbon dioxide laser treatment of cervical stenosis. Fertil Steril 1987;48:24–28.

Baggish MS, Barash F, Noel Y, Brooks M: Comparison of thermal injury zones in loop electrical and laser cervical excisional conization. Am J Obstet Gynecol 1992;166:545.

Baggish MS, Campion MJ, Ferenczy AS, Richart R: Ways of using LEEP for external lesions. Contemp Obstet Gynecol Surg 1992;37:138.

Baggish MS, Dorsey JH: Carbon dioxide laser for the treatment of vulva carcinoma in situ. Obstet Gynecol 1981;57:371.

Baggish MS, Dorsey JH: Vaginal intraepithelial neoplasia: II. Indications and technique for total vaginectomy with split thickness graft replacement. Colposc Gynecol Laser Surg 1984;1:149.

Baggish MS, Dorsey JH: The CO_2 laser combination conization. Am J Obstet Gynecol 1985;151:23.

Baggish MS, Dorsey JH, Adelson MD: A ten-year experience treating cervical intraepithelial neoplasia with the carbon dioxide laser. Am J Obstet Gynecol 1989;161:60–68.

Baggish MS, Ferenczy A, Reid R, Richart R: Laser therapy for lower genital tract lesions. Contemp Obstet Gynecol Surg 1989:1–15.

Baggish MS, Gerbie M, Ferenczy A, Richart R: Potential complications of loop excision. Contemp Obstet Gynecol Surg 1994;39:93–107.

Baggish MS, Karram MM: Atlas of Pelvic Anatomy and Gynecologic Surgery. Philadelphia, WB Saunders, 2001.

Baggish MS, Kooyman D, Woodruff JD: The cryostat cone for rapid diagnosis in carcinoma of the uterine cervix. Md State Med J 1970;19:64.

Baggish MS, Miklos J: Vulvar pain syndrome: A review. Obstet Gynecol Surv 1995;50:618.

Baggish MS, Noel Y, Brooks M: Electrosurgical thin loop conization by selective double excision. J Gynecol Surg 1991;7:83.

Baggish MS, Robinson D, Passman B: Stilbestrol induced muellerian cervix: A colposcopic study. J Gynecol Oncol 1976;4: 20–32.

Baggish MS, Sze EHM: Subdermal decadron and bupivacaine to treat symptomatic lichen sclerosus. J Gynecol Surg 1995;11:245.

Baggish MS, Sze EHM, Adelson MD, et al: Quantitative evaluation of the skin and accessory appendages in vulvar carcinoma in situ. Obstet Gynecol 1989;74:169–174.

Baggish MS, Sze EHM, Johnson R: Urinary oxalate excretion and its role in vuvlar pain syndrome. Am J Obstet Gynecol 1997;177:507.

Baggish MS, Valle R, Barbot J: Diagnostic and operative hysteroscopy. pp 106–122, 2nd ed. St. Louis, Mosby, 1999.

Baggish MS, Woodruff JD: Adenoid basal carcinoma of the cervix. Obstet Gynecol 1966;28:213.

Baggish MS, Woodruff JD: Adenoid basal lesions of the cervix. Obstet Gynecol 1971;37:807–819.

Balas C: A novel optical imaging method for the early detection, quantitative grading, and mapping of cancerous and precancerous lesions of cervix. Trans Biomed Eng 2001;48:96–104.

Baldauf JJ, Dreyfus M, Ritter J, et al: Cytology and colposcopy after loop electrosurgical excision: Implications for follow-up. Obstet Gynecol 1998;92:124–130.

Baldauf JJ, Dreyfus M, Ritter J, et al: Cervicography: Does it improve cervical cancer screening? Acta Cytol 1997;41:295–301.

Baldauf JJ, Dreyfus M, Ritter J, Philippe E: An analysis of the factors involved in the diagnostic accuracy of colposcopically directed biopsy. Acta Obstet Gynecol Scand 1997;76:468–473.

Bandieramonte G, Lomonico S, Quattrone P, et al: Laser conization assisted by crypt visualization for cervical intraepithelial neoplasia. Obstet Gynecol 1998;91:263–269.

Bar-Am A, Daniel Y, Ron IG, et al: Combined colposcopy, loop conization, and laser vaporization reduces recurrent abnormal cytology and residual disease in cervical dysplasia. Gynecol Oncol 2000;78:47–51.

Barrasso K, Coupez F, Ionesco M, DeBrux J: Human papilloma viruses and cervical intraepithelial neoplasia: The role of colposcopy. Gynecol Oncol 1987;27:197–207.

Bauer HM, Ting Y, Greer CE, et al: Genital human papillomavirus infection in female university students as determined by a PCR-based method. JAMA 1991;264:472–477.

Beckwith BA, Abu-Jawdeh GM, Burke L, Wang HH: Lack of utility of Pap smears obtained at colposcopy with tissue sampling. J Gynecol Surg 1995;11:85–89.

Bellina JH: The use of the carbon dioxide laser in the management of condyloma acuminatum with eight-year follow-up. Am J Obstet Gynecol 1983;147:375–378.

Beresford JM, McFaul SM, Moher D: Laser treatment of cervical intraepithelial neoplasia and the endocervical button. J Gynecol Surg 1990;6:111–114.

Bergeron C, Ferenczy A, Shah KV, Naghashfar Z: Multicentric human papillomavirus infections of the female genital tract: Correlation of viral types with abnormal mitotic figures, colposcopic presentation, and location. Obstet Gynecol 1987;69: 736–742.

Bergeron C, Jeannel D, Poveda J, et al: Human papillomavirus testing in women with mild cytologic atypia. Obstet Gynecol 2000;95(6 Pt 1):821–827.

Berget A, Lenstrup C: Cervical intraepithelial neoplasia: Examination, treatment and follow-up. Obstet Gynecol Surv 1985;40: 545–552.

Bernstein A, Harris B: The relationship of dietary and serum vitamin A to the occurrence of cervical intraepithelial neoplasia in sexually active women. Am J Obstet Gynecol 1984;148:309–312.

Bernstein SG, Kovacs BR, Townsend DE, Morrow CP: Vulvar carcinoma in situ. Obstet Gynecol 1983;61:304–307.

Bigrigg MA, Codling BW, Pearson P, et al: Colposcopic diagnosis and treatment of cervical dysplasia at a single clinic visit: Experience of low-voltage diathermy loop in 1000 patients. Lancet 1990;336:229–231.

Bjerre H, Eliasson G, Linell F, et al: Conization as the only treatment of carcinoma in situ of the uterine cervix. Am J Obstet Gynecol 1976;125:143.

Bolten KA: Practical colposcopy in early cervical and vaginal cancer. Clin Obstet Gynecol 1967;10:808.

Bolten KA, Jacques WE: Introduction to Colposcopy. New York, Grune and Stratton, 1960.

Borgatta L, Lopatinsky I, Shaw FM: Overcoming unsatisfactory colposcopy: Use of osmotic dilators. J Reprod Med 1997;42: 271–275.

Borgo G, Feyles E, Gaglio A, et al: Villoglandular papillary adenocarcinoma of the uterine cervix: Report of a case. Tumori 1998;84:717–719.

Boyle CA, Lowell DM, Kelsey JL, et al: Cervical intraepithelial neoplasia among women with *Papillomavirus* infection compared to women with *Trichomonas* infection. Cancer 1989;64:168–172.

Branca M, Rossi E, Alderisio M, et al: Performance of cytology and colposcopy in diagnosis of cervical intraepithelial neoplasia (CIN) in HIV-positive and HIV-negative women. Cytopathology 2001;12:84–93.

Brewer CA, Wilczynski SP, Kurosaki T, et al: Colposcopic regression patterns in high-grade cervical intraepithelial neoplasia. Obstet Gynecol 1997;90(4 Pt 1):617–621.

Broders AC: Carcinoma in situ contrasted with benign penetrating metaplasia. JAMA 1932;99:1670–1674.

Brown BH, Tidy JA, Boston K, et al: Relation between tissue structure and imposed electrical current flow in cervical neoplasia. Lancet 2000;355(9207):892–895.

Brown JV, Fu YS, Berek JS: Ovarian metastases are rare in stage I adenocarcinoma of the cervix. Obstet Gynecol 1990; 76:623–626.

Brown M, Mira J, Husseinzadeh N: Adenoid basal carcinoma of the cervix after subtotal hysterectomy. J Gynecol Surg 2000;16:125–127.

Bruner JM, Rosebrook LE, Crushhman GW: Photographic records of the cervix uteri. Am J Obstet Gynecol 1937; 34:1027–1029.

Burghardt E: Über dei atypische umwandlungszone. Geburtshilfe Frauenheilkd 1959;19:676.

Burghardt E: Early histological diagnosis of cervical cancer. Stuttgart, Thieme, 1973.

Burghardt E: Spezielle Gynakologie und Geburtshilfe. New York, Springer, 1985.

Burghardt E: Colposcopy: Cervical Pathology. Stuttgart, Thieme, 1991.

Burghardt E, Bajardi F: Ergebnisse der früherfassung des collumcarcinoms mittels cytologie und kolposkopie an der Universitäts-Frauenklinik Graz. Arch Gynakol 1956;1987:621.

Burghardt E, Coupez F, Dexeus S, et al: A European proposal for a classification of colposcopic findings. Cervix 1989;7:251–254.

Burghardt E, Holzer E: Diagnosis and treatment of microinvasive carcinoma of the cervix. Obstet Gynecol 1977;49:641.

Burghardt E, Holzer E: Treatment of carcinoma in situ: Evaluation of 1609 cases. Am J Obstet Gynecol 1980;55:539–545.

Burke L: Is laser surgery superior to cryosurgery for the treatment of high grade CIN? J Gynecol Surg 1991;7:53–55.

Burke L, Antonioli S, Rosen S: Vaginal and cervical squamous cell dysplasia in women exposed to diethylstilbestrol in utero. Am J Obstet Gynecol 1978;132:537.

Caglar H, Tamer S, Hreshchyshyn MM: Vulvar intraepithelial neoplasia. Obstet Gynecol 1982;60:346–349.

Callaway P, Frisch L: Does a family physician who offers colposcopy and LEEP need to refer patients to a gynecologist? J Fam Pract 2000;49:534–536.

Campion MJ, Singer A, McCance DJ, et al: Subclinical penile human papillomavirus infection in consorts of women with cervical neoplasia: A clue to the high-risk male. Colposc Gynecol Laser Surg 1987;3:11–22.

Campion MJ, Hacker NF: Vulvar intraepithelial neoplasia and carcinoma. Semin Cutan Med Surg 1998;17:205–212.

Cantor SB, Mitchell MF, Tortolero-Luna G, et al: Obstet Gynecol 1998;91:270–277.

Cardosi RJ, Arango HA, Phillips R, et al: Atypical squamous cells of undetermined significance: Do we need colposcopy? J Gynecol Surg 1999;15:13–17.

Carmichael JA, Maskens PD: Cervical dysplasia and human papillomavirus. Am J Obstet Gynecol 1989;160:916–918.

Cartier R: Practical Colposcopy. Paris, Laboratoire Cartier, 1984.

Chang T, Bova C, Wong F: Adenocarcinoma in situ of the uterine cervix progressing to invasive adenocarcinoma. Aust N Z J Obstet Gynaecol 1996;36:218–220.

Chang TC, Lai CH, Tseng CJ, et al: Prognostic factors in surgically treated small cell cervical carcinoma followed by adjuvant chemotherapy. Cancer 1998;83:712–718.

Chang WC, Matisic JP, Zhou C, et al: Cytologic features of villoglandular adenocarcinoma of the uterine cervix: Comparison with typical endocervical adenocarcinoma with a villoglandular component and papillary serous carcinoma. Cancer 1999;87:5–11.

Chang Chien CC, Lin H, Leung SW, et al: Effect of acetic acid on telomerase activity in cervical intraepithelial neoplasia. Gynecol Oncol 1998;71:99–103.

Charlton A, Kirker JA, Robertson AK, Jones RW: Vaginal adenosis with adenocarcinoma in situ in a woman with no recognized antecedent factors. Aust N Z J Obstet Gynaecol 2001;41:97–99.

Chin AB, Bristow RE, Korst LM, et al: The significance of atypical glandular cells on routine cervical cytologic testing in a community-based population. Am J Obstet Gynecol 2000;182: 1278–1282.

Choo K, Pan C, Liu M, et al: Presence of episomal and integrated human papillomavirus DNA sequences in cervical carcinoma. J Med Virol 1987;21:101–107.

Christopherson WM, Gray LA, Parker JE: Role of punch biopsy in subclinical lesions of the uterine cervix. Obstet Gynecol 1967;30:806.

Cohn DE, Peters WA III, Muntz HG, et al: Adenocarcinoma of the uterine cervix metastatic to lymph nodes. Am J Obstet Gynecol 1998;178:1131–1137.

Collins RJ, Wong LC: Adenocarcinoma of the uterine cervix with beta-hCG production: A case report and review of the literature. Gynecol Oncol 1989;33:99–107.

Conley LJ, Ellerbrock TV, Bush TJ, et al: HIV-1 infection and risk of vulvovaginal and perianal condylomata acuminata and intraepithelial neoplasia: A prospective cohort study. Lancet 2002;359(9301):108–113.

Cook-Glenn CL, Keyhani-Rofagha S: Adenocarcinoma of the uterine cervix associated with pregnancy: A retrospec-tive 10-year investigative study. Diagn Cytopathol 1998;18:393–397.

Coppleson M: The new colposcopic terminology. J Reprod Med 1976;16:214.

Coppleson M, Pixley E, Reid B: Colposcopy. Springfield, Ill, Charles C Thomas, 1971.

Coppleson M, Reid B: A colposcopic study of the cervix during pregnancy and the puerperium. J Obstet Gynecol Br Commonwealth 1966;73:575.

Costa S, Sideri M, Syrjanen K, et al: Combined Pap smear, cervicography and HPV DNA testing in the detection of cervical intraepithelial neoplasia and cancer. Acta Cytol 2000;44:310–318.

Cox JT: ASCCP practice guidelines: Endocervical curettage. J Lower Genital Tract Dis 1997;1:251–256.

Cox SM, Kaufman RH, Kaplan A: Recurrent carcinoma in situ of the vulva in a skin graft. Am J Obstet Gynecol 1986; 155:177–179.

Craigo J, Hopkins M, DeLucia A: Uterine cervix adenocarcinoma with both human papillomavirus type 18 and tumor suppressor gene p53 mutation from a woman having an intact hymen. Gynecol Oncol 1995;59:423–426.

Cronje HS, van Rensburg E, Niemand I, et al: Screening for cervical neoplasia during pregnancy. Int J Gynaecol Obstet 2000;68:19–23.

Crozier M, Morris M, Levenback C, et al: Pelvic exenteration for adenocarcinoma of the uterine cervix. Gynecol Oncol 1995;58: 74–78.

Cruickshank ME, Kitchener HC: The problem with low-grade Pap smears. Contemp Obstet Gynecol 1996;44:80–93.

Crum CP, Egawa K, Barron B, et al: Human papilloma virus infection (condyloma) of the cervix and cervical intraepithelial neoplasia: A histopathologic and statistical analysis. Gynecol Oncol 1983;15:88–94.

Crum CP, Levine RU: Human papillomavirus infection and cervical neoplasia: New perspectives. Int J Gynecol Pathol 1984;3: 376–388.

Crum CP, Nagal N, Levine RU, Silverstein S: In situ hybridization analysis of HPV 16 DNA sequences in early cervical neoplasia. Am J Pathol 1986;123:174–182.

Cullimore JE, Rollason TP, Luesley DM, et al: Invasive cervical cancer after laser vaporization for cervical intraepithelial neoplasia: A ten-year experience. J Gynecol Surg 1990;6:103–110.

Curtis MG: The use of the loop electrosurgical excision procedure (LEEP) in relieving stenosis of the external cervical os. J Gynecol Surg 1996;12:201–203.

Das SS, Elias AH: Diagnosis and treatment of cervical intraepithelial neoplasia in a single visit. Aust N Z J Obstet Gynaecol 1998;38:246–250.

Datta CK: Well-differentiated papillary villoglandular adenocarcinoma of the uterine cervix. W V Med J 1997;93:186–188.

Demopoulos RI, Horowitz LF, Vamvakas EC: Endocervical gland involvement by cervical intraepithelial neoplasia grade III: Predictive value for residual and/or recurrent disease. Cancer 1991;68:1932–1936.

Denise-Zielinski G, Snijders PJ, Rosendaal L, et al: High-risk HPV testing in women with borderline and mild dyskaryosis: Long-term follow-up data and clinical relevance. J Pathol 2001;195:300–306.

Denny L, Kuhn L, Pollack A, Wright TC Jr: Direct visual inspection for cervical cancer screening: An analysis of factors influencing test performance. Cancer 2002;94:1699–1707.

DeSutter PH, Coibion M, Vosse M, et al: A multicentre study comparing cervicography and cytology in the detection of cervical intraepithelial neoplasia. Br J Obstet Gynaecol 1998;105:613–620.

Diakomanolis E, Rodolakis A, Michalas S: Diagnostic conization for cervical neoplasia during pregnancy using the CO_2 laser. J Gynecol Surg 1999;15:197–202.

Diakomanolis E, Stefanidis K, Rodolakis A, Sakellaropoulos G: Local vasoconstrictive effect of ornipressin (POR8) in laser conization of the cervix: A randomized study. J Gynecol Surg 1997;13:187–196.

Diakomanolis E, Stefanidis K, Solomou E, et al: Local vasoconstrictive effect of ornipressin (POR8) in loop excision of the cervix: A randomized study. J Gynecol Surg 1998;14:75–79.

Dietrich CS III, Yancey MK, Miyazawa K, et al: Risk factors for early cytologic abnormalities after loop electrosurgical excision procedure. Obstet Gynecol 2002;99:188–192.

Dixit S, Singhal S, Vyas R, et al: Adenoid cystic carcinoma of the cervix. J Postgrad Med 1993;39:211–215.

Dorsey JH: Understanding CO_2 laser surgery of the vulva. Colposc Gynecol Laser Surg 1984;1:205–213.

Dorsey JH, Baggish MS, Sharp EF, Jordan JA: Multifocal vaginal intraepithelial neoplasia with uterus in situ: Proceedings of the 15th Study Group of the RCOG. Ithaca, New York, Perinatology Press, 1986:173–179.

Draeby-Kristiansen J, Garsaae M, Bruun M, Hansen K: Ten years after cryosurgical treatment of cervical intraepithelial neoplasia. Am J Obstet Gynecol 1991;165:43–45.

Dudding N, Sutton J, Lane S: Koilocytosis: An indication for conservative management. Cytopathology 1996;7:32–37.

Duggan B, Muderspach LI, Roman LD, et al: Cervical cancer in pregnancy: Reporting on planned delay in therapy. Obstet Gynecol 1993;82(4 Pt 1):598–602.

Duggan MA, McGregor SE, Stuart GC, et al: Predictors of co-incidental CIN II/III amongst a cohort of women with CIN I detected by a screening pap test. Eur J Gynaecol Oncol 1998;19:209–214.

Eger RR, Peipert JF: Risk factors for non-compliance in a colposcopy clinic. J Reprod Med 1996;41:671–674.

Epperson JWW, Hellman LM, Galvin GA, Busby T: The morphological changes in the cervix during pregnancy, including intraepithelial carcinoma. Am J Obstet Gynecol 1951;61:50.

Eskridge C, Begneaud WP, Landwehr C: Cervicography combined with repeat Papanicolaou test as triage for low-grade cytologic abnormalities. Obstet Gynecol 1998;92:351–355.

Etherington IJ, Dunn J, Shafi MI, et al: Video colpography: A new technique for secondary cervical screening. Br J Obstet Gynaecol 1997;104:150–153.

Etherington IJ, Luesley DM, Shafi MI, et al: Observer variability among colposcopists from the West Midlands region. Br J Obstet Gynaecol 1997;104:1380–1384.

Evans AS, Monaghan JM, Anderson MC: A nuclear deoxyribonucleic acid analysis of normal and abnormal vulvar epithelium. Obstet Gynecol 1987;69:790–793.

Falcone T, Ferenczy A: Cervical intraepithelial neoplasia and condyloma: An analysis of diagnostic accuracy of post-treatment follow-up methods. Am J Obstet Gynecol 1986;154:260–264.

Favalli G, Lomini M, Schreiber C, et al: The use of carbon-dioxide laser surgery in the treatment of intraepithelial neoplasia of the uterine cervix. Przegl Lek 1999;56:58–64.

Ferenczy A: Using the laser to treat vulvar condylomata acuminata and intraepidermal neoplasia. Can Med Assoc J 1983;128:135–137.

Ferenczy A: Comparison of 5-fluorouracil and CO_2 laser for treatment of vaginal condylomata. Obstet Gynecol 1984;64:773–778.

Ferenczy A: Evaluation and management of male partners of condyloma patients. Colposc Gynecol Laser Surg 1986;2:15–24.

Ferenczy A, Choukroun D, Falcone T, Franco E: The effect of cervical loop electrosurgical excision on subsequent pregnancy outcome: North American experience. Am J Obstet Gynecol 1995;172:1246–1250.

Ferenczy A, Choukroun D, Arseneau J: Loop electrosurgical excision procedure for squamous intraepithelial lesions of the cervix: Advantages and potential pitfalls. Obstet Gynecol 1996;87:332–337.

Ferenczy A, Mitao M, Nagai N, et al: Latent papillomavirus and recurring genital warts. N Engl J Med 1985;313:784–788.

Ferguson JH, Brown GC: Cervical conization during pregnancy. Surgery 1960;111:603.

Ferris DG, Schiffman M, Litaker MS: Cervicography for triage of women with mildly abnormal cervical cytology results. Am J Obstet Gynecol 2001;185:939–943.

Flannelly G, Bolger B, Fawzi H, et al: Follow-up after LLETZ: Could schedules be modified according to risk of recurrence? Br J Obstet Gynaecol 2001;108:1025–1030.

Flannelly G, Langhan H, Jandial L, et al: A study of treatment failures following large loop excision of the transformation zone for the treatment of cervical intraepithelial neoplasia. Br J Obstet Gynaecol 1997;104:718–722.

Fluhmann CF: The cervix uteri and its diseases. Philadelphia, WB Saunders, 1961.

Fowler JM, Davos I, Leuchter RS, Lagasse LD: Effect of CO_2 laser conization of the uterine cervix on pathologic interpretation of cervical intraepithelial neoplasia. Obstet Gynecol 1992;79:693–698.

Fraser IS, Lahteenmaki P, Elomaa K, et al: Variations in vaginal epithelial surface appearance determined by colposcopic inspection in healthy, sexually active women. Hum Reprod 1999;14:1974–1978.

Freeman-Wang T, Walker P, Linehan J, et al: Anxiety levels in women attending colposcopy clinics for treatment for cervical intraepithelial neoplasia: A randomized trial of written and video information. Br J Obstet Gynaecol 2001;108:482–484.

Friedman-Kien AE, Eron LJ, Conant M, et al: Natural interferon alfa for treatment of condylomata acuminata. JAMA 1988;259:533–538.

Fruchter RG, Maiman M, Sedlis A, et al: Multiple recurrences of cervical intraepithelial neoplasia in women with the human immunodeficiency virus. Obstet Gynecol 1996;87:338–344.

Fujii T, Crum CP, Winkler B, et al: Human papillomavirus infection and cervical intraepithelial neoplasia: Histopathology and DNA content. Obstet Gynecol 1984;63:99–104.

Fukushima M, Yamakawa Y, Shimano S, et al: The physical state of human papillomavirus 16 DNA in cervical carcinoma and cervical intraepithelial neoplasia. Cancer 1990;66:2155–2161.

Furber SE, Weisberg E, Simpson JM: Progression and regression of low-grade epithelial abnormalities of the cervix. Aust N Z J Obstet Gynaecol 1997;37:107–112.

Gabriel G, Thin RNT: Treatment of anogenital warts: Comparison of trichloracetic acid and podophyllin versus podophyllin alone. Br J Vener Dis 1983;59:124–126.

Gal D, Friedman M, Mitrani-Rosenbaum S: Transmissibility and treatment failures of different types of human papillomavirus. Obstet Gynecol 1989;73:308–311.

Galloway CE: Photography of the uterine cervix. JAMA 1938;111:1996–1998.

Gallup DG, Stock RJ, Talledo OE: Current management of non-squamous carcinoma of the cervix. Oncology 1989;3:95–102; discussion 104, 106.

Ganse R: Kolpototogramme zur einfuhrung in die kolposkopie. Berlin, Akademie Verlag 1953.

Gardeil F, Turner MJ: A study of treatment failures following large loop excision of the transformation zone for the treatment of cervical intraepithelial neoplasia. Br J Obstet Gynaecol 1997;104:1325; discussion 1326.

Geier CS, Wilson M, Creasman W: Clinical evaluation of atypical glandular cells of undetermined significance. Am J Obstet Gynecol 2001;184:64–69.

Geisler JP, Hiett AK, Geisler HE, et al: Papillary serous carcinoma of the cervix: Ultrasonographic findings. Eur J Gynaecol Oncol 1998;19:519–521.

Gentry DJ, Baggish MS, Brady K, et al: The effects of loop excision of the transformation zone on cervical length: Implications for pregnancy. Am J Obstet Gynecol 2000;182:516–520.

Gerber S, DeGrandi P, Petignat P, et al: Colposcopic evaluation after a repeat atypical squamous cells of undetermined significance (ASCUS) smear. Int J Gynaecol Obstet 2001;75:251–255.

Giacalone PL, Laffargue F, Aligier N, et al: Randomized study comparing two techniques of conization: Cold knife versus loop excision. Gynecol Oncol 1999;75:356–360.

Giles JA, Gafar A: The treatment of CIN: Do we need lasers? Br J Obstet Gynaecol 1991;98:3–6.

Glatthaar E: Kolposkopie in Biologie und Patholigie des Weibes: 2 Aufl Band III s. Berlin, Urban und Schwarzenberg, 1955:911–980.

Goette DK: Review of erythroplasia of Queyrat and its treatment. Urology 1976;8:311–315.

Golbang P, Scurry J, DeJong S, et al: Investigation of 100 consecutive negative cone biopsies. Br J Obstet Gynaecol 1997;104:100–104.

Gomez-Irizarry FL, Helm CW, Hartman G, Barton DPJ: Unilateral invasive adenosquamous carcinoma of the cervix in a uterus didelphys. J Gynecol Surg 1996;12:213–216.

Gonzalez DI Jr, Zahn CM, Retzloff MG, et al: Recurrence of dysplasia after loop electrosurgical excision procedures with long-term follow-up. Am J Obstet Gynecol 2001;184:315–321.

Goodman HM, Buttlar CA, Niloff JM, et al: Adenocarcinoma of the uterine cervix: Prognostic factors and patterns of recurrence. Gynecol Oncol 1989;33:241–247.

Gordon HK, Duncan ID: Effective destruction of cervical intraepithelial neoplasia (CIN) 3 at 100°C using the Semm cold coagulator: 14 years experience. Br J Obstet Gynaecol 1991;98:14–20.

Grayson W, Taylor LF, Cooper K: Adenoid cystic and adenoid basal carcinoma of the uterine cervix: Comparative morphologic, mucin, and immunohistochemical profile of two rare neoplasms of putative "reserve cell" origin. Am J Surg Pathol 1999;23:448–458.

Green RR, Peckham BM: Preinvasive cancer of the cervix and pregnancy. Am J Obstet Gynecol 1958;75:551.

Gross G, Hagedorn M, Ikenberg H, et al: Bowenoid papulosis: Presence of human papillomavirus (HPV) structural antigens and of HPV 16-related DNA sequences. Arch Dermatol 1985;121:858–863.

Gross G, Roussaki A, Schöpf E: Successful treatment of condylomata acuminata and bowenoid papulosis with subcutaneous injections of low-dose recombinant interferon-α. Arch Dermatol 1985;122:749.

Grunebaum AN, Sedlis A, Sillman F, et al: Association of human papillomavirus infection with cervical intraepithelial neoplasia. Obstet Gynecol 1983;62:448–455.

Guerra B, DeSimone P, Gabrielli S, et al: Combined cytology and colposcopy to screen for cervical cancer in pregnancy. J Reprod Med 1998;43:647–653.

Guijon FB, Paraskevas M, Brunham R: The association of sexually transmitted diseases with cervical intraepithelial neoplasia: A case-control study. Am J Obstet Gynecol 1985;151:185–190.

Gupta JW, Gupta PK, Rosenshein N, Shah KV: Detection of human papillomavirus in cervical smears: A comparison of in situ hybridization, immunocytochemistry and cytopathology. Acta Cytol 1987;31:387–396.

Gupta J, Pilotti S, Shah KV, et al: Human papillomavirus-associated early vulvar neoplasia investigated by in situ hybridization. Am J Surg Pathol 1987;11:430–434.

Haffenden DK, Bigrigg A, Codling BW, Read MD: Pregnancy following large loop excision of the transformation zone. Br J Obstet Gynaecol 1993;100:1059–1060.

Hallam NF, West J, Harper C, et al: Large loop excision of the transformation zone (LLETZ) as an alternative to both local ablative and cone biopsy treatment: A series of 1000 patients. J Gynecol Surg 1993;9:77–82.

Hamm RM, Loemker V, Reilly KL, et al: A clinical decision analysis of cryotherapy compared with expectant management for cervical dysplasia. J Fam Pract 1998;47:193–201.

Hartman KE, Nanda K, Hall S, Myers E: Technologic advances for evaluation of cervical cytology: Is newer better? Obstet Gynecol Surv 2001;56:765–774.

Hartz LE, Fenaughty AM: Management choice and adherence to follow-up after colposcopy in women with cervical intraepithelial neoplasia 1. Obstet Gynecol 2001;98:674–679.

Held E, Schreiner WE, Oehler I: Bedeutung der kolposkopie und cytologie zur erfassung des genitalkarzinoms. Schweiz Med Wochenschr 1954;84:856.

Henderson BR, Thompson CH, Rose BR, et al: Detection of specific types of human papillomavirus in cervical scrapes, anal scrapes, and anogenital biopsies by DNA hybridization. J Med Virol 1987;21:381–393.

Henriksen HM: The cryosurgical treatment of intraepithelial neoplasia. Acta Obstet Gynecol Scand 1979;58:271.

Herbst AL, Cole P, Norusis MJ, et al: Epidemiologic aspects and factors related to survival in 384 registry cases of clear cell adenocarcinoma of the vagina and cervix. Am J Obstet Gynecol 1979;135:876.

Herbst AL, Kurman RJ, Scully RE, Poskanzer DC: Clear cell adenocarcinoma of the genital tract in young females. N Engl J Med 1972;284:1259.

Herbst AL, Pickett KE, Follen M, Noller KL: The management of ASCUS cervical cytologic abnormalities and HPV testing: A cautionary note. Obstet Gynecol 2001;98:849–851.

Herbst AL, Ulfelder U, Poskanzer DC: Adenocarcinoma of the vagina. N Engl J Med 1971;284:878.

Herod JJ, Shafi MI, Rollason TP, et al: Vulvar intraepithelial neoplasia: Long term follow-up of treated and untreated women. Br J Obstet Gynaecol 1996;103:446–452.

Hinselmann H: Verbesserung der inspektionsmöglichkeit von vulva, vagina, and portio. Munch Med Wochenschr 1925;72:1733.

Hinselmann H: Der begriff der umwandlungszone der portio. Arch Gynakol 1927;131:422.

Hinselmann H: Zur kenntnis der präekanzerösen veränderungen der portio. Zentralbl Gynakol 1927;51:901.

Hinselmann H: Das klinische bild der indirekten metaplasie der ektopischen zylinderzellenschleimhaut der portio. Arch Gynakol 1928;133:64–69.

Hinselmann H: Beitrag zur ordnung ableitung der leukoplakien des weiblichen geschlecttraktes. Z Geburtshilfe Gynakol 1932;101:142.

Hinselmann H: Ausgewählte gesichtspunkte zur beurteilung des zusammenhanges der "matrixbezirke" und des karzinoms der sichtbaren abschnitte des weiblichen ganitaltraktes. Z Geburtshilfe 1933;104:228.

Hinselmann H: Einführung in die kolposkopie. Hamburg, Paul Hartung, 1933.

Hinselmann H: Die klinische und mikroskopische frühdiagnose des portiokarzinoms. Arch Gynakol 1934;156:239.

Hinselmann H: Die essigsäureprobe ein bestandteil der erweiterten kolposkopie. Dtsch Med Wochenschr 1938;vol 64:40.

Hinselmann H: In welchem stadium möchten wir das portiokarzinom klinisch diagnostizieren? Munch Med Wochenschr 1938;35:1071–1073.

Hinselmann H: Der nachweis der aktiven ausgestaltung der gefässe beim jungen portiokarzinom als neues differential diagnostisches hilfsmittel. Zentralbl Gynakol 1940;64:1810.

Hinselmann H: Die kolposkopie. Wuppertal, Germany, Girardet, 1954.

Hinselmann H: Aktuelle probleme der praktischen und wissenschaftlichen kolposkopie. Jena, Germany, VEB Gustav Fischer, 1956.

Hirai Y, Takeshima N, Haga A, et al: A clinicocytopathologic study of adenoma malignum of the uterine cervix. Gynecol Oncol 1998;70:219–223.

Hocking GR, Hayman JA, Ostor AG: Adenocarcinoma in situ of the uterine cervix progressing to invasive adenocarcinoma. Aust N Z J Obstet Gynaecol 1996;36:218–220.

Hoepfner I, Löning T: Human papillomavirus (HPV) infection of cervical lesions detected by immunohistochemisty and in situ hybridization. Cancer Detect Prev 1986;9:293–301.

Hoffman MS, Finan M, Wallach P, et al: Use of the cytobrush in postmenopausal women. J Gynecol Surg 1991;7:23–25.

Hogenmiller JR, Smith ML, Stephens LC, McIntosh DG: Patterns of pap smear screening in women diagnosed with invasive cervical cancer. J Gynecol Surg 1994;10:247–253.

Hollingworth J, Kotecha K, Dobbs SP, et al: Cervical disease in women referred to colposcopy following inadequate smears. Cytopathology 2000;11:45–52.

Hollyhock VE, Chanen W: Electrocoagulation therapy for the treatment of cervical dysplasia and carcinoma in situ. Obstet Gynecol 1976;47:196.

Hopman EH, Kenemans P, Helmerhorst TJ: Positive predictive rate of colposcopic examination of the cervix uteri: An overview of literature. Obstet Gynecol Surv 1998;53:97–106.

Houghton SJ, Shafi MI, Rollason TP, Luesley DM: Is loop excision adequate primary management of adenocarcinoma in situ of the cervix? Br J Obstet Gynaecol 1997;104:325–329.

Howe DT, Vincenti AC: Is large loop excision of the transformation zone (LLETZ) more accurate than colposcopically directed punch biopsy in the diagnosis of cervical intraepithelial neoplasia? Br J Obstet Gynaecol 1991;98:588–591.

Howells RE, Dunn PD, Isasi T, et al: Is the provision of information leaflets before colposcopy beneficial? A prospective randomized study. Br J Obstet Gynaecol 1999;106:528–534.

Howells RE, O'Mahony F, Tucker H, et al: How can the incidence of negative specimens resulting from large loop excision of the cervical transformation zonc (LLETZ) be reduced? An analysis of negative LLETZ specimens and development of a predictive model. Br J Obstet Gynaecol 2000;107:1075–1082.

Howells RE, Tucker H, Millinship J, et al: A comparison of the side effects of prilocaine with felypressin and lignocaine with adrenaline in large loop excision of the transformation zone of the cervix: Results of a randomized trial. Br J Obstet Gynaecol 2000;107:28–32.

Hurt WG, Silverberg SG, Frable WJ, et al: Adenocarinoma of the cervix: Histopathologic and clinical features. Am J Obstet Gynecol 1977;129:304–315.

Husniye-Dilek F, Kucukali T: Mucin production in carcinoma of the uterine cervix. Eur J Obstet Gynecol Reprod Biol 1998;79:149–151.

Ikenberg H, Gissmann L, Gross G, et al: Human papillomavirus type-16 related DNA in genital Bowen's disease and in bowenoid papulosis. Int J Cancer 1983;32:563–565.

Ishii K, Hosaka N, Toki T, et al: A new view of the so-called adenoma malignum of the uterine cervix. Virchows Arch 1998;432:315–322.

Ishikawa H, Nakanishi T, Inoue T, Kuzuya K: Prognostic factors of adenocarcinoma of the uterine cervix. Gynecol Oncol 1999;73:42–46.

Ismail SM, Colclough AB, Dinnen JS, et al: Reporting cervical intraepithelial neoplasia (CIN): Intra- and interpathologist variation and factors associated with disagreement. Histopathology 1990;16:371–376.

Jaworski RC: Endocervical glandular dysplasia, adenocarcinoma in situ, and early invasive (microinvasive) adenocarcinoma of the uterine cervix. Semin Diagn Pathol 1990;7:190–204.

Jenson AB, Lim LY, Lancaster WD: Role of papilloma virus in proliferative squamous lesions. Surv Synth Pathol Res 1985;4:8–13.

Jobling TW, Shepherd JH, Curtis P, Lowe DG: Squamous cell carcinoma arising in a human amnion neovagina. J Gynecol Surg 1993;9:53–57.

Johnson DB, Rowlands CJ: Diagnosis and treatment of cervical intraepithelial neoplasia in general practice. BMJ 1989;299:1083–1086.

Johnson JC, Burnett AF, Willet GD, et al: High frequency of latent and clinical human papillomavirus cervical infections in immunocompromised human immunodeficiency virus-infected women. Obstet Gynecol 1992;79:321–327.

Johnson N, Brady J: Dilating the cervix medically to overcome an unsatisfactory colposcopy: 5 year follow-up. Eur J Obstet Gynaecol Reprod Biol 1996;69:125–127.

Jones HW III: Should conization by hot loop or laser replace cervical biopsy? J Gynecol Surg 1991;7:195.

Jones HW III: Clinical treatment of women with atypical squamous cells of undetermined significance or atypical glandular cells of undetermined significance cervical cytology. Clin Obstet Gynecol 2000;43:381–393.

Jones HW III, Buller RE: The treatment of cervical intraepithelial neoplasia by cone biopsy. Am J Obstet Gynecol 1980;137:882.

Jones MW, Silverberg SG, Kurman RJ: Well-differentiated villoglandular adenocarcinoma of the uterine cervix: A clinicopathological study of 24 cases. Int J Gynecol Pathol 1993;12:1–7.

Kadish AS, Burk RD, Kress Y, et al: Human papillomaviruses of different types in precancerous lesions of the uterine cervix: Histologic, immunocytochemical and ultrastructural studies. Hum Pathol 1986;17:384–392.

Kaferle JE, Malouin JM: Evaluation and management of the AGUS papanicolaou smear. Am Fam Physician 2001;63: 2239–2244.

Kaku T, Kamura T, Sakai K, et al: Early adenocarcinoma of the uterine cervix. Gynecol Oncol 1997;65:281–285.

Kaku T, Kamura T, Shigematsu T, et al: Adenocarcinoma of the uterine cervix with predominantly villoglandular papillary growth pattern. Gynecol Oncol 1997;64:147–152.

Kaku T, Kirakawa T, Kamura T, et al: Angiogenesis in adenocarcinoma of the uterine cervix. Cancer 1998;83:1384–1390.

Kaufman RH, Adam E: Is human papillomavirus testing of value in clinical practice? Am J Gynecol Surg 1999;180: 1049–1053.

Kaufman RH, Adam E: Findings in female offspring of women exposed in utero to diethylstilbestrol. Obstet Gynecol 2002;99: 197–200.

Kaufman RH, Conner JS: Cryosurgical treatment of cervical dysplasia. Am J Obstet Gynecol 1971;109:1167.

Kaufman RH, Faro S: Benign Diseases of the Vulva and Vagina, 2nd ed. St. Louis, Mosby, 1994.

Kavanagh AM, Simpson JM: Predicting non-attendance for colposcopy clinic follow-up after referral for an abnormal Pap smear. Aust N Z J Public Health 1996;20:266–271.

Keijer KGG, Kenemans P, van der Zanden P, et al: Diathermy loop excision in the management of cervical intraepithelial neoplasia: Diagnosis and treatment in one procedure. Am J Obstet Gynecol 1992;166:1281–1287.

Kennedy AW, Salmieri SS, Wirth SL, et al: Results of the clinical evaluation of atypical glandular cells of undetermined significance (AGCUS) detected on cervical cytology screening. Gynecol Oncol 1996;63:14–18.

Kevorkian AY, Younger PA: Contemporary means of evaluation of the uterine cervix. Clin Obstet Gynecol 1963;6:334.

Kilgore LC, Helm CW: Adenocarcinoma of the uterine cervix. Clin Obstet Gynecol 1990;33:863–871.

Kim JJ, Wright TC, Goldie SJ: Cost-effectiveness of alternative triage strategies for atypical squamous cells of undetermined significance. JAMA 2002;287:2382–2390.

Kirby AJ, Spiegelhalter DJ, Day NE, et al: Conservative treatment of mild/moderate cervical dyskaryosis: Long-term outcome. Lancet 1992;339:828–831.

Kishi Y: Individualized electrosurgical excision of cervical intraepithelial neoplasia of the uterus. J Gynecol Surg 2000;16:25–32.

Kjaer SK, Brinton LA: Adenocarcinoma of the uterine cervix: The epidemiology of an increasing problem. Epidemiol Rev 1993;15:486–498.

Kohan S, Beckman EM, Bigelow B, et al: The role of colposcopy in the management of cervical intraepithelial neoplasia during pregnancy and postpartum. J Reprod Med 1980;25:279–284.

Koller O: The vascular patterns of cervical cancer. Acta Un Int Cancer 1989;15:375.

Kolstad P: Vascularisation, oxygen tension and radiocurability in cancer of the cervix. Oslo, Universitetsforlaget, 1963.

Kolstad P: The colposcopical picture of trichomonas vaginitis. Acta Obstet Gynecol Scand 1964;43:388.

Kolstad P: Intercapillary distance, oxygen tension and local recurrence in cervix cancer. Scand J Clin Lab Invest 1968;22:145 (suppl 106).

Kolstad P: Diagnosis and management of precancerous lesions of the cervix uteri. Int J Gynaecol Obstet 1970;8:551.

Kolstad P, Klem V: Long-term follow-up of 1121 cases of carcinoma in situ. Obstet Gynecol 1976;48:125–129.

Kolstad P, Stafl A: Atlas of Colposcopy. Baltimore, University Park Press, 1972.

Korhorn MO, Kaufman RH, Roberts D, et al: Carcinoma in situ of the vulva: The search for viral particles. J Reprod Med 1982;27:746–748.

Korn AP, Abercrombie PD, Foster A: Vulvar intraepithelial neoplasia in women infected with human immunodeficiency virus-1. Gynecol Oncol 1996;61:384–386.

Koss LG: Concepts of genesis and development of carcinoma of the cervix. Obstet Gynecol Surv 1969;24:850.

Koss LG, Stewart FW, Foote FW, et al: Some histological aspects of behavior of epidermoid carcinoma in situ and related lesions of the uterine cervix: A long-term prospective study. Cancer 1963;16:1160–1211.

Koutsky LA, Ault KA, Wheeler CM, Brown DR, Barr E, Alvarez FB, Chiacchierini LM, Jansen KU: A controlled trial of a human papillomavirus type 16 vaccine. N Engl J Med 2002;347: 1645.

Kraatz H: Farbfiltervorschaltung zur leichteren erlernung der kolposkopie. Zentralbl Gynakol 1939;63:2307–2309.

Krebs HB: Combination of laser plus 5-fluorouracil for the treatment of extensive genital condylomata acuminata. Lasers Surg Med 1988;8:135–138.

Krebs HB, Wheelock JB: The CO_2 laser for recurrent and therapy-resistant condylomata acuminata. J Reprod Med 1985;30:489–492.

Krumholz BA: Colposcopy in pregnancy: Directed brush cytology compared with cervical biopsy. Obstet Gynecol 1999;94:1054–1055.

Kumar L, Tanwar RK, Singh SP: Intracranial metastases from carcinoma of the cervix and review of literature. Gynecol Oncol 1992;46:391–392.

Kuppers V, Stiller M, Somville T, Bender HG: Risk factors for recurrent VIN: Role of multifocality and grade of disease. J Reprod Med 1997;42:140–144.

Kurian K, Nafussi A: Relation of cervical glandular intraepithelial neoplasia to microinvasive and invasive adenocarcinoma of the uterine cervix: A study of 121 cases. J Clin Pathol 1999;52:112–117.

Kurinczuk JJ, Burton P: Cervical intraepithelial neoplasia in women with renal allografts. BMJ 1989;298:598.

Kurman D, Kurman RJ: The Bethesda System. New York, Springer-Verlag, 1994.

Kurman RJ, Sanz LE, Jenson AB, et al: Papillomavirus infection of the cervix: I. Correlation of histology with viral structural antigens and DNA sequences. Int J Gynecol Pathol 1982;1:17–28.

Kurman RJ: Blaustein's Pathology of the Female Genital Tract, 4th ed. New York, Springer-Verlag, 1994.

Kurman RJ, Henson DE, Herbst AL, et al: Interim guidelines for management of abnormal cervical cytology: For the 1992 National Cancer Institute Workshop. JAMA 1994;271:1866–1869.

Lancaster WD, Castellano C, Santos C, et al: Human papillomavirus deoxyribonucleic acid in cervical carcinoma from primary and metastatic sites. Am J Obstet Gynecol 1986;154: 115–119.

Larsson G: Conization for cervical dysplasia and carcinoma in situ: Long-term follow-up of 1013 women. Ann Chir Gynaecol 1981;70:79.

Lee KE, Koh CF, Watt WF: Comparison of the grade of CIN in colposcopically directed biopsies with that in outpatient loop electrosurgical excision procedure (LEEP) specimens: A retrospective review. Singapore Med J 1999;40:694–696.

Lee KR, Darragh TM, Joste NE, et al: Atypical glandular cells of undetermined significance (AGUS): Interobserver reproducibility in cervical smears and corresponding thin-layer preparations. Am J Clin Pathol 2002;117:96–102.

Lee MF, Chang MC, Wu CH: Detection of human papillomavirus types in cervical adenocarcinoma by the polymerase chain reaction. Int J Gynaecol Obstet 1998;63:265–270.

Lee SS, Collins RJ, Pun TC, et al: Conservative treatment of low-grade squamous intraepithelial lesions (LSIL) of the cervix. Int J Gynaecol Obstet 1988;60:35–40.

Leuchter RS, Townsend DE, Pretorius RG, et al: Treatment of vulvar carcinoma in situ with the CO_2 laser. Gynecol Oncol 1984;19:314–322.

Leveque J, Laurent JF, Burtin F, et al: Prognostic factors of the uterine cervix adenocarcinoma. Eur J Obstet Gynecol Reprod Biol 1998;80:209–214.

Levine RU, Crum CP, Herman E, et al: Cervical papillomavirus infection and intraepithelial neoplasia: A study of male sexual partners. Obstet Gynecol 1984;64:16–20.

Lewis P, Lashgari M: A comparison of cold knife, CO_2 laser, and electrosurgical loop conization in the treatment of cervical intraepithelial neoplasia. J Gynecol Surg 1994;10:229–234.

Lifton RJ: The Nazi Doctors. New York, Basic Books, 1986.

Lonky NM, Sadeghi M, Tsadik GW, Petitti D: The clinical significance of the poor correlation of cervical dysplasia and cervical malignancy with referral cytologic results. Am J Obstet Gynecol 1999;181:560–566.

Lorincz AT, Reid R, Jenson AB, et al: Human papillomavirus infection of the cervix: Relative risk associations of 15 common anogenital types. Obstet Gynecol 1992;79:328–337.

Lotmar W, Wespi HJ: Stereo-kolpophotographie. Geburtshilfe Frauenheilkd 1955;15:22–27.

Luesley DM, Cullimore J, Redman CWE, et al: Loop diathermy excision of the cervical transformation zone in patients with abnormal cervical smears. BMJ 1990;300:1690–1693.

Lungu O, Wei Sun X, Felix J, et al: Relationship of human papillomavirus type to grade of cervical intraepithelial neoplasia. JAMA 1992;267:2493–2496.

McCance DJ, Campion MJ, Clarkson PK, et al: Prevalence of human papillomavirus type 16 DNA sequences in cervical intraepithelial neoplasia and invasive carcinoma of the cervix. Br J Obstet Gynaecol 1985;92:1101–1105.

McClintock J, Hoffman MS, Fiorica JV, Cavanagh D: Vulvar melanoma: A retrospective review of prognostic factors and outcomes. J Gynecol Surg 1998;14:25–26.

McGonigle KF, Berek JS: Early-stage squamous cell and adenocarcinoma of the cervix. Curr Opin Obstet Gynecol 1992;4:109–119.

Mann CH, Steele JC, Burton A, et al: LLETZ: Evidence of its efficacy against HPV infection. Gynecol Oncol 2001;81:125–127.

Manos MM, Kinney WK, Hurley LB, et al: Identifying women with cervical neoplasia: Using human papillomavirus DNA testing for equivocal Papanicolaou results. JAMA 1999;281:1605–1610.

Marana HR, Andrade JM, Duarte G, et al: Colposcopic scoring system for biopsy decisions in different patient groups. Eur J Gynaecol Oncol 2000;21:368–370.

Massad LS: The performance of colposcopy for women with atypical and low-grade cervical cytologic abnormalities. Gynecol Oncol 1999;74:527.

Massad LS, Collins YC, Meyer PM: Biopsy correlates of abnormal cervical cytology classified using the Bethesda system. Gynecol Oncol 2001;82:516–522.

Massad LS, Halperin CJ, Bitterman P: Correlation between colposcopically directed biopsy and cervical loop excision. Gynecol Oncol 1996;60:400–403.

Masterson BJ, Krantz KE, Calkins JW, et al: The carbon dioxide laser in cervical intraepithelial neoplasia: A five-year experience

in treating 230 patients. Am J Obstet Gynecol 1981;139:565.

Mathoulin-Portier MP, Penault-Liorca F, Labit-Bouvier C, et al: Malignant mullerian tumor of the uterine cervix with adenoid cystic component. Int J Gynecol Pathol 1998;17:91–92.

Matsuura Y, Kawagoe T, Toki N, et al: Early cervical neoplasia confirmed by conization: Diagnostic accuracy of cytology, colposcopy and punch biopsy. Acta Cytol 1996;40:241–246.

Meanwell CA, Blackledge G, Cox MF, Maitland NJ: HPV 16 DNA in normal and malignant cervical epithelium: Implications for the aetiology and behaviour of cervical neoplasia. Lancet 1987;(8535):703–707.

Meisels A, Fortin R, Roy M: Condylomatous lesions of the cervix: 2. Cytologic, colposcopic and histopathologic study. Acta Cytol 1977;21:379.

Mencaglia L, Gilardi G: Conservative treatment of CIN: A review. J Gynecol Surg 1990;6:237–255.

Mene A, Buckley CH: Involvement of the vulval skin appendages by intraepithelial neoplasia. Br J Obstet Gynaecol 1985;92:634–638.

Meyer R: Die epithelentwicklung der cervix und portio vaginalis uteri und die pseudoerosio congenita. Arch Gynakol 1910;91:579.

Mitchell MF, Schottenfeld D, Tortolero-Luna G, et al: Colposcopy for the diagnosis of squamous intraepithelial lesions: A meta-analysis. Obstet Gynecol 1988;91:626–631.

Mohammed DK, Lavie O, de B-Lopes A, et al: A clinical review of borderline glandular cells on cervical cytology. Br J Obstet Gynaecol 2000;107:605–609.

Moniak CW, Kutzner S, Adam E, et al: Endocervical curettage in evaluating abnormal cervical cytology. J Reprod Med 2000;45:285–292.

Mor-Yosef S, Lopes A, Pearson S, Monaghan JM: Loop diathermy cone biopsy: Instruments and methods. Obstet Gynecol 1990;75:884–886.

Moss TR: Cervical cytology and colposcopy in young patients attending genitourinary medicine clinics: Invalid intrusion or preventive opportunity and definitive audit? Cytopathology 1999;10:2–7.

Nafussi A, Rebello G, Yusif R, McGoogan E: The borderline cervical smear: Colposcopic and biopsy outcome. J Clin Pathol 2000;53:439–444.

Naghashfar Z, Sawada E, Kutcher MJ, et al: Identification of genital tract papillomavirus HPV-6 and HPV-16 in warts of the oral cavity. J Med Virol 1985;17:313–324.

Nahhas WA, Marshall ML, Ponziani J, Jagielo JA: Evaluation of urinary cytology of male sexual partners of women with cervical intraepithelial neoplasia and human papillomavirus infection. Gynecol Oncol 1986;24:279–285.

Naumann RW, Crispens MA, Alvarez RD, et al: Treatment of cervical dysplasia with large loop excision of the transformation zone: Is endocervical curettage necessary? South Med J 1996;89:961–965.

Nguyen GK, Daya D: Cervical adenocarcinoma and related lesions: Cytodiagnostic criteria and pitfalls. Pathol Annu 1993;28(Pt 2):53–75.

Nguyen GK, Daya D: Exfoliate cytology of papillary serous adenocarcinoma of the uterine cervix. Diagn Cytopathol 1997;16:548–550.

Nieminen P, Soares VRX, Aho M, et al: Cervical human papillomavirus deoxyribonucleic acid and cytologic evaluations in gynecologic outpatients. Am J Obstet Gynecol 1991;164:1265–1269.

Novak ER, Woodruff JD: Novak's Gynecologic and Obstetric Pathology, 7th ed. Philadelphia, WB Saunders, 1974.

Novotny DB, Ferlisi P: Villoglandular adenocarcinoma of the cervix: Cytologic presentation. Diagn Cytopathol 1997;17: 383–387.

Obermair A, Wanner C, Bilgi S, et al: The influence of vascular space involvement on the prognosis of patients with stage IB cervical carcinoma: Correlation of results. Cancer 1998;82: 689–696.

Ong S, Lees DA: A study of treatment failures following large loop excision of the transformation zone for the treatment of cervical intraepithelial neoplasia. Br J Obstet Gynaecol 1997;104: 718–722.

Osborne NG: Mucopurulent cervicitis: Antibiotic management. J Gynecol Surg 1997;14:197–198.

Ostergard DR: Cryosurgical treatment of cervical intraepithelial neoplasia. Obstet Gynecol 1980;56:231.

Ott F, Eichenberger-DeBeer H, Storck H: The local treatment of precancerous skin conditions with 5-fluorouracil ointment. Dermatologica 1970;140(Suppl I):109–113.

Oyesanya OA, Amerasinghe CN, Manning EAD: Outpatient excisional management of cervical intraepithelial neoplasia: A prospective, randomized comparison between loop diathermy excision and laser excisional conization. Am J Obstet Gynecol 1993;168:485–488.

Ozsaran AA, Ates T, Dikmen Y, et al: Evaluation of the risk of cervical intraepithelial neoplasia and human papilloma virus infection in renal transplant patients receiving immunosuppressive therapy. Eur J Gynaecol Oncol 1999;20:127–130.

Palit A, McDowell H, Carty H, et al: Endometroid adenocarcinoma of the cervix in a 9-year old girl. Br J Radiol 1998;71:1093–1095.

Palle C, Bangsboll S, Andreasson B: Cervical intraepithelial neoplasia in pregnancy. Acta Obstet Gynecol Scand 2000;79: 306–310.

Papanicolau GN, Traut HF: Diagnosis of uterine cancer by the vaginal smear. New York, Commonwealth Fund, 1943.

Paraskevaidis E, Jandial L, Mann EMF, et al: Pattern of treatment failure following laser for cervical intraepithelial neoplasia: Implications for follow-up protocol. Obstet Gynecol 1991;78:80–83.

Paraskevaidis E, Koliopoulos G, Paschopoulos M, et al: Effects of ball cauterization following loop excision and follow-up colposcopy. Obstet Gynecol 2001;97:617–620.

Parham GP, Andrews NR, Lee ML: Comparison of immediate and deferred colposcopy in a cervical screening program. Obstet Gynecol 2000;95:340–344.

Parkkinen S, Mäntyjärvi R, Syrjänen K, Ranki M: Detection of human papillomavirus DNA by the nucleic acid sandwich hybridization method from cervical scraping. J Med Virol 1986;20:279–288.

Pater MM, Hughes GA, Hyslop DE, et al: Glucocorticoid-dependent oncogenic transformation by type 16 but not type 11 human papilloma virus DNA. Nature 1988;335: 832–835.

Patni S, Hutchon DJ: A prospective follow-up study of women with colposcopically unconfirmed positive cervical smears. Br J Obstet Gynaecol 1999;106:1232.

Pederson E, Hoeg K, Kolstad P: Mass screening for cancer of the uterine cervix in Ostfold County, Norway: An experiment. Second report of the Norwegian Cancer Society. Acta Obstet Gynecol Scand 1971; vol 50(suppl 11).

Pete I, Toth V, Bosze P: The value of colposcopy in screening cervical carcinoma. Eur J Gynaecol Oncol 1998;19:120–122.

Pickel H, Winter R: Colposcopic diagnosis: Clinical aspects and experiences. Clin Exp Obstet Gynecol 1999;26:120–122.

Piura B, Dgani R, Yanai-Inbar I, et al: Adenocarcinoma of the uterine cervix: A study of 37 cases. J Surg Oncol 1996;61:249–255.

Pogue BW, Kaufman HB, Zelenchuk A, et al: Analysis of acetic acid-induced whitening of high-grade squamous intraepithelial lesions. J Biomed Opt 2001;6:397–403.

Powell CB, Sedlacek TV, Riva JM, Mangan C: Multicentricity of human papillomavirus infections in the female genital tract. J Gynecol Surg 1990;6:39–42.

Powell JL: Pitfalls in cervical colposcopy. Obstet Gynecol Clin North Am 1993;20:177–188.

Poynor EA, Barakat RR, Hoskins WJ: Management and follow-up of patients with adenocarcinoma in situ of the uterine cervix. Gynecol Oncol 1995;57:158–164.

Prendiville W: Large loop excision of the transformation zone. Clin Obstet Gynecol 38:622–639.

Prendiville W, Cullimore J, Norman S: Large loop excision of the transformation zone (LLETZ): A new method of management for women with cervical intraepithelial neoplasia. Br J Obstet Gynaecol 1989;96:1054–1060.

Pretorius RG, Belinson JL, Zhang WH, et al: The colposcopic impression: Is it influenced by the colposcopist's knowledge of the findings on the referral Papanicolaou smear? J Reprod Med 2001;46:724–728.

Raab SS: The cost-effectiveness of cervical-vaginal rescreening. Am J Clin Pathol 1997;108:525–536.

Rader AE, Rose PG, Rodriguez M, et al: Atypical squamous cells of undetermined significance in women over 55: Comparison with the general population and implications for management. Acta Cytol 1999;43:357–362.

Raio L, Ghezzi F, DiNaro E, et al: Duration of pregnancy after carbon dioxide laser conization of the cervix: Influence of cone height. Obstet Gynecol 1997;90:978–982.

Reagan JW, Hamonic MH: The cellular pathology in carcinoma in situ: A cytohistopathological correlation. Cancer 1956;9:385.

Redman CW: Does histological incomplete excision of cervical intraepithelial neoplasia following large excision of the transformation zone increase recurrence rates? A six year cytological follow-up. Br J Obstet Gynaecol 2001;108:771–772.

Reich O, Lahousen M, Pickel H, et al: Cervical intraepithelial neoplasia: III. Long-term follow-up after cold knife conization with involved margins. Obstet Gynecol 2002;99:193–196.

Reid R: Papillomavirus and cervical neoplasia: Modern implications and future prospects. Colposc Gynecol Laser Surg 1984;1:3–34.

Reid R: Superficial laser vulvectomy: III. A new surgical technique for appendage-conserving ablation of refractory condylomas and vulvar intraepithelial neoplasia. Am J Obstet Gynecol 1985;152: 504–509.

Reid R: Understanding HPV infection: The key to rational triage. Colposc Gynecol Laser Surg 1987;3:37–43.

Reid R, Laverty CR, Coppleson M, et al: Non-condylomatous cervical wart virus infection. Obstet Gynecol 1980;55:476–483.

Reid R, Scalzi P: Genital warts and cervical cancer: VII. An improved colposcopic index for differentiating benign papillomaviral infections from high-grade cervical intraepithelial neoplasia. Am J Obstet Gynecol 1985;153:611–618.

Reid R, Elfont EA, Zirkin RM, Fuller TA: Superficial laser vulvectomy: The anatomic and biophysical principles permitting accurate control over the depth of dermal destruction with the carbon dioxide laser. Am J Obstet Gynecol 1985;152:261–271.

Reid R, Greenberg M, Jenson AB, et al: Sexually transmitted papillomaviral infections: I. The anatomic distribution and pathologic grade of neoplastic lesions associated with different viral types. Am J Obstet Gynecol 1987;156:212–222.

Reid WA, Nafussi AI, Rebello G, Williams AR: Effect of using templates on the information included in histopathology reports on specimens of uterine cervix taken by loop excision of the transformation zone. J Clin Pathol 1999;52:825–828.

Rettenmaier MA, Berman ML, DiSaia PJ: Skinning vulvectomy for the treatment of multifocal vulvar intraepithelial neoplasia. Obstet Gynecol 1987;69:247–250.

Richart RM: The correlation of Schiller positive areas on the exposed portion of the cervix with intraepithelial neoplasia. Am J Obstet Gynecol 1964;90:697.

Richart RM: Natural history of cervical intraepithelial neoplasia. Clin Obstet Gynecol 1967;10:748.

Richart RM: A theory of cervical carcinogenesis. Obstet Gynecol Surv 1969;24:874.

Richart RM, Sciarra JJ: Treatment of cervical dysplasia by outpatient electrocauterization. Am J Obstet Gynecol 1968;101:200.

Richart RM, Townsend DE, Crips W, et al: An analysis of "long-term" follow-up results in patients with cervical intraepithelial neoplasia treated by cryotherapy. Am J Obstet Gynecol 1980;137:823.

Roberts JM, Gurley AM, Thurloe JK, et al: Evaluation of the ThinPrep Pap test as an adjunct to the conventional pap smear. Med J Aust 1997;167:466–469.

Robertson JH, Woodend BE, Crozier EH, Hutchinson J: Risk of cervical cancer associated with mild dyskaryosis. BMJ 1988;297:18.

Rokyta Z: Diagnostic reliability of prebioptic methods in the prediction of a histological basis of cervical lesions and its correlation with accuracy of colposcopically directed biopsy in patients with cervical neoplasia. Eur J Gynaecol Oncol 2000;21:484–486.

Ross MJ, Ehrmann RL: Histologic prognosticators in stage I squamous cell carcinoma of the vulva. Obstet Gynecol 1987;70:774–784.

Rossetti D, Gerli S, Saab JC, Di-Renzo GC: Atypical squamous cells of undetermined significance (ASCUS), low-grade squamous intraepithelial lesion (LSIL), high-grade squamous intraepithelial lesion (HSIL) and histology. J Med Liban 2000;48:127–130.

Roteli-Martins CM, Alves VA, Santos RT, et al: Value of morphological criteria in diagnosing cervical HPV lesions confirmed by in situ hybridization and hybrid capture assay. Pathol Res Pract 2001;197:677–682.

Rubinstein E: Probably virus induced epithelial lesions in preinvasive cervical cancer. Acta Obstet Gynecol Scand 1980;59:529–534.

Sadeghi SB, Hsieh EW, Gunn SW: Prevalence of cervical intraepithelial neoplasia in sexually active teenagers and young adults: Results of data analysis of mass Papanicolaou screening of 796,337 women in the United States in 1981. Am J Obstet Gynecol 1984;148:726–729.

Saigo PE, Cain JM, Kim WS, et al: Prognostic factors in adenocarcinoma of the uterine cervix. Cancer 1986;57:1584–1593.

Sammour MB, Shahwan AA, Iskander SG: Mucopolysaccharide activity in intraepithelial neoplasia of the cervix: 7th International Congress of Cytology, Munich, May 1980. Program 185:135.

Sankaranarayanan R, Shyamalakumary B, Wesley R, et al: Visual inspection with acetic acid in the early detection of cervical cancer and precursors. Int J Cancer 1999;80:161–163.

Santin AD, Hermonat PL, Ravaggi A, et al: Secretion of vascular endothelial growth factor in adenocarcinoma and squamous cell carcinoma of the uterine cervix. Obstet Gynecol 1999;94:78–82.

Saunders NJSG, Sharp F, Nottingham J, Lambourne C: Alcian blue staining of cone specimens: A guide to complete excision of the transformation zone. J Gynecol Surg 1989;5:375–379.

Schauenstein WW: Histologische untersuchungen Über atypisches plattenepithel an der portio und an der innenfläche der cervix uteri. Arch Gynakol 1908;85:576–581.

Schellhas HF: Laser surgery in gynecology. Surg Clin North Am 1978;58:151.

Schiffman MH: Latest HPV findings: Some clinical implications. Contemp Obstet Gynecol 1993; 38(10):27–40.

Schiffman MH, Herrero R, Hildesheim A, et al: HPV DNA testing in cervical cancer screening: Results from women in a high-risk province of Costa Rica. JAMA 2000;283:87–93.

Schiller W: Zur histologischen frÜhdiagnose des portiokarzinom. Zentralbl Gynakol 1928;52:1562.

Schiller W: Zur klinischen frÜhdiagnose des portiokarzinoms. Zentralbl Gynakol 1928;52:1886–1892.

Schneider A, Kraus H, Schuhmann R, Gissmann L: Papillomavirus infection of the lower genital tract: Detection of viral DNA in gynecological swabs. Int J Cancer 1985;35:443–448.

Schneider A, Hoyer H, Lotz B, et al: Screening for high-grade cervical intraepithelial neoplasia and cancer by testing for high-risk HPV, routine cytology or colposcopy. Int J Cancer 2000;89:529–534.

Schneppenheim P, Hamperl H, Kaufmann C, Ober KG: Die beziehungen des schleimepithels zum plattenepithel an der cervix uteri im lebenslauf der frau. Arch Gynakol 1958;190:303.

Scholl SM, Kingsley Pillers EM, Robinson RE, Farrell PJ: Prevalence of human papillomavirus type 16 DNA in cervical carcinoma samples in East Anglia. Int J Cancer 1985;35:215–218.

Schottländer J, Kermauner F: Zur kenntnis des uteruskarzinoms. Berlin, Karger, 1912.

Scott JW, Brass P, Seckinger D: Colposcopy plus cytology. Am J Obstet Gynecol 1969;103:925.

Scott JW, Vence CA: Colposcopy, cytology and biopsy in the office diagnosis of uterine malignancy. Cancer Cytol J 1963;5:5.

Scott JW, Welch WB, Blake TF: Bloodless technique of cold knife conization (ring biopsy). Am J Obstet Gynecol 1960;79:62.

Sedlacek TV: Colposcopic guidance for LOOP. J Reprod Med 1999;44:313–314.

Seidl ST: Praxis der kolposkopie: EinfÜhrung in methode und techn. Gynakol Prax 1986;10:673–682.

Semple D, Saha A, Maresh M: Colposcopy and treatment of cervical intraepithelial neoplasia: Are national standards achievable? Br J Obstet Gynaecol 1999;106:351–355.

Sen C, Brett MT: Outcome of women referred to colposcopy for persistently inadequate smears. Cytopathology 2000;11:38–44.

Senzaki H, Osaki T, Uemura Y, et al: Adenoid basal carcinoma of the uterine cervix: Immunohistochemical study and literature review. Jpn J Clin Oncol 1997;27:437–441.

Shackelford DP, Griffin D, Hoffman MK, Jones DE: Influence of specialty on pathology resource use in evaluation of cervical dysplasia. Obstet Gynecol 1999;94(5 Pt 1):709–712.

Shafi MI, Luesley DM, Jordan JA, et al: Randomized trial of immediate versus deferred treatment strategies for the management of minor cervical cytological abnormalities. Br J Obstet Gynaecol 1997;104:590–594.

Shah K, Kashima H, Polk BF, et al: Rarity of cesarean delivery in cases of juvenile-onset respiratory papillomatosis. Obstet Gynecol 1986;68:795–799.

Shatz P, Bergeron C, Ferenczy A: Anatomy of vulvar skin with emphasis on the pilosebaceous unit and subcutaneous fat. J Gynecol Surg 1989;5:183–191.

Sherman AI, Goldrath M, Berlin A, et al. Cervical-vaginal adenosis after in utero exposure to synthetic estrogens. Obstet Gynecol 1974;44:531–545.

Sherman ME, Schiffman M, Cox JT: Effects of age and human papilloma viral load on colposcopy triage: Data from the randomized atypical squamous cells of undetermined significance/low-grade squamous intraepithelial lesion triage study (ALTS). J Natl Cancer Inst 2002;94:102–107.

Sherman ME, Tabbara SO, Scott DR, et al: "ASCUS, rule out HSIL": Cytologic features, histologic correlates, and human papillomavirus detection. Mod Pathol 1999;12:335–342.

Shlay JC, Dunn T, Byers T, et al: Prediction of cervical intraepithelial neoplasia grade 2-3 using risk assessment and human papillomavirus testing in women with atypia on Papanicolaou smears. Obstet Gynecol 2000;96:410–416.

Shylasree T, Ashraf M, Jayawickrama N: Retrospective audit of standards and quality in colposcopy services in a district hospital. J Qual Clin Pract 2001;21:22–24; discussion 25.

Sianturi MH: Dense acetowhite: A high grade lesion? J Obstet Gynaecol Res 1997;23:79–83.

Sideri M, Schettino F, Spolti N, et al: Loop diathermy to replace conization in the conservative treatment of in situ cancer of the uterine cervix. J Gynecol Surg 1994;10:235–239.

Silbar EL, Woodruff JD: Evaluation of biopsy, cone and hysterectomy sequence in intraepithelial carcinoma of the cervix. Obstet Gynecol 1966;27:89.

Sillman FH, Sedlis A, Boyce JG: A review of lower genital intraepithelial neoplasia and the use of topical 5-fluorouracil. Obstet Gynecol Surv 1985;40:190–220.

Simsir A, Loffe OB, Bourquin P, et al: Repeat cervical cytology at the time of colposcopy: Is there an added benefit? Acta Cytol 2001;45:23–27.

Sincock AM: Semi-automated diagnosis of cervical intraepithelial neoplasia grade 2 by the measurement of acid labile DNA in cytologically normal nuclei. Cancer 1986;58:83–86.

Singer A, Jordan JA: The Cervix. Philadelphia, WB Saunders, 1961.

Smith KT, Campo MS: The biology of papillomaviruses and their role in oncogenesis. Anticancer Res 1985;5:31–48.

Smith KT, Campo MS: Papillomaviruses and their involvement in oncogenesis. Biomed Pharmacother 1985;39:405–414.

Smotkin D, Berek JS, Fu YS, et al: Human papillomavirus deoxyribonucleic acid in adenocarcinoma and adenosquamous carcinoma of the uterine cervix. Obstet Gynecol 1986;68:241–244.

Sokoll WC, Creasman WT: Is laser surgery superior to cryosurgery for the treatment of high grade CIN? J Gynecol Surg 1991;7:57–59.

Solomon D, Schiffman M, Tarone R: Comparison of three management strategies for patients with atypical squamous cells of undetermined significance: Baseline results from a randomized trial. J Natl Cancer Inst 2001;93:293–299.

Soloman D, Davey D, Kurman R, et al: The 2001 Bethesda system: Terminology for reporting results of cervical cytology. JAMA 2002;287:2114.

Spitzer M, Krumholz BA, Seltzer VL: The multicentric nature of disease related to human papillomavirus infection of the female lower genital tract. Obstet Gynecol 1989;73:303–307.

Stafl A: The clinical diagnosis of early cervical cancer. Obstet Gynecol Surv 1969;24:976.

Stafl A: New nomenclature for colposcopy. Obstet Gynecol 1976;48:123.

Stafl A: Cervicography: A new method for cervical cancer detection. Am J Obstet Gynecol 1981;139:815–825.

Stafl A, Linhartová A, Dohnal V: Das kolposkopische bild der felderung und seine pathogenese. Arch Gynakol 1963:199:223.

Stafl A, Mattingly RF: Colposcopic diagnosis of cervical neoplasia. Obstet Gynecol 1973:41:168.

Stafl A, Mattingly RF: Vaginal adenosis: A precancerous lesion? Am J Obstet Gynecol 1974;120:666.

Stafl A, Mattingly RF: Angiogenesis of cervical neoplasia. Am J Obstet Gynecol 1975;121:845.

Stafl A, Wilkinson EJ, Mattingly RF: Laser treatment of cervical and vaginal neoplasia. Am J Obstet Gynecol 1977;128:128.

Stefanon B, DePalo G: Is vulvoscopy a reliable diagnostic technique for high-grade vulvar intraepithelial neoplasia? Eur J Gynaecol Oncol 1997;18:211.

Steren A, Nguyen HN, Averette HE, et al: Radical hysterectomy for stage IB adenocarcinoma of the cervix: The University of Miami experience. Gynecol Oncol 1993;48:355–359.

Stockton D, Cooper P, Lonsdale RN: Changing incidence of invasive adenocarcinoma of the uterine cervix in East Anglia. J Med Screen 1997;4:40–43.

Sundfor K, Lyng H, Rofstad EK: Oxygen tension and vascular density in adenocarcinoma and squamous cell carcinoma of the uterine cervix. Acta Oncol 1998;37:665–670.

Sutton GP, Stehman FB, Ehrlich CE, Roman A: Human papillomavirus deoxyribonucleic acid in lesions of the female genital tract: Evidence of type 6/11 in squamous carcinoma of the vulva. Obstet Gynecol 1987;70:564–568.

Syrjänen K, Parkkinen S, Mäntyjärvi R, et al: Human papillomavirus (HPV) type as an important determinant of the natural history of HPV infections in uterine cervix. Eur J Epidemiol 1985;1:180–187.

Syrjänen S, Syrjänen K, Mäntyjärvi R, et al: Human papillomavirus (HPV) DNA sequences demonstrated by in situ DNA hybridization in serial paraffin-embedded cervical biopsies. Arch Gynakol 1986;239:39–48.

Sze EHM, Rosenzweig BA, Birenbaum DL, et al: Excisional conization of the cervix uteri: A five-part review. J Gynecol Surg 1989;5:235–268, 325–341.

Tabbara S, Saleh ADM, Andersen WA, et al: The Bethesda classification for squamous intraepithelial lesions: Histologic, cytologic, and viral correlates. Obstet Gynecol 1992;79:338–346.

Tabor A, Berget A: Cold-knife and laser conization for cervical intraepithelial neoplasia. Obstet Gynecol 1990;76:633–635.

Teale GR, Moffitt DD, Mann CH, Luesley DM: Management guidelines for women with normal colposcopy after low-grade cervical abnormalities: Population study. BMJ 2000;320(7251):1693–1696.

Thomas DB, Ray RM: Oral contraceptives and invasive adenocarcinoma and adenosquamous carcinomas of the uterine cervix: The World Health Organization Collaborative Study of Neoplasia and Steroid Contraceptives. Am J Epidemiol 1996;144:281–289.

Toki T, Shiozawa T, Hosaka N, et al: Minimal deviation adenocarcinoma of the uterine cervix has abnormal expression of sex steroid receptors, CA125, and gastric mucin. Int J Gynecol Pathol 1997;16:111–116.

Toms C: ASCUS in postmenopausal women. Acta Cytol 2002;46:68–69.

Torashima M, Yamashita Y, Hatanaka Y, et al: Invasive adenocarcinoma of the uterine cervix: MR imaging. Comput Med Imaging Graph 1997;21:253–260.

Townsend DE: Cryosurgery. Obstet Gynecol 1975;4:331.

Townsend DE: Vaginal adenosis, adenocarcinoma and diethylstilbestron. In Morrow CP and Townsend DE: Synopsis of gynecologic oncology 3rd ed. New York, Churchill Livingston, 1987:45–55.

Townsend DE, Levine RU, Richart RM, et al: Management of vulvar intraepithelial neoplasia by carbon dioxide laser. Obstet Gynecol 1982;60:49–52.

Townsend DE, Richart RM, Marks E, Nielsen J: Invasive cancer following outpatient evaluation and therapy for cervical disease. Obstet Gynecol 1981;57:145.

Tseng CJ, Horng SG, Soong YK, et al: Conservative conization for microinvasive carcinoma of the cervix. Am J Obstet Gynecol 1997;176:1009–1010.

van Beurden M, van der Vange N, de Craen AJ, et al: Normal findings in vulvar examination and vulvoscopy. Br J Obstet Gynaecol 1997;104:320–324.

van Niekerk WA, Dunton CJ, Richart RM, et al: Colposcopy, cervicography, speculoscopy, and endoscopy: International Academy of Cytology Task Force summary. Diagnostic Cytology Towards the 21st Century: An International Expert Conference and Tutorial. Acta Cytol 1988;42:33–49.

van Vliet W, van Loon AJ, ten Hoor KA, Boonstra H: Cervical carcinoma during pregnancy outcome of planned delay in treatment. Eur J Obstet Gynecol Reprod Biol 1998;79:153–157.

von Franqué O: Das beginnende portiokankroid und die ausbreitungswege des gebärmutterhalskrebses. Z Geburtshilfe 1901;44:173.

von Franqué O: Leukoplakia und carcinoma vaginae et uteri. Z Geburtshilfe 1907;60:237.

Vaccher E, Tirelli U: Invasive cervical cancer after treatment for cervical intraepithelial neoplasia. Lancet 1997;349(9069):1909–1910.

Valentine BH, Arena B, Green E: Laser ablation of recurrent Paget's disease of the vulva and perineum. J Gynecol Surg 1992;8:21–24.

Vecchia C, Franceschi S, Decarli A, et al: Sexual factors, venereal diseases, and the risk of intraepithelial and invasive cervical neoplasia. Cancer 1986;58:935–941.

Vermund SH, Kelley KF, Klein RS, et al: High risk of human papillomavirus infection and cervical squamous intraepithelial lesions among women with symptomatic human immunodeficiency virus infection. Am J Obstet Gynecol 1991;165:392–400.

Vessey MP: Epidemiological studies of the effects of diethylstilbesterol. IARC Sci Pub 1989;96:335–348.

Vessey MP, Grice D: Carcinoma of the cervix and oral contraceptives: Epidemiological studies. Biomed Pharmacother 1989;43:157–160.

Vesterinnen E, Meyer B, Purola E, et al: Treatment of vaginal flat condyloma with interferon cream. Lancet 1984;1:157.

Villani C, Inghirami P, Pietrangeli D, Pace S: Today's stage in differential diagnosis between cervical condyloma and CIN. Clin Exp Obstet Gynecol 1986;13:26–32.

Visvalingam S, Blumenthal N, Clarke A, Kench J: Vaginal melanoma masquerading as adenocarcinoma based on cervical cytology: A case report and review of the literature. Aust N Z J Obstet Gynaecol 2000;40:466–467.

Wagner D, Ikenberg H, Boehm N, Gissmann L: Identification of human papillomavirus in cervical swabs by deoxyribonucleic acid in situ hybridization. Obstet Gynecol 1984;64:767–772.

Walker EM, Dodgson J, Duncan ID: Is colposcopy of teenage women worthwhile? An 11-year review of teenage referrals in Dundee. J Gynecol Surg 1989;5:385–388.

Walsh JT Jr, Flotte TJ, Anderson RR, Deutsch TF: Pulsed CO_2 laser tissue ablation: Effect of tissue type and pulse duration on thermal damage. Lasers Surg Med 1988;8:108–118.

Ward JW, Clifford WS, Monaco AR, Bicherstaff HJ: Fatal systemic poisoning following podophyllin treatment of condyloma acuminatum. South Med J 1954;47:1204.

Watts KC, Husain OAN, Campion MJ, et al: Quantitative DNA analysis of low-grade cervical intraepithelial neoplasia and human papillomavirus infection by static and flow cytometry. BMJ 1987;295:1090–1092.

Wespi HJ: Erfahrungen mit der systematischen kolposkopie an der zürcher frauenklinik. Zentralbl Gynakol 1938;82:1762–1776.

Wespi HJ: Entstehung und Früherfassung des portiokarzinoms. Basel, Benno Schwabe, 1946. Translated by M. Schiller: Early Carcinoma of the Uterine Cervix: Pathogenesis and Detection. New York, Grune and Stratton, 1949.

Wespi HJ: Kolpophotographic. Gynaecologia 1951;131:65–73.

Wespi HJ: Altersverteilung und Latenzzeit beim portiokarzinom. Gynaecologia 1952;133:169–178.

Wespi HJ: Die rolle der kolposkopie zum ausschluss des karzinoms im portiobereich in gynaecologia 1952;34:111–121.

Wespi HJ: Colposcopic-histologic correlation in the benign acanthotic non-glycogenated squamous epithelium. Colposc Gynecol Laser Surg 1986;2:147–158.

Wespi HJ: Enhancement of the colposcopic image of the uterine cervix by salicyclic alcohol and metacresol sulphonic acid. The cervix and l.f.g.t. 1986;4:139–148.

Wespi HJ: 50 years colposcopy. Annali di Obstetricia e Ginecologia Medicina Perinatal 1988 CIX (109):319–350.

Wespi HJ, Sauter H: Der einfluss von alter und geburtenzahl auf die entstehung des genitalcarcinoms. Z Krebsforsch 1943;53:347–357.

Wickenden C, Coleman DV, Malcolm ADB: Cross-hybridisation of human papillomavirus DNA on filters. J Virol Methods 1987;15:249–255.

Widrich T, Kennedy AW, Myers TM, et al: Adenocarcinoma in situ of the uterine cervix: Management and outcome. Gynecol Oncol 1996;61:304–308.

Wolcott HD, Gallup DG: Wide local excision in the treatment of vulvar carcinoma in situ: A reappraisal. Am J Obstet Gynecol 1984;150:695–698.

Wright CV, Davis E, Riopelle MA: Laser cylindrical excision to replace conization. Am J Obstet Gynecol 1984;150:704.

Wright CV, Davis E: Laser surgery for vulvar intraepithelial neoplasia: Principles and results. Am J Obstet Gynecol 1987;156:374–378.

Wright TC Jr, Gagnon S, Richart RM, Ferenczy A: Treatment of cervical intraepithelial neoplasia using the loop clcctrosurgical excision procedure. Obstet Gynecol 1992;79:173–178.

Wright TC Jr, Cox JT, Massad LS, et al: 2001 consensus guidelines for the management of women with cervical cytological abnormalities. JAMA 2002;287:2120–2129.

Yabroff KR, Kerner JF, Mandelblatt JS: Effectiveness of interventions to improve follow-up after abnormal cervical cancer screening. Prev Med 2000;31:429–439.

Yandell RB, Hannigan EV, Dinh TV, Buchanan VS: Avoiding conization for inadequate colposcopy: Suggestions for conservative therapy. J Reprod Med 1996;41:135–139.

Yang YJ, Gordon GB: Cervical adenoid cystic carcinoma co-existing with multiple human papillomavirus-associated genital lesions: A common etiology? Gynecol Obstet Invest 1999;47:272–277.

Yeh IT, LiVolsi VA, Noumoff JS: Endocervical carcinoma. Pathol Res Pract 1991;187:129–144.

Yoshida M, Jimbo H, Shirai T, et al: A clinicopathological study of postoperatively upgraded early squamous-cell carcinoma of the uterine cervix. J Obstet Gynaecol Res 2000;26:259–264.

Yost NP, Santoso JT, McIntire DD, Iliya FA: Postpartum regression rates of antepartum cervical intraepithelial neoplasia II and III lesions. Obstet Gynecol 1999;93:359–362.

Young LS, Bevan IS, Johnson MA, et al: The polymerase chain reaction: A new epidemiological tool for investigating cervical human papillomavirus infection. BMJ 1989;298:14–18.

Young RH, Scully RE: Atypical forms of microglandular hyperplasia of the cervix simulating carcinoma: A report of five cases and review of the literature. Am J Surg Pathol 1989;13:50–56.

Young RH, Scully RE: Invasive adenocarcinoma and related tumors of the uterine cervix. Semin Diagn Pathol 1990;7: 205–227.

Zheng T, Holford TR, Ma Z, et al: The continuing increase in adenocarcinoma of the uterine cervix: A birth cohort phenomenon. Int J Epidemiol 1996;25:252–258.

Zhou C, Gilks CB, Hayes M, Clement PB: Papillary serous carcinoma of the uterine cervix: A clinicopathologic study of 17 cases. Am J Surg Pathol 1998;22:113–120.

Zinser HK: Zur gynäkologischen krebsvorsorgeuntersuchung. GBK-Mitteilungsdienst Nr 1985;45:12–18.

Zinser HK, Rosenbauer KA: Untersuchungen über die angioarchitektonik der normalen und pathologisch veränderten cervix uteri. Arch Gynakol 1960;194:73.

SECTION VI
Index

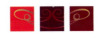

Index

Note: Page numbers followed by f indicate figures; those followed by t indicate tables.